Doctor Mom Chung
of the Fair-Haired Bastards

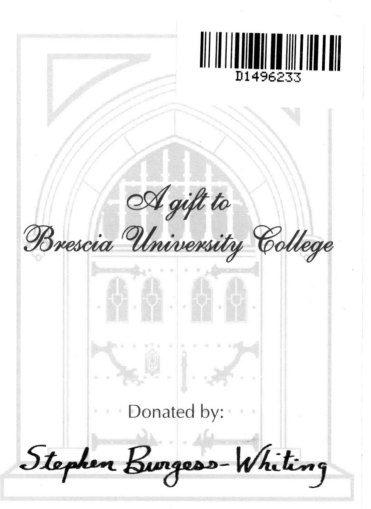

D1496233

A gift to
Brescia University College

Donated by:

Stephen Burgess-Whiting

Brescia University College

Doctor Mom Chung of the Fair-Haired Bastards

The Life of a Wartime Celebrity

Judy Tzu-Chun Wu

UNIVERSITY OF CALIFORNIA PRESS
Berkeley · Los Angeles · London

University of California Press
Berkeley and Los Angeles, California

University of California Press, Ltd.
London, England

Library of Congress Cataloging-in-Publication Data

Wu, Judy Tzu-Chun.
   Doctor Mom Chung of the fair-haired bastards : the
life of a wartime celebrity / Judy Tzu-Chun Wu.
      p.   cm.
   Includes bibliographical references and index.
   ISBN 0-520-24143-6 (cloth : alk. paper)
      1. Chung, Margaret, 1889–1959. 2. Chinese
American physicians—Biography. 3. Women
physicians—United States—Biography. 4. Chinese
American women—United States—Biography. I. Title
R154.C3345W8   2005
610'.92—dc22   2004012680

Manufactured in the United States of America
14   13   12   11   10   09   08   07   06   05
10   9   8   7   6   5   4   3   2   1

For my parents
Betty Chao-Hua Huang Wu
and John Yu-Pu Wu

For my life partner
Mark

And for Konrad
for transforming me into a mom

Contents

Introduction

During World War II, Mom Chung's was *the* place to be in San Francisco. Soldiers preparing for departure to the Pacific arena of war or on leave from their duties went to eat good comfort food there. They consumed vast quantities of BBQ ribs, red beans, and chocolate cake, making up for the dreariness of military fare. They swapped stories with each other over drinks at the bar. They also caught glimpses of and actually talked with some of the foremost celebrities of their time: John Wayne, Ronald Reagan, Tennessee Williams, Helen Hayes, Sophie Tucker, Tallulah Bankhead, and many others. At Mom Chung's, they met prominent politicians and military leaders like Kentucky senator and future commissioner of baseball "Happy" Chandler and U.S. Navy fleet admiral Chester W. Nimitz.

Mom Chung's was not a restaurant or a nightclub. It was the private residence of Dr. Margaret Jessie Chung, the first known American-born woman of Chinese descent to become a physician. She hosted these weekly Sunday parties for seventy-five to a hundred people in her modest-sized home. Then in her fifties, she cooked the food herself and made the rounds to ensure that her guests felt welcome. After all, almost all of them were members of her adopted family. The celebrities, the politicians, the highly ranked, and the common soldiers were bound to each other through her, their surrogate mother. Their ties stemmed not from blood connection but from their mutual affection for one another and their common dedication to the Allied cause.

Chung's family, which grew to approximately fifteen hundred members, served as a vital political resource during the international conflicts of the 1930s and 1940s. She claimed to have recruited pilots from among her "sons" for the Flying Tigers, the American volunteer force that fought in support of China during the Sino-Japanese War. Once the United States formally entered World War II, she used her contacts to lobby for the creation of WAVES, the Women's Naval Reserve. Described as a serious, commanding, almost regal, person, Chung nevertheless had a bawdy sense of humor. Because she never married and could offer no legitimate father figure for her mostly white and male children, they became known as Mom Chung's "Fair-Haired Bastards."

Despite her pioneering achievements and colorful style, Margaret Chung has all but disappeared from historical memory.[1] This biography seeks to refocus public attention on her life by exploring two questions: How did Chung accomplish what she did in her professional, political, and personal life? And, how do her experiences provide insight into the historical transformation of American norms regarding race, gender, and sexuality over the course of her lifetime?

Born in Santa Barbara, California, in 1889, Chung was the eldest child in a large impoverished family. Raised as a Christian by her immigrant parents, she aspired to serve as a medical missionary in China so she could offer both physical and spiritual healing to her ancestral people. Prevailing racial and gender barriers, in addition to her family's poverty, posed serious challenges to this dream, however. Just seven years before her birth, the U.S. Congress passed the Chinese Exclusion Act of 1882.[2] Reflecting the widespread hostility toward people of Chinese ancestry, the legislation barred Chinese laborers from entering the country and denied all immigrants from China the right to obtain citizenship through naturalization. Born on U.S. soil, Chung automatically qualified as a member of the American polity. Her parents, who had arrived in the 1870s, would remain perpetual aliens. Furthermore, residing in a state known for its virulent anti-Chinese politics would remind all members of the Chung family of their vulnerable status as unwanted outsiders. They, along with other Chinese in the United States, experienced segregation and other forms of discrimination on a daily basis. As a result, the overwhelming majority of Chinese Americans worked in low-status, labor-intensive occupations.[3]

In addition, Victorian gender norms subscribed to the concept of separate spheres, which assigned men and women different responsibilities on the basis of "inherent" gender differences.[4] Men, presumed to have more rational minds and a will to dominate, occupied the public world; women, credited with innate moral purity and nurturing instincts, occupied the private realm of home and family. Becoming a medical doctor entailed transgressing these gender norms.

By the time of Chung's death in 1959, these racial and gender outlooks had been challenged, although not completely eclipsed, by more egalitarian values. In contrast to the rigid and hierarchical social structures associated with the Victorian era, modern society was beginning to celebrate the breaking of barriers and the seemingly limitless potential of individuals, regardless of race, gender, or nationality. The trajectory of Chung's life provides an opportunity to explore this transition from Victorian to modern America. Her experiences do not indicate an unbroken linear progression from segregation and hierarchy to integration and equality. Rather, Chung's strategies for advancement indicate the coexistence of contradictory norms, each with its own constraints as well as advantages. As much as she embraced modern changes, Chung also appropriated Victorian roles as she made and remade herself during various phases of her life.

Living through a period of such dramatic transition provided opportunities for Chung to fashion and refashion her identity. She transformed herself from a medical professional who adopted masculine clothing to a glamorous and feminine mother figure. She assimilated into mainstream and even elite American society but remained a symbol of China, a country that she never visited. She became a respectable public figure, yet she lived an unconventional private life that included developing romantic relationships with other women. Of course Chung did not have unlimited choice in creating her identities. However, by crafting multiple personas that catered to conflicting social expectations, Chung could challenge certain norms by affirming others. That is, she achieved acceptance because she demonstrated a dual ability to traverse social barriers and yet personify the immutability of social difference. By being all things to all people—Victorian and modern, maternal and masculine, asexual and transgressive, exotically different and mainstream—Chung symbolized and fulfilled the broader society's desire for transformation as well as stability, change as well as continuity.

NARRATING A LIFE

This biography presents the life of Margaret Chung in three acts.[5] Part 1 examines the influence of Christian missionaries on her professional aspirations. During the late nineteenth century, white Protestant female reformers in the American West assisted in the adaptation of Chinese immigrants and promoted the medical training of Chinese women. Rather than reject the notion of inherent gender difference, female missionaries embraced the belief that women were naturally more moral and nurturing; medical training for women, in their view, would expand women's protective maternal influence over the broader society.[6] The white reformers also subscribed to the cultural superiority of Western religion and education. However, instead of advocating for racial exclusion, they sought to expose Chinese people to the benefits of American society. Steeped in these benevolent yet unequal relationships, Margaret Chung adopted the Christian missionary belief system to help her obtain a professional education during the early decades of the twentieth century.

Part 2 explores Chung's efforts to establish a sense of professional and personal belonging. Following her graduation from medical school in 1916, she relocated to Chicago. There, she came into contact with Progressive reformers, who used their scientific expertise to remedy the social problems of urban America. Chung returned to Southern California in the late 1910s and became a celebrity physician within the nascent Hollywood industry. She eventually settled in San Francisco, which boasted the largest Chinese neighborhood outside of China as well as an emerging "queer" subculture. During this period of her life, Chung traversed both geographic and social boundaries to gain entry into various communities. Despite her desire to serve people of her own ancestry and gender, Chung increasingly discovered greater acceptance among non-Chinese and men. Her friends, colleagues, and supporters tended to come from marginalized backgrounds due to their ethnicity, gender, or sexuality. Like Chung, they engaged in a struggle to gain social entitlement. However, they also embraced her out of desire to fulfill their fantasies about the exotic Orient and the comforting nurturance of women.

Part 3 examines the emergence and significance of Chung's surrogate maternal identity during the 1930s and 1940s. She initially created her family of "Fair-Haired Bastards" in the context of the Great Depression and the Sino-Japanese conflicts of the 1930s. As the United States officially entered World War II, Chung achieved national and even international fame as a symbol of U.S.-China unity. Her new celebrity status granted her access to the inner circles of American political power. Her respectability as a dedicated mother of the Allied fighting forces offered some protection from allegations concerning her sexuality. However, Chung's experiences at the height of her popularity also reveal limitations to her strategy of gaining influence and acceptance by capitalizing on her Chinese ancestry and motherly persona.

Finally, an epilogue analyzes the legacy of Margaret Chung and examines why she received so little public or scholarly attention following World War II.

In this biography, I use the words "strategies" and "roles" to highlight Chung's efforts to create identities that satisfied her aspirations as well as the social norms of acceptability. To obtain insight into another person's consciousness is not an easy task, even when that individual writes an autobiography and leaves her imprint on historical records.[7] Like all people, Chung was selective in what she chose to present about her life. However, the variety, if not the completeness, of sources provides fragmented insights into her efforts to craft possibilities for herself.

To capture how historical forces shaped the choices as well as the constraints on Chung's life, this biography juxtaposes microscopic and macroscopic perspectives. The lens shifts back and forth between a focus on her and a broader portrayal of her times. In developing this depiction of Margaret Chung, I am cognizant of my role in highlighting certain experiences and shading others. Undoubtedly, another biographer would discover different aspects of her identity. It strikes me as particularly fitting that this should be so. After all, Margaret Chung's ability to perform multiple identities to diverse audiences goes a long way toward explaining her life accomplishments and makes her a particularly fascinating subject for study.

PART ONE

Religion and Medicine

CHAPTER I

"The Medical Lady Missionary"

I was born on the soil, drank the water, and breathed the air
that is America. . . . I am particularly grateful to be a citizen
of the United States with all of its privileges because my
parents and my forefathers were Chinese, and had I been born
in China I probably would have been thrown down the
Yangtze River for I was the oldest of eleven children and most
of us were girls. . . . Fortunately for me, both my parents were
Christian and, therefore, believed in giving their daughters an
equal opportunity to go to school.

To America and to Christianity, I owe all that I am, and ever
hope to be.

Margaret Chung, "Autobiography"

Margaret Chung was born into a family, a country, and an era pro-
foundly influenced by Christianity. Her mother, Ah Yane, and her father,
Chung Wong, emigrated separately from China to the United States in
the mid-1870s. In California, both converted under the influence of
Presbyterian missionaries. The assistance offered by these white and
mostly female reformers enabled Ah Yane and Chung Wong to survive
and adapt in a new country. Furthermore, the Christian faith laid the
foundation for their daughter's aspiration to become a medical missionary among the Chinese people.

Margaret Chung's chosen vocation reveals the influence of the largest
women's movement in the United States at the turn of the twentieth century, the missionary enterprise. White, middle-class, American-born women
constituted the overwhelming majority of the many thousands of female
missionaries and their 3 million supporters.[1] However, the movement
also sought to empower immigrants and nonwhites, especially women

of color, both in the United States and abroad. Enlisting the services of so-called native women benefited conversion efforts in two ways. First, "native" wives and mothers who converted could build Christian homes and raise Christian children. Second, a select few could be trained as missionary physicians. In that capacity, regardless of their marital or maternal status, they could gain access to "heathen" families by offering "healing for the body in one hand and healing for the soul in the other."[2]

The missionary movement both relied upon and challenged Victorian practices of gender separatism, immigration restriction, and segregation. The reformers justified women's entry into male professions such as medicine, as well as their travels across racial and national boundaries, by drawing on Victorian belief in woman's maternal nature. The missionary role was portrayed as a natural expansion of women's inclination to nurture, protect, and keep watch over the moral and physical well-being of her charges. Fears concerning racial mixing were minimized by emphasizing the ultimate goal of training "native helpers" who could then serve people of their own ancestry. The missionaries believed in the inherent goodness of their offerings. They sought to educate, elevate, and improve those they considered in need of instruction. While the missionary project imposed Western religious values and furthered the interests of American empire-building, it also provided opportunities for immigrant, especially female immigrant, advancement.

ARRIVING IN A CHRISTIAN LAND

Chung's parents came to the United States in the 1870s as part of the initial wave of Chinese immigration, which lasted from the 1840s until the passage of the 1882 Chinese Exclusion Act. Propelled by economic and political instability in their homeland and lured by promises of opportunity and adventure in the developing American West, nearly three hundred thousand Chinese from the Canton (Guangdong) region arrived in Hawaii and the continental mainland during this period. The scant surviving sources on Chung's parents suggest that their lives mirrored the experiences of other Chinese in America, especially those of uncertain economic standing.

One of just nine thousand Chinese women to immigrate prior to 1882, five-year-old Ah Yane arrived in the United States in 1874.[3] The small numbers of female immigrants, constituting approximately 3 to 5 percent of the Chinese American population, resulted from a combination of factors. Migration commonly represented a group decision. In order to obtain resources to support an ailing family economy, a representative traveled abroad to earn and remit income. For cultural and economic reasons, Chinese kinship networks overwhelmingly sent male representatives overseas. Traditional cultural values emphasized women's confinement to the home and their responsibility for taking care of the daily needs of the family. Women who did participate in the wage economy found opportunities more readily in China than in the United States. Finally, Chinese families hoped to ensure the return of their sons from far-away places by holding their wives and children "hostage."

In addition to these self-imposed reasons for limiting female migration, external factors also obstructed and eventually prevented Chinese women's entry into the United States. The racial hostility that Chinese immigrants faced, especially on the West Coast, discouraged them from establishing permanent roots in America. Capitalists initially welcomed Chinese workers as a form of "cheap labor" to develop the economic and transportation infrastructure of the West. In response, the white working class targeted Chinese immigrants, accusing them of undercutting their livelihoods. Middle-class Victorian Christian society also expressed disdain toward the practitioners of what they saw as a heathen culture. Thus, a wide spectrum of the American public regarded the Chinese as a temporary work force and not as permanent members of their society. Due to this combination of external and internal factors, few females came to the United States during the initial period of Chinese immigration.

The women who did migrate to the United States primarily came as prostitutes to serve the sexual needs of the overwhelmingly male Chinese population. In San Francisco, which had approximately thirty thousand Chinese residents in 1870, about 70 percent of all Chinese women worked in the sex trade. By 1880, the numbers had declined to 20 to 50 percent as a result of the passage of the 1875 Page Law, which prohibited the entry of women for "criminal or demoralizing purposes."[4] If Chung's mother had arrived after 1875, immigrant officials most likely would have denied her entry. They enforced the Page Law so strictly that all Chinese women were considered immoral until proven otherwise.[5] In addition, Ah Yane was very likely a prostitute-in-training.

Despite her youth, Ah Yane apparently arrived unaccompanied by family members.[6] Around the age of eleven—six years after her initial entry to the United States—she was arrested in a San Francisco brothel on 12 October 1880 and placed in the Presbyterian Chinese Mission Home.[7] Her early years in the United States were harsh. Margaret Culbertson, the first superintendent of the mission home, recalled Ah Yane's initial arrival there: she was "small of stature, miserably clad in dirty garments, and in her flight had lost one of her shoes. . . . She [also] was suffering from a severe cough and a catarrhal difficulty." Because of her youth, her size, and her grubby appearance, Ah Yane most likely served as a *mui tsai,* or servant girl, to the two older women who were arrested with her and who claimed to be her "mothers, No. 1 and No. 2."[8]

As Margaret Chung reveals in the opening paragraph of her unpublished autobiography, poor families in China sometimes resorted to infanticide, abandonment, or selling their children in order to survive times of extreme distress.[9] Because Chinese society valued sons for their ability to carry on the family lineage, parents tended to sell their daughters, either as domestic servants or as prostitutes. Being sold as a servant, or *mui tsai,* then, represented a "form of charity for impoverished girls."[10] The deed of sale usually stipulated their release at the age of eighteen. However, during their servitude, girls received no wages, did not have liberty to leave, and had no legal recourse against mistreatment, rape, or forced marriage.

In the United States, *mui tsai* frequently worked as domestic servants in wealthy Chinese households or in brothels. While some owners treated their *mui tsai* well, providing education as well as arranging marriages, others exploited the vulnerable girls. In fact, "Brothel owners often purchased young girls from China with the intention of using them first as domestic servants and then as prostitutes when they became older, thus maximizing their investment."[11] Ironically, the small numbers of Chinese women in the United States increased the demand for and economic value of *mui tsai.* The Presbyterian Chinese Mission Home reported in 1882 that "since the advance in the price of young girls, from $300 and $400 to $1000, they are guarded most jealously by their owners."[12]

With such a heavy financial investment in Ah Yane, her owners refused to release her without a struggle. The Presbyterian missionaries appeared in court five times to obtain legal guardianship of Ah Yane. Her experiences were not unique. During the same year that she arrived at the mission home, the Society for Prevention of Cruelty to Children also placed seven other young girls there. From the perspective of the reformers, these girls had been betrayed by both their biological parents and their surrogate guardians in the Chinese community. Consequently, the mission home, with the support of the American legal system, provided alternative maternal figures and an alternative family.

In contrast to the dramatic account of Ah Yane's arrival at the Presbyterian Chinese Mission Home in San Francisco, there is little information on Chung Wong's early experiences in the United States. Born between 1860 and 1862, he was an adolescent at the time of his immigration in 1875. The dialect that he and Ah Yane spoke suggests that they both came from the Sze Yup region, an impoverished area of Canton.[13] He may have left China to earn money to help sustain a family farm. He may have traveled in the company of a family member. At the time of his death in 1917, however, his children had no knowledge of his relations in China.[14] Chung Wong most likely first arrived in San Francisco, the primary entryway for Chinese immigrants.

By the late 1880s, Chung Wong was reported as residing in Southern California and was listed as a member of the Presbyterian Church. In his 1887 annual report, Reverend Ira M. Condit, a missionary stationed in Los Angeles, described Chung Wong as "one of the [Sabbath] school's faithful scholars" and the only Chinese immigrant to be "baptized & received into the Communion" for the year of 1886:

> He was a constant attendant on our church, receiving here all his instruction & preparation for entering the church. But before the time came he went to Santa Barbara, where he opened a store & is doing quite a successful business as a Chinese merchant. But he took his religion with him, & at once identified himself with our work there, & was received into our church in Santa Barbara.[15]

That Chung Wong established his business eleven years after his arrival in the United States indicates that he did not immigrate with the capital but instead accumulated it in California.

CHRISTIAN MATERNALISM AND THE ASSIMILABLE CHINESE

For both Ah Yane and Chung Wong, the Presbyterian missionaries mitigated the harshness of immigrant life by providing resources that facilitated their adaptation to American society. For Ah Yane, the mission home offered shelter, education, and a surrogate family. Established in 1874, the institution represented a concrete manifestation of maternalist reform ideology. Like most of the nineteenth-century female reformers, the founders and supporters of the mission home subscribed to Victorian values of "true womanhood." They believed in women's inherent purity and sought to expand their motherly authority over the broader society. In San Francisco, these benevolent women targeted what they called "Chinese slave girls" for rescue. In order to combat members of the Chinese and white communities who profited from the sex trade, the reformers worked with social service agencies and law enforcement to draw attention to and provide solutions for female subjugation. For example, Margaret Culbertson developed the technique of raiding brothels and homes to physically remove Chinese women from their subjugation. She cultivated relationships with the San Francisco police and the Society for the Prevention of Cruelty to Children to assist in these raids. She also oversaw the general operation of the mission home, which provided these women with an alternative place to live and work.[16]

Although the mission home reformers wanted to help all Chinese "slave girls," they preferred saving the younger servant girls. The older prostitutes, "accustomed to making money, disdainful of housework, and as a rule too old for school, were generally more critical of the Home than other groups of residents."[17] Consequently, the missionaries explained that "while our doors are closed against none who seek our protection, we are always especially glad to receive the children, for good seed sown in the fertile soil of childhood, gives promise of fruit in after years."[18]

A preference for admitting younger charges facilitated the white reformers' efforts to develop surrogate familial relationships. The Presbyterian Chinese Mission Home, like other female missionary institutions, wanted to create an ideal Christian home. Due to their belief in the superior moral authority of women, their family was not led by a male patriarch but by the purity and love of a maternal figure. The superintendent of the home, or "matron," was called "mother." The Chinese residents generally referred to one another as "sisters." Trusted "native" assistants eventually could ascend to the title of "auntie," but never "mother."[19] The use of familial language served multiple purposes. From the perspective of the matrons, most of whom were single women, their status as surrogate mothers justified their professional and missionary responsibilities as an extension of traditional gender roles. Furthermore, the rhetoric of family acknowledged racial and cultural hierarchies between white Christian "mothers" and their Chinese, "heathen" "daughters," yet also softened these hierarchies by emphasizing the emotional bonds between family members. From the perspective of the Chinese women, the use of familial terms to describe unequal relationships of obligation and reciprocity resonated with Chinese practices of social protocol. Furthermore, the "rescued" women recognized the value of cultivating surrogate family ties with white female missionaries, who had access to the economic, cultural, and legal resources of American society.

While some Chinese women chafed under the maternal supervision of the Presbyterian Chinese Mission Home, Ah Yane appeared to blossom under the guidance of her "rescuers." On the night of her arrival, she not only showed signs of physical illness and mistreatment, but she also was emotionally overwrought. One of her mission home "sisters" recalled that "Ah Yane . . . cried very hard," but after one of the assistants brought her some cakes, "she stopped crying, and played with us."[20] Three years after her arrival, the missionaries reported a transformation of Ah Yane's physical, mental, and spiritual health:

> What a change of three years of home care and comfortable living have made. In looking at her tall, well-rounded figure and intelligent face, fresh with the glow of health, one can scarcely recall a vestige of the unpromising little waif that sought shelter with us one dark October night in 1880. She speaks English very sweetly, reads, writes and sings well, and is studying music, under the direction of her teacher. Ah Yane publicly professed her faith in Christ, and was received into the Church at the last Communion season.[21]

The Presbyterian missionaries certainly had reason to exaggerate Ah Yane's progress; yet her own words and actions reveal that the portrayal was not an inaccurate one. The 1885 *Occidental Board Report* featured a letter from Ah Yane thanking the secretary of the Society for the Prevention of Cruelty to Children for rescuing her.

> My Dear Mr. Hunter,
> If it were not for you, to bring me in the Mission Home, I don't know where I would be now. . . . I have learned how to read and write, and to keep house. I am studying geography and arithmetic. I hope God will help you to bring more little girls to the Home, so they can be happy and learn about Jesus. May God bless you, and give you more strength to work for Him, and reward you when you leave this earth.
> *Your Chinese friend,*
> *Ah Yane.*[22]

These expressions of gratitude represented a form of payment that the "rescued" women could provide for their "rescuers."[23] However, for Ah Yane, her articulations of obligation did not stem solely from calculation, but also from a sincere conversion to Christianity. When one of her fellow mission home "sisters" became terminally ill from consumption, Ah Yane comforted her with promises of religious salvation:

> [Ah Yute] was able to talk with Ah Yane, to whom she expressed sorrow for all the care she had occasioned her teachers and friends during her illness, and for a moment expressed a fear that God might not accept her. Ah Yane assured her that if she was truly sorry for her sins, and asked Him to forgive them, He *surely would*, for He had *promised this*.[24]

The transformation of Ah Yane allowed her to become a "native helper," a term applied to "one of a handful of ethnic minority women who [were] selected by home mission women to serve as trusted assistants."[25] She served as the secretary to the "Tong Oke," or Light House Band, a missionary society organized by residents of the mission home to support proselytizing work abroad and at home.[26] Ah Yane also assisted in the efforts to rescue other Chinese women by serving as an interpreter. In this capacity, she accompanied Margaret Culbertson and other mission home reformers on visits to prisons and courts throughout California.[27] These rescue missions were emotionally trying endeavors. Frequently, the owners of prostitutes attempted to thwart the rescuers by employing legal maneuvers and threatening physical abuse. In addition, traveling outside the secure confines of the mission home also attracted the hostile attention of some white Americans. Ah Yane apparently faced these tense circumstances with poise. The missionaries reported that while serving as an interpreter in Sacramento, she "made a favorable impression upon the court by her ladylike ingenuous manner, [with] the Judge himself expressing his pleasure at her intelligence."[28] During Ah Yane's residence in the mission home, she gained the skills and confidence not only to challenge abusive conditions in the Chinese sex trade but also to navigate the legal and social institutions of white America.

The Presbyterian missionaries also provided Chung Wong with resources to adapt to American society, imparting cultural skills needed to function in late nineteenth-century Protestant America. The Bible class that he attended in Los Angeles taught not only religious scripture but also the English language and American customs. The missionary reformers themselves viewed their work as efforts to acculturate the Chinese immigrants to a Christian vision of America. When asked by a stranger about the purpose of the mission work among the Chinese, Culbertson reported that "we hope to Christianize them . . . [as] a step towards Americanizing [them]."[29] The ability to adapt to a Christian nation became increasingly important as racial hostility toward Chinese immigrants intensified during the 1870s and 1880s, culminating in widespread violence as well as the passage of discriminatory legislation. The Presbyterian missionaries themselves noted the correlation between religious conversion and anti-Chinese movements of the late nineteenth century: "The greatest prosperity of the mission has come in the years of the exclusion-law handicap."[30] If Chinese immigrants, who were accused of being inassimilable, could acquire American language, customs, and religion, the animosity directed toward them might be lessened.

PLANTING CHRISTIAN CHINESE HOMES

Presbyterian missionaries sought to Christianize and thereby Americanize the Chinese, but at the same time they emphasized and fostered the importance of immigrant ties to their own people. The Presbyterian missionary board in California, known as the Occidental Board, began under the auspices of the Foreign Missionary Society, an international organization, and resisted all efforts to transfer their work to the domestic branch of the Presbyterian Church. In a petition to the church's General Assembly, the missionary reformers explained that they viewed their work among the Chinese in the United States as intricately connected with their work in China, the central site of overseas missionary activity:[31]

> Our work is but a *branch* of the great work in China. They are *intimately* & *inseparably* connected. The Chinese here all expect to return to their own land to live. They are continually going & coming, so that Christian Chinese converted both in *China* & *here,* are at one time under *our care,* & at another under the care of Missionaries *in China.* The Chinese are not allowed to become citizens of our country, but are regarded & treated by our Government as *aliens.* The Chinese know & feel this. And when they become Christians they feel that it means going back to China, in a short time, & becoming part of *the same work* there under the *same* Board of Missions.[32]

Recognizing the racial resistance to the incorporation of Chinese immigrants as full members of American society, Presbyterian missionaries attempted to capitalize on the sojourner status of the Chinese by converting them into missionaries for their own people. Those not returning immediately to China could serve as role models and missionaries to the Chinese in the United States.

In this plan of chain conversion, Presbyterian reformers emphasized the importance of women's roles, especially in their capacity as biological or surrogate mothers. To the missionaries, the low status of Chinese women signified the lack of spiritual and social advancement of the country. As Margaret Culbertson explained, "When a daughter is born to Chinese parents, she is not accorded the joyous welcome that a son receives. . . . They are denied education and looked down upon by the sterner sex as being inferior to themselves. A certain writer has said that 'a nation cannot rise above its women.' If this statement be true, and we believe it is, China will not advance till women are allowed the privileges of education."[33]

For the missionaries, elevating the position of women represented the key to converting and elevating an entire society. As mothers and wives, Christian women provided moral guidance for their families. As one missionary publication explains, "Plant Christian Chinese homes and educate their women, and ere long we shall see the walls of heathenism falling down before the advance of the Gospel, and 'coming generations will arise up and call you blessed.'"[34]

To promote the development of Chinese Christian families, Presbyterian missionaries played the role of matchmaker. Given the imbalanced gender ratio among Chinese immigrants, "rescued" women under the guidance of the San Francisco mission home became highly desirable marriage partners. Although the white reformers believed in the value of "companionate" marriages based on mutual affection, they nevertheless sought to increase chances of compatibility by screening potential suitors.[35] The missionaries preferred Chinese men who had converted to Christianity and who could financially support a middle-class household. In all likelihood, that is how Ah Yane, who resided in the Northern California city of San Francisco, met and married the respected Christian merchant Chung Wong in the Southern California town of Santa Barbara.

Margaret Chung's parents apparently succeeded in fulfilling the goal of creating a Christian home and serving as role models for other Chinese Americans. In December 1888, Ah Yane wrote to inform Occidental Board members of her marriage and new home in Santa Barbara:

> My Dear President, Mrs. Browne, and Ladies of Occidental Board:
> I want to write a few lines to thank you ladies. I was married November 14th, 1888, to Cheaung Wong. We have a very pleasant home here. . . . I shall always remember what was done for me when I was in the Home, and the teachings that I received. . . . I cannot reward all you dear ladies for all the kindness that you have shown me, but I can pray God to bless you all and give you all many years to work for Him, and at last give you all a bright crown in heaven above. I hope we can be stars in your crown. . . .
>
> *Yours gratefully,*
> Ah Yane.[36]

Ah Yane maintained contact with the mission home after her marriage. The board reported that the newlyweds "have a pleasant Christian home there, and are much respected by a large circle of Chinese and American friends."[37] Just over a year after the marriage, a missionary publication announced the birth of their first child, Margaret Chung, on 2 October 1889, and her baptism soon after.[38] An 1893 report revealed the continued religious participation of the Chung family, noting that "the only Christian Chinese woman in Santa Barbara was educated at the Home in San Francisco and she, her husband and little girl are present regularly at Sabbath school.[39] Margaret's recollections also indicate the importance of religion in her family:

> My father & mother were devout Christians, who lived their religion. Mother played the organ for church services, in the little Presbyterian church in Santa Barbara. . . . My father always said "grace" before each meal, even tho the meal might only have consisted of coffee & sandwiches—each night before our bedtime father would gather us in front of the fireplace and sing hymns which he dearly loved—and even now, a wave of nostalgia sweeps over me when I hear the old time church hymns. . . . He lived his Christianity—when neighbors saw him coming up the street, they would say "Here comes a saint!"[40]

WOMAN'S MEDICAL MISSIONS

While Ah Yane chose to fulfill her missionary promise by forming a Christian home, the religious reformers also advocated professional work as an alternative method for women to promote Christian conversion. Presbyterian publications consistently called for the service of female missionaries, especially those trained in medicine. The interest in providing Western medical care was motivated by practical as well as religious concerns. The earliest Western missionaries sought to sidestep "China's anti-Christianity policy" by engaging "in a variety of activities rather than focusing on overtly evangelical work."[41] The effort to introduce Western medicine was not a secular alternative to the religious mission but rather an integral part of it. Missionaries viewed traditional Chinese medicine as "superstition," an indication of the culture's "intellectual darkness."[42] In their eyes, fraudulent beliefs about medical healing correlated with fallacious beliefs about religion. One publication explained: "The Medical Missionary strikes at the foundations of superstition. The conjurer with his evil spirits, the quack with his absurd nostrums, the priest with his charms and incantations, flee before the light of science, the gospel of fresh air, improved homes, sanitary laws."[43] The introduction of Western science represented an extension of missionary efforts to introduce Western culture, especially Protestantism. As the same publication went on to explain, "The *Medical* Missionary['s] . . . ultimate aim is to reach the soul by ministering to the body."

Reformers encouraged both men and women to serve as medical missionaries. However, the "medical lady missionary" was especially desirable because of her potential to access other women: "We would emphasize the importance of Woman's Medical Missions. Woman with her quick intuitions, her exquisite tact, her tender sympathies, is welcomed as a ministering angel by her suffering sisters in those countries whose customs forbid the presence of a male physician."[44] This passage demonstrates the use of traditional gender roles to justify women's entry into the male realm of professional medicine. Female physicians are characterized by their nurturing and moral qualities and not by their rational, scientific minds. Furthermore, women doctors are necessary for societies that practice strict separation of the sexes. In other words, becoming a "medical lady missionary" was not a departure from but rather an extension of traditional female responsibilities.

Missionary conversion strategies, based upon Victorian gender roles and the religious significance of medical service, encouraged increasing numbers of single professional women to serve abroad.[45] Western reformers also established opportunities for educational and professional training for "native" women, especially in the realm of medicine. During the late nineteenth and early twentieth centuries, missionaries founded female academies, medical schools, and hospitals throughout Asia. Furthermore, they also encouraged exceptional "native" converts to obtain religious and professional training in the United States. In fact, the first Chinese female students to arrive in America all came to study medicine.[46] Their status as students technically exempted them from the Chinese Exclusion Act, which targeted laborers for exclusion. However, it was their connections with American missionaries that smoothed their entry into the United States and created opportunities for medical training. All of these Chinese female physicians eventually returned to their homeland to serve as medical missionaries and engage in social reform. The combined efforts of establishing educational institutions in Asia and sponsoring the professional training of Asian women in the United States contributed to a sizable population of Asian female physicians. In China alone, women physicians constituted 12 percent of the profession by 1920, more than double the percentage of female physicians in the United States.[47]

White missionaries also promoted professional opportunities for racialized women in the United States. Just as female reformers on the East Coast supported the education of Susan La Flesche, the first Native American woman doctor, the staff at the San Francisco mission home repeatedly conveyed the importance of female medical missionaries to their Chinese charges.[48] Almost all the publications by the Occidental Board contained references to the contributions of women doctors to missionary efforts. Toward the end of Ah Yane's stay at the mission home, the home school even began teaching physiology.[49] Shortly after Ah Yane's departure from the home in 1888, the annual reports reveal that a Dr. Minnie Worley volunteered her services at the home and trained some of the residents in basic medical care.[50] Mission home residents also contributed to the work of female physicians in China. In 1890, members of Ah Yane's former missionary society, the "Tong Oke," raised $137.46 to purchase medical instruments for a woman doctor stationed in Suchow, China.[51]

The high status accorded to female medical missionaries is demonstrated by an account published in the Occidental Board annual report. Culbertson described the last wishes of a former resident who returned to the mission home when she realized how seriously ill she was: "Her one prayer had been to live to reach the Home with her children, Margaret and Henry, and just before passing away she committed them with all her belongings to our care, wishing that Margaret might become a medical missionary, and Henry a minister of the gospel."[52] The dying mother's request suggests that she viewed the role of medical missionary as the most honorable position for women, equal to that of minister for men. This particular resident had named her daughter after Margaret Culbertson, who was most likely the namesake for Margaret Chung as well.

Ah Yane apparently developed similar aspirations for her daughter. Through her efforts to rescue other Chinese women and convert them to Christianity, Ah Yane had engaged in missionary work herself. She explained that "before we came to the Mission Home we were taught to pray to idols, but now we have learned about the true God and we want our sisters in China to know about Him too."[53] Ah Yane's beliefs may have inspired her choice of Americanized names for herself and her children. After she left the mission home, she changed her name to Minnie, probably after Minnie Berry, a missionary who served in China and among Chinese in the United States, or Dr. Minnie G. Worley, the medical doctor who ministered to the residents of the mission home.

The Presbyterian missionaries who played such important roles in shaping the lives of the Chung family used traditional notions of gender and race relations to justify the expansion of women's roles and the partial incorporation of Chinese immigrants into American society. The reformers subscribed to Victorian values about women's inherent morality and nurturing capacity, marshaling these beliefs to justify the global expansion of women's social responsibility and authority. The missionaries clearly viewed their religion, science, and culture as superior to the native customs and beliefs of the Chinese. However, their belief that the Chinese could be transformed and uplifted undergirded their attempts to counter racial hostility toward these immigrants. Just as missionaries abroad espoused a form of "humane" imperialism, so missionaries in the United States practiced a "benevolent" form of racial hierarchy. The use of traditional attitudes about gender and race relations to justify social advances operated in a delicate balance within the world of the Presbyterian missions. However, the contradictions embedded in the missionary worldview came into sharper focus for the Chung family as they sought to establish themselves in Southern California.

CHAPTER 2

Living Their Religion

When I announced at the age of 10 that I was going to be
a medical missionary, my mother answered, "I hope you can,
Daughter!" . . . In spite of all the poverty and illnesses and
deaths, I don't think it ever occurred to my parents that
I would not become a doctor.

My early childhood was very sad.

Margaret Chung, *"Autobiography"*

Margaret Chung's parents began their marriage with much promise. As
Christians and as members of the merchant class, they would serve as
beacons both to fellow Chinese in this country and to those many white
Americans who viewed Chinese as unassimilable. Nevertheless, during
their twenty-six-year marriage, they faced racism, poverty, and ill health.
Margaret was born in the small town of Santa Barbara in 1889, but her
family, ever searching for the means of survival, relocated to sparsely
populated Ventura County in 1899 and then to Los Angeles shortly after
the turn of the century. Their precarious existence reflected the lives of
other Chinese in Southern California in the early twentieth century. For
help in facing these challenges, the Chung family held fast to their
religious faith.

The United States formally annexed California in 1848, following
the Mexican War. As Anglo settlers moved into the state, they sought to
supplant the existing society, which was deeply influenced by Catholicism and based upon a pastoral economy of ranching and subsistence
agriculture. To stimulate capitalist enterprises, white American develop-
ers promoted the rural regions as ripe for agribusiness and the urban areas
as sites for manufacturing and tourism. Under the terms of the Treaty of
Guadalupe-Hidalgo, Mexicans who remained in areas that became U.S.
land would have the right to U.S. citizenship and their property would
be protected under American law. However, the combination of Anglo

squatters, new taxes, and high legal fees eventually led to the economic demise of the large Mexican ranchos. Former peasants who owned land and pursued a variety of economic activities increasingly relied upon wage labor for their livelihoods. To make room for the new Anglo settlers, Mexican Americans were relocated and increasingly segregated into "barrios." Many of their adobe homes were destroyed, with wood or brick homes constructed in their place. The ghettoization or "barriorization" of Mexican Americans not only ensured their cultural and social separation from Anglos; it also made it easier to gerrymander voting districts to minimize their political power.[1]

As Anglos developed new business ventures, the Chinese also came to seek opportunities and initially provided essential labor in industries such as railroad construction, mining, and fishing. However, as growing numbers of native-born white Americans and European immigrants settled in Southern California, they organized anti-Chinese movements that initiated vigilante violence and demanded the removal and exclusion of their economic competitors. In both Santa Barbara and Los Angeles, riots targeting the Chinese took place in the 1870s. Like Mexican Americans, Chinese Americans increasingly resided in ethnic enclaves. In fact, these Chinatowns were frequently located in undesirable areas adjacent to Mexican barrios and vice districts. While some Chinese, like the Chungs, adopted religious and cultural practices that facilitated their interactions with the Protestant Anglo population, the Chinese remained a separate racial group with a status akin to the increasingly segregated and proletarianized Mexican Americans.

CHRISTIAN MERCHANT OR CHINESE LABORER?

Chung Wong and Minnie arrived in Santa Barbara after the worst of the racial violence had already occurred and just as the coastal town was experiencing an economic and population boom. The railroad connection between Los Angeles and Santa Barbara was completed in 1887. The greater ease in travel promoted tourism, and the number of residents nearly doubled, from 3,460 in 1890 to 6,587 in 1900. As in other frontier towns, the dirt streets were crowded with horses, livestock, and wagons. Saloons, stables, banks, and general stores catered to both residents and visitors. The architecture in Santa Barbara reflected the cultural and economic mixture of the population, ranging from crumbling adobes and wooden buildings with false fronts to impressive multi-leveled Victorian structures.

Margaret Chung's first home was in the back of a store located on the edge of Santa Barbara Chinatown and Pueblo Viejo, the Mexican barrio. The 1888 city directory listed Chung Wong's business as a "Chinese Bazaar—Dealer in Chinese and Japanese Fancy Goods, Silks and Chinaware, Ladies' Underwear, Etc."[2] The merchandise available for purchase, the placement of the advertisement, and the use of English indicate that he sought to attract non-Chinese customers interested in purchasing exotic goods associated with the Orient. The location of his store in the Chinatown district likely added to the appeal of the products. The several hundred Chinese in Santa Barbara occupied a two-block area and created a community to service the needs of its residents.[3] The neighborhood featured boarding homes, a joss house for traditional religious observances, a Chinese language school, gambling establishments, and even opium dens. Attracted by the exotic and even dangerous reputation of Chinatown, tourists became interested in visiting the area and purchasing mementos of their experience. Chung Wong, a merchant who was acculturated enough to advertise his business in English and known in the Santa Barbara community for his Protestant Christian beliefs, served as a "safe" supplier of curios for the curious.[4]

Chung Wong's career as a merchant of Oriental goods did not last long. The Chinese Bazaar did not appear in the next extant city directory. Instead, the 1893 publication indicates that he became an agricultural merchant by operating a "Hay and Grain" business.[5] "Chung Wong & Co" was located a block away from the previous enterprise but still on the edge of Chinatown and the Mexican barrio. This venture also folded rather quickly, not appearing in the 1894 Collector of Customs survey of Chinese merchants in Santa Barbara.[6] The reasons for Chung Wong's business failures are probably varied. It is possible that he did not have a good head for commerce. Margaret recalled, "My father, who was a good, honest, decent, God-fearing Christian, tried very hard to make a living for his large family. . . . [but I don't think] he ever made more than 45.00 a month in his whole life."[7] Given that most Chinese in the United States were channeled toward low-paying, manual jobs, Chung Wong's financial woes also likely reflected the economic difficulties facing racially despised groups.

On the basis of an interview with Margaret Chung, a Santa Barbara newspaper recounted that her father turned to growing and selling vegetables to support his family: "Dr. Chung's parents were poor, even by Chinese standards, when they lived in Santa Barbara. Her father failed to make a success as the proprietor of one of the city's first Chinese china and art stores and joined others of his race who kept Santa Barbara in fresh vegetables. . . . He worked in his gardens early and late and peddled their products during the day, for the small profits that maintained his rapidly-growing family."[8] Chung Wong's participation in small-scale commercial growing and selling, otherwise known as "truck gardening," reflects Chinese dominance of the occupation during the era following the anti-Chinese movements. As new urban communities like Santa Barbara and Los Angeles developed, the demand for fresh produce created a niche for the Chinese. No longer desired in the more lucrative trades of mining and railroad construction, they turned to the task of feeding the Anglo settlers. In Los Angeles alone, nearly half of the Chinese population engaged in truck farming in the 1880s and were responsible for nearly 90 percent of all the vegetables consumed in the city.[9]

As a vegetable peddler, Chung Wong occupied an uncertain class position. While nominally recognized as a merchant, since he sold his own produce, Chung Wong could also be considered a farm laborer. The ambiguity of his occupation was reflected in the birth certificates of his children. The document for Paul Chung, born 18 February 1897, identifies the occupation of his father as a laborer, while the certificate for Andrew Chung, born 6 April 1898, identifies the father as a merchant.[10]

The distinction between the two occupations, merchant and laborer, held great significance for Chinese immigrants during the late nineteenth and early twentieth centuries. The 1882 Chinese Exclusion Act prevented the entry of Chinese laborers but exempted merchants. As a merchant, Chung Wong could travel in and out of the United States as well as sponsor the migration of his family members. Furthermore, the occupation of merchant carried a positive social status among Chinese and white Americans. Merchants, with their contacts with the broader society and their economic resources, could provide opportunities for employment and social services for other Chinese immigrants. White Americans also recognized the higher status of Chinese merchants and considered them as more deserving of respect and acceptance. In other words, Chung Wong's status as a merchant reinforced the roles that the Presbyterian missionaries had prescribed for him, that of leader and representative of Chinese Americans.

During his early years in Santa Barbara, Chung Wong functioned as a respected intermediary between the white and Chinese American communities. He appears in an official survey on Chinese merchants in Santa Barbara which sought to identify and verify the status of Chinese residents for the purposes of administering immigration legislation. Although Chung Wong was no longer a merchant in 1894, the report indicates his prior activities. Chung's name surfaces three times in the document. In one instance, Quan Quong, identified as a pastry cook for the Arlington Hotel in Santa Barbara, claimed that he qualified as a merchant and was therefore eligible for reentry into the country, because he owned an interest in the store of Chung Wong & Co. prior to his departure from the United States in July 1892.[11] In two other cases, Chung played a more active role in verifying the status of Chinese immigrants. In July and August of 1893, he requested that the firm of Burson and Lamb issue certificates authenticating the merchant standing of Yee Tong Jong and Yee June.[12]

As these cases indicate, members of the Santa Barbara Chinese and white American communities respected Chung Wong. The immigrants who either claimed partnership with him or sought his assistance in verifying their merchant status believed that he would be an asset to their cases. Their belief appears to have been well founded. The testimonies of Burson and Lamb indicate that they accepted Chung Wong's word regarding his friends. His ability to serve as an intermediary between Chinese and white Santa Barbarans, however, depended upon his status as an established merchant. As a vegetable peddler, even though he interacted daily with white Americans in selling produce, his statements regarding the position of other Chinese Americans would hold less value due to perceptions of his laborer status. Furthermore, the increasing transience of the Chung family, a by-product of their economic instability, would make it difficult for him to establish local connections.

Class status and religious affiliation could mediate but not prevent racial discrimination, since under the Chinese Exclusion Act neither merchants nor laborers were eligible for U.S. citizenship. In Southern California, as in other parts of the country, racial harassment of Chinese was endemic. William A. Edwards, who grew up in Santa Barbara during the turn of the century, recalled that the Chinese population worked in occupations that depended on the patronage of white residents. The close, daily interactions between Chinese and white Santa Barbarans did not lessen the perception of cultural difference, however. Although the Edwards family employed a Chinese cook, a common practice among white families, he emphasizes that the Chinese, "coming from a quite different civilization from ours, . . . brought their customs with them; and their language, clothing and habits kept them apart." These outward indications of "alienness" sometimes evoked negative reactions from the white residents of Santa Barbara: "Their oriental dress and 'Pidgin English' made them a natural prey for small boys and toughs who took delight in pestering them, with rocks and frightening their horses as they went about their daily business." Edwards himself was not above ridiculing Chinese Santa Barbarans. He recalled attending grade school with Margaret Chung, the only Chinese girl in his class, whom he mistakenly describes as the daughter of a launderer:

> It happened one afternoon that I was leaving school alone. When I reached the street her father drove up in his delivery wagon and on learning that his daughter was in my class he asked me if I would tell the teacher that her father was outside and wanted to take her home. Like an obliging boy I went to the class, but instead of giving the message as requested I opened the door a little and shouted, "Can Margaret Chung Wung be excused?" The class all thought it very funny and for a few days I heard no end of it.[13]

Margaret's presence in school demonstrates that her parents subscribed to Presbyterian views about the importance of education for girls. In fact, Christian missionaries organized the first schools open to Chinese children in Santa Barbara. Margaret's status as the only Chinese girl in the class suggests that she gained exposure to mainstream American culture and interacted daily with non-Chinese Americans. It is unclear how many of Chung's classmates were Mexican Americans. They constituted approximately 20 percent of the Santa Barbara population, a community double to quadruple the size of the Chinese. However, residents of Mexican ancestry objected to the English-only instruction in public schools and preferred parochial schools, which not only offered bilingual education but also instruction on Catholicism.[14] As perhaps one of just a few non-Anglo students in the school, Margaret became the subject of jokes and pranks. Edwards' account suggests that the dominant American society simultaneously needed and stigmatized the Chinese in Santa Barbara.

IMMIGRANT DOMESTICITY

The Presbyterian missionaries who selected Christian merchants as husbands for their charges recognized that material resources were necessary to fulfill the ideal of a Victorian, middle-class, companionate marriage. As Chung Wong's status declined from merchant to laborer,

Minnie and the rest of the family clung to middle-class aspirations but also assumed roles more typical of working-class, immigrant families.

It must have been quite a culture shock for Minnie to move from the Presbyterian Chinese Mission Home to Santa Barbara. At the mission home, she was secluded in a protective, all-female environment. In her new home, Minnie was a minority within a minority, in terms of both gender and race. Few Chinese women, let alone families, lived among the overwhelmingly male population. At the same time, Minnie faced the challenge of learning how to be a wife and mother. It is likely that she knew Chung Wong only slightly, if at all, before their marriage. Whatever her anxieties may have been, though, her daughter remembered that Chung Wong "loved his family devotedly—and adored his wife."[15]

Life must have been difficult for Minnie. During her marriage to Chung Wong, she endured relentless poverty and debilitating illness. She bore eleven children, seven of whom survived.[16] Throughout, Minnie never abandoned her early Presbyterian roots, turning to religion for much-needed emotional and spiritual comfort. And, although her ties to the mission home became more tenuous following the departure of Margaret Culbertson in 1897, Minnie continued her participation in Christian communities.[17] The Chung family regularly attended the Santa Barbara First Presbyterian Church as well as its affiliated Chinese mission. A newspaper clipping from December of 1898 reported that nine-year-old Margaret performed in a Christmas pageant at the mission that year.[18]

In addition, Minnie kept in contact with her "sisters" from the Presbyterian Chinese Mission Home. Like her, other Chinese women had left the mission home to marry and create Christian homes of their own. Minnie kept photographs of her sisters and maintained her close friendship with Chin Mooie, who, like Minnie, married a merchant and moved to Santa Barbara in the early 1890s.[19] Chin Mooie's papers indicate that she corresponded, exchanged photographs, and sent clothes to former mission home residents. One letter, written by a mission home "sister," reports the changes in the lives of other residents:

> My Dear Sister
> Your letter was received. Glad to hear from you . . . Ah Mooie has another baby girl. Sing Chouie has a girl too and [illegible] has a boy. . . . I had a letter from Miss Culbertson she was feeling better. Give my kind regards to your husband and all the children also to Mrs. Chung Wong. Hopefully you are all well. . . .
>   *Your sister*
>   *Chun Fah*[20]

The letter, as well as the photographs and newspaper clippings that Chin Mooie and Minnie Chung collected, suggests that a support network existed among the Chinese American women who formerly resided at the Presbyterian Chinese Mission Home.

Many of these women, inspired by Christian missionary ideals, helped to establish community service organizations in the areas where they resided. Chin Mooie eventually moved to Bakersfield, where she was "reputedly the first Chinese Christian woman" and "one of the founders of the Chinese Congregational mission."[21] Chun Fah, whose husband, the Rev. Ng Poon Chew, founded the influential Chinese American newspaper *Chung Sai Yat Po,* helped launch the YWCA in San Francisco Chinatown in 1916.[22] Thus the rescue efforts of the Presbyterian Chinese Mission Home resulted in a network of Chinese Christian women who in turn formed a core of middle-class families and shaped the development of religious reform institutions in various cities throughout the West.[23]

Minnie participated in this network. At the same time, however, she and the older children in the family needed to work in order to survive. Even though Chung Wong advertised his businesses under his name, they most likely functioned as family enterprises. The Santa Barbara city directory lists the Chinese Bazaar's address as a residence as well as a store, a common practice among Chinese merchants. Thus, while Victorian social norms supported separate gender spheres—and husbands of the Chinese merchant class, in particular, sought to seclude their wives from the predominantly male immigrant population— Minnie almost certainly worked alongside her husband. Such work did not meet the Victorian ideal for middle-class family life, but it was necessary for many if not most immigrants. After all, "women of leisure were but a small proportion of immigrant wives in the late nineteenth century. [The lives] of most wives [were] marked by constant toil."[24] Minnie's social skills, honed in the mission home, no doubt served as valuable assets in interactions with potential customers, especially female shoppers interested in silks, "Chinaware," and intimate apparel.[25] Having the store and household integrated under one roof also probably facilitated Minnie's efforts to combine housekeeping, child rearing, and business responsibilities.

The Chungs' economic circumstances continued to worsen, and when they moved to Ventura County in 1899, Minnie and the children found work related to Chung Wong's agricultural occupation. Located between Santa Barbara and Los Angeles, the entire county of Ventura contained the same number of Chinese as the city of Santa Barbara.[26] Most likely through his business and/or religious connections, Chung Wong became ranch manager at the Rancho Guadalasca, one of the large Mexican ranchos in the county that had devolved to Anglo ownership after the 1848 conquest.[27] Despite his new position, the labor of the entire family was needed to survive. Margaret recalled that "in order to eat, we would plant potatoes, yams, and other vegetables. . . . My mother and the children and I would go up to Mower park and pit apricots. We got nine cents for pitting fifty pound lug boxful of apricots."[28]

Because the family relied on their ability to perform physical labor to earn wages, illness had a devastating impact on their economic welfare. When Margaret's father became "bedridden with rheumatism," she earned money by mowing hay and hauling freight. At ten years old, she was "too small to reach the horses' necks with the harness," so she pulled them "alongside of a large packing case." To cut down on expenses, Margaret also "learned to half-sole the shoes for my brothers and sisters, for even though the shoes cost only about ninety-five cents or a dollar a pair they would wear out fast and there wasn't even enough money to get them half-soled."[29]

In addition to working outside the home, Margaret and Anna, the two eldest daughters, assisted their mother in raising their siblings. Years later, Margaret explained her responsibilities: "I had to wash the diapers for all of them, feed them—usually there were at least two on diapers and two on milk bottles. . . . I would have to do the cooking and the cleaning and take care of my mother as best as a little child of that age could."[30] Minnie desperately needed her daughters' assistance because she suffered from tuberculosis, a common disease among immigrants and the poor. She very likely had the illness when she first arrived at the mission home with a severe cough. Good care ameliorated some of the symptoms. However, living in poverty and experiencing numerous pregnancies worsened her condition. Minnie's sufferings traumatized her young daughter, Margaret: "I remember when I was about five, watching with horror as my mother leaned over an ashcan, haemorrhaging from the lungs as a result of tuberculosis. About every month I would stand at the foot of her bed all night long giving her teaspoonsful of salt which is what the doctors at the time ordered in an effort to stop the haemorrhage. For twenty-six long years, each month there would be several nights that I would stand, agonized with terror, watching her die a little at a time."[31]

PATHS TO A HIGHER CALLING

Margaret's early experience with poverty, as well as the missionary ethos imparted to her by her mother, prepared her to work for a living. In fact, her early exposure to manual work motivated her to pursue a more elevated occupation. Margaret declared her goal of becoming a medical missionary around age ten, the same time that she was assuming greater responsibility for the family's welfare and engaging in arduous agricultural work in Ventura County. Despite the difficulties that the Chungs faced, she received encouragement to fulfill her perceived calling. Her mother, in particular, served as a role model. Margaret had great respect for her father, whom she described as "inventive." However, she viewed her mother as "the more brilliant of the two" and "very modern." Minnie "spoke English without a trace of accent . . . [and] there were very few subjects that she could not discuss intelligently."[32] Despite being "an invalid most of her life," Minnie fueled her daughter's desire to learn.

The Chungs' economic and racial status, however, affected their ability to educate their children. Like other poor families, they moved rather frequently, looking for work. As a result, Margaret's early education was repeatedly interrupted. In June of 1899, her name appears in the records of the San Buena Ventura school district in Ventura County as a fourth-grade pupil. Unlike most of the other students, who received instruction for nine to ten months during that school year, Chung only attended fifty-two-and-a-half days—less than two months.[33] She most likely joined the school late in the academic year, since that is when her family moved into the county. In a combination third- and fourth-grade class of thirty-four students, she was again the only one of Asian ancestry; there were two pupils with Spanish last names.[34]

Margaret did not attend fifth grade until two years after she first appeared in the school records as a fourth grader. She was enrolled in the Ocean View District of Ventura County for nine months in 1900–1901.[35] Reflecting the sparse population in the region, the school listed a total of twenty-one students ranging from first through seventh grade. This time, she appeared to be the only non-Anglo pupil. Her younger siblings were not yet old enough to join her.

The Chungs decided to move to Los Angeles shortly after Margaret completed fifth grade just after the turn of the century. The Chung family arrived in Los Angeles as part of a larger population explosion. The population went from one hundred thousand in 1900 to over three hundred thousand in 1910, and then nearly doubled, reaching nearly six hundred thousand in 1920.[36] Due to immigration restriction and the continuing predominance of males, the Chinese population remained steady at approximately two thousand during the first two decades of the twentieth century. However, increases in the numbers of Japanese, African, and Mexican Americans kept pace with the general growth of the city.[37] These groups were joined by white migrants from the Midwest as well as European immigrants from abroad. Unlike cities in the East, where four out of five residents were native to their respective locations, half of the Los Angeles population in 1930 had been there less than five years, and nine out of ten had been there less than fifteen years.[38]

The demographic diversity of Los Angeles shaped the development of educational institutions in the city. In her autobiography, Margaret Chung characterized education as a privilege available to all Americans, explaining that "I was educated on the taxes of free men whose foresight it was that everyone in this country should be literate and enlightened."[39] The idea of universal public education actually took hold during the late nineteenth and early twentieth centuries, an era described as "the incorporation of America."[40] As the economy became dominated by large-scale industries, new types of labor and educational training became necessary. Formal schooling helped to prepare the middle class for the emerging managerial and technical occupations. For members of the working class, who increasingly came from racialized and immigrant backgrounds, education served as a mechanism to instill American cultural norms and good work habits. Reflecting these ideas of social uplift as well as social control, working-class children discovered opportunities for advancement but also experienced stigmatization that reinforced their marginal social status. For example, in Los Angeles, "the increased application of I.Q. testing, always administered in English, invariably segregated Mexican children in special classes for the mentally inferior or mentally retarded."[41] Furthermore, schools located in predominantly working-class, immigrant, and racialized communities tended to develop courses that integrated citizenship classes with vocational training, associating Americanization with learning appropriate skills for manual labor.

Margaret Chung very likely attended these schools that channeled "undesirable" students toward less intellectually rigorous courses. Although her Los Angeles school records are not available, her family lived in working-class ethnic neighborhoods. Following his departure from Ventura County, Chung Wong worked on a dairy in Vernon, an area southeast of the Los Angeles downtown and adjacent to the East Adams area, known as a farming and produce center for Chinese Americans.[42] The 1910 census indicates that the family had moved again, this time closer to the San Pedro district, where just the year before, Chinese, Japanese, and European immigrants, as well as American-born peddlers, opened the City Market to sell fruits and vegetables grown on nearby farmlands. Chung Wong resumed his work as a vegetable peddler there. The family's neighbors were a stockyard on one side and a household of four Chinese men who also worked as vegetable peddlers on the other. However, the most dominant ethnic group in the neighborhood consisted of working-class Mexican Americans. Shortly after the 1910 census, the family moved near the central Plaza area. Formerly a commercial market and gathering place for the Mexican community, it became the primary Chinatown in Los Angeles.[43] Still, Chinese Americans did not become the predominant residents of the area. The region surrounding the Plaza was known as the most ethnically diverse neighborhood in Los Angeles, home to over twenty different groups, including Mexican, Japanese, Italian, Jewish, and African Americans.[44] The Chung family subsequently returned to the San Pedro Market area in the mid-1910s, when plans for an impending redevelopment project threatened relocation from the Plaza area.[45]

Dorothy, the youngest child in the Chung family, recalled that even when they resided in areas with few Chinese Americans, Chung Wong and Minnie took their children to Chinatown to visit friends and "family," most likely Minnie's "sisters" from the mission home. The Chungs also attended Chinese church (a Christian institution with a Chinese congregation). When they lived close enough to a Chinese school, Chung Wong and Minnie sent their children in the afternoons, after attending public school, to improve their Chinese and learn about the history and culture of their ancestral country. According to Dorothy, her parents encouraged their children to speak Cantonese at home, a practice they abandoned after Minnie and Chung Wong died. It is likely that Margaret did not enroll in Chinese school herself, because she worked in the afternoons to help support her family. However, at least two of her younger sisters attended, suggesting that the parents honored their Chinese heritage.[46]

Being part of a cosmopolitan urban environment shaped Margaret's educational experiences and vocational aspirations. She discovered new forms of employment, which both positively and negatively influenced her ambitions. Because of the large population of Chinese in Los Angeles, there was a thriving ethnic service sector. As she recalled, "While in the seventh and eighth grades in grammar school, I went to work in a chop suey restaurant in order to help out with the family finances. After school I would go to this restaurant and clean the tables, fill the salt and peppers, mop the floor, wait on tables, and sometimes would do a little cooking in the kitchen. For all of this work from 3:30 in the afternoon until 3:00 in the morning seven days a week, I received the sum of six dollars a week."[47] Working at the restaurant provided benefits aside from wages. Margaret recalled that "the manager of a restaurant would sometimes gives us trimmings from ham and bacon rind. My sister, Anna, and I would use these to flavor whatever vegetables we could get hold of. . . . As necessity is the mother of invention so my sister and I became very good cooks because we had learned in the years of poverty to make very common ordinary things tasty."[48] Such benefits, however, did not outweigh the long hours, low pay, and grueling physical work, and Margaret set her sights beyond the restaurant to other employment opportunities.

Following her graduation from grammar school, Margaret obtained a position in the Central Department Store in Los Angeles. Both restaurant and retail work were considered female occupations, and hence subject to low wages and little prestige. However, the opportunity to work in a department store that catered to mainstream Americans seemed glamorous to the young woman and most likely provided slightly better pay as well. In contrast to the family-owned businesses in ethnic and rural communities, these new consumer palaces sold standardized goods featured in mass advertising campaigns. And, although immigrant labor no doubt created the products sold in both ethnic restaurants and mainstream department stores, their contributions were rendered invisible in the latter. Native-born white women were more likely to work as clerks and sale assistants in department stores, while immigrant and racialized women found positions in ethnic businesses and factories. The few who were lucky enough to secure jobs at department stores tended to be placed in positions that required little public interaction.

It is not clear how Chung obtained employment at the Central Department Store or what she did there. In any case, this job inspired her to become an entrepreneur. At the time, the law did not require school attendance beyond age fourteen; thus only 15 percent of Los Angeles youth were enrolled in high school in 1900.[49] Following her graduation from eighth grade, Margaret sought to "fit herself for business life" and attempted to gain a scholarship to attend the local Brownsberger Business College. Very likely, her ambitions were fueled by the accomplishments of Mansie Kim, a recent graduate of Browns-berger and the daughter of Chin Mooie, who had resided at the mission home with Margaret's mother.[50] Like other women with middle-class aspirations, Mansie and Margaret sought to prepare themselves for white-collar professions in the entrepreneurial world.[51]

It is unclear why Margaret chose not to enter business college but instead returned to her original goal of becoming a medical missionary. Perhaps the decision resulted from her inability to obtain financial support for business school and her success in winning a scholarship to attend the Preparatory Academy, which was affiliated with the University of Southern California. While these historical accidents and financial considerations no doubt played a role, her life experiences and religious upbringing also guided her decision to become a physician.

Minnie's struggles with her health likely influenced Margaret's career choice. Many female doctors cite "a childhood or adolescent encounter with illness—either their own or that of a close friend or relative" as a motivation for pursuing medicine as a profession.[52] Given Margaret's memories of helplessness while watching her mother suffer and eventually die from tuberculosis, she may have envisioned the possibility of playing a more heroic role in curing her mother's illness.

Her mother's confinements and poor health also provided opportunities for Margaret to gain exposure to physicians. The birth certificates for two of her siblings indicate that Minnie was attended by one of the first female physicians in Santa Barbara.[53] Margaret also recalled admiring "the gentleness, the goodness and the ability of the family doctor who made his visits on a bicycle" during their stay in Ventura County.[54] Not only did the physician's compassion impress the young child, but the novelty of the bicycle as a mode of transportation reinforced the sense of social prestige and independence associated with the medical profession.

Furthermore, by becoming a medical missionary, Margaret could fulfill the religiously inspired goal of offering physical healing for those in spiritual need. Despite the hardships experienced by the Chung family, they persisted in their religious faith. When young Margaret announced her desire to be a "medical missionary," not just a physician, she proclaimed the importance of Christianity in her life.

Finally, because most physicians established their own practices, Margaret could pursue her interest in becoming an independent businesswoman while also fulfilling her desire to serve in an altruistic religious capacity. In fact, she relied on her entrepreneurial skills to win a scholarship to pursue secondary education. In exchange for selling the most number of subscriptions for the *Los Angeles Times,* the newspaper provided funds to support her enrollment at a private high school. Her entry into this elite world offered opportunities to fulfill a purpose higher than mere survival.

CHAPTER 3

Where Womanhood
and Childhood Meet

Any woman surgeon . . . bucks heavy odds of lay prejudice
and professional resentment at usurpation of what many
consider to be a man's undisputed field and when that woman
is an American of Chinese descent she is granted even fewer
mistakes and less leisure.

Margaret Chung, Los Angeles Times, 1939

In the fall of 1907, Margaret enrolled in the Preparatory Academy, which was affiliated with the University of Southern California (USC). Reflecting the recurring delays to her education, she was nearly eighteen years old when she entered ninth grade. Her desire to become a medical missionary most likely influenced her academic plans. Established by the Methodist Episcopal Church in 1881, USC took its religious charge seriously. The school expected all students to attend daily chapel exercises and regular church services. Those who intended to pursue a religious profession or who were children of ministers received reductions in their tuition.[1] The USC College of Physicians and Surgeons, located near the San Pedro and Plaza Chinatown communities, accepted students with high school diplomas who could demonstrate their ability to undertake medical study.[2] Attending the USC Preparatory Academy enhanced Chung's chances of gaining admission to medical school without a college education, and indeed she entered the College of Physicians and Surgeons in 1911, graduating in 1916.

At the USC Preparatory Academy, Chung entered a world that sharply contrasted with her childhood experiences of poverty and uprootedness. The chance to gain a college preparatory education and professional training represented an opportunity to remake herself. Aside from the potential to obtain skills that could improve her economic status, her education also exposed her to the more intangible elements of middle-class identity. The socialization experience would allow her to develop appropriate cultural mannerisms and a new set of peers.

In this new environment, however, Chung's Chinese ancestry, class background, and gender marked her as an outsider. Her classmates were overwhelmingly white and very likely well-to-do. Although female pupils constituted nearly half of the Preparatory Academy student body, they represented a tiny minority in medical school. During the nine years that Chung attended USC, from 1907 to 1911 in the academy and 1911 to 1916 in medical school, she experimented with extracurricular activities, intellectual interests, and even her appearance to establish a niche for herself. Her efforts demonstrate a particular enthusiasm for adopting various gender and cultural personas. Creating these malleable identities allowed her to pursue a dual strategy of assimilation and separatism. On the one hand, she attempted to blend in to the social mainstream. On the other hand, unable to erase completely her femaleness or her Chinese ancestry, she capitalized on her "otherness" to obtain support and recognition.

Chung's twofold approach was a response to the uneasy coexistence of divergent social values during this era of transformation. During the early decades of the twentieth century, American norms increasingly shifted away from Victorian beliefs in inherent gender and racial differences to modern values of equality and cosmopolitanism. As a member of this transitional generation, Chung promoted gender and racial integration.[3] However, modern reforms in the education system and the field of medicine actually decreased the numbers of women and people of color admitted into the profession. Furthermore, a minimally coeducational and racially mixed setting did not necessarily promote social equality. The persistence and even strengthened intensity of discrimination encouraged "sex solidarity" and "race consciousness" even among those who asserted their individuality and rejected the Victorian notion that biology was destiny.

THE FEMINIZATION OF EDUCATION

In deciding to enroll in a private high school, Chung chose an unusual path for someone of her race and economic background, but not necessarily for her sex. Female students constituted nearly half, approximately 44 percent, of her class.[4] By the early twentieth century, primary, secondary, and even most higher institutions of learning accepted the principle of coeducation.[5] The presence of women in these schools represented a victory for advocates of female education. Previously, conservatives had argued that teaching girls, particularly in mixed settings, defeminized these young women and rendered them unfit for motherhood. Supporters countered that education helped girls to reach their full female potential. For much of the nineteenth century, women interested in pursuing secondary and college education attended gender-segregated academies, where their uniquely feminine qualities could be nurtured. By the end of the century, however, women's successful efforts to enter traditionally male institutions had resulted in increasing numbers of coeducational schools. This movement met with greater receptivity in the Midwest and West, where many institutions, like USC, enrolled women from the outset. The newness of these schools, relative to those in the South and the East, combined with the smaller pool of potential students, favored more open admission standards.

Coeducational schools, however, did not imply a belief in gender equality or a commitment to coeducation as it is understood today. In fact, precisely because young women and men attended the same institution, administrators and teachers carefully considered how to instruct and monitor their pupils. Some schools separated girls and boys into different classes or required them to sit in separate sections of the same classroom. It is unclear if the USC Preparatory Academy instituted these practices. However, the academy school catalogues and yearbooks reveal that gender differences were structured into many areas of the academic experience. Young men and women organized segregated literary, religious, and service organizations. In school photographs, the girls posed together as a group; the boys posed either opposite or around the girls. Perhaps as an indication of her marginalization, Chung tended to stand at the outermost edge of these pictures. Differentiations based on gender also extended to the instructional staff. Professors affiliated with the USC College of Liberal Arts taught academy students to prepare them for university-level instruction. Although women constituted approximately 38 percent of the faculty, most of them served in the lower ranks of assistant professors and teaching assistants.

The persistence of gender-based distinctions did not prevent all forms of female advancement. Some young women played active leadership roles in coeducational settings. For example, Chung's first-year class elected three girls and one boy to serve as class officers. Although two of the young women served in the lower status positions of secretary and treasurer, one assumed the position of president.

Margaret herself participated in both gender-segregated organizations and coeducational activities at the Preparatory Academy. During her sophomore year, she became a member of the Willard Literary Society, a women's organization that met weekly to discuss and recite literature. Her participation reveals her interest in cultivating a refined sensibility associated with a classical Victorian education. The curriculum at the academy sought to prepare students not only scholastically but also socially to participate as members of an educated elite. Students were required to take courses in science, literature, Latin, and modern European languages. The Willard Literary Society provided a venue for Chung to develop her cultural tastes and establish friendships with those of similar interests.

While in some ways she aspired to be a Victorian lady, Chung also experimented with modern forms of female behavior. During her junior year, the academy established an interscholastic girls' basketball team. Although she does not appear in the annual photograph, Chung claimed to have played on the team.[6] Female participation in athletics, especially in organized competition, challenged older notions of gender-appropriate behavior. The Victorian lady was characterized by placidity and gentility, whereas the "new woman" took pleasure in physical exertion and in experimenting with traditionally "male" forms of recreation. While USC decided to endorse this new model of athletic womanhood, the public Los Angeles High School actually banned interscholastic competition. Instead, they encouraged female students to participate as cheerleaders at male athletic competitions.[7] By playing basketball, Chung joined the "sports craze" that consumed modern women during the early decades of the twentieth century.

The ability to experiment and develop new skills in gender segregated environments prepared Chung to succeed in coeducational settings. During her first year at the Preparatory Academy, she entered the Declamation Contest. She did not receive an award for her recitation, but she persevered in her public-speaking efforts.[8] After a year in the Willard Literary Society, where she practiced her speaking skills with other women, Margaret went on to win a schoolwide coeducational oratorical contest during her junior year. For winning the USC Academy competition, she represented her school at an interscholastic contest, competing against speakers from three other local high schools. She was the only woman and the only Chinese American to participate. Chung won second honors at the event, gaining recognition as well as a scholarship to complete her high school education.[9]

WOMEN IN A MASCULINE PROFESSION

When Margaret entered the USC College of Physicians and Surgeons in 1911, she continued to find support in women's separatist communities, but she also developed new strategies to establish a niche among her male classmates. In contrast to the Preparatory Academy, the medical school enrolled only a small fraction of women. During Chung's first year, there were three other female students out of a total of forty.[10] In subsequent years, she had at most one other female classmate. Aside from one woman professor, who taught during Chung's first year of medical school, all of the faculty were men.

Chung's experience reflects broader changes in medical education. Elizabeth Blackwell first broke the American gender barrier in 1847 by successfully enrolling in and graduating from the Geneva Medical College in upstate New York. However, as late as 1890, one year after Chung's birth, two thirds of all female physicians received their training at women's medical colleges.[11] In fact, the first Native American, the first three African American, and three of the earliest Chinese women physicians all graduated from women's schools.[12] In response to the continued resistance to admitting female students into traditionally male institutions, seventeen women's medical colleges were created during the second half of the nineteenth century.[13]

By 1910, however, just a year before Chung entered medical school, all but one of the women's schools had closed and more than 80 percent of female students were receiving their training in coeducational institutions.[14] This revolution in medical education stemmed from broader changes in the profession. During the nineteenth century, a variety of schools provided training in a diversity of health-care approaches, including herbal medicine, midwifery, homeopathy, and other eclectic forms of treatment. Most physicians adopted a holistic and community-based approach to medical care.[15] They established practices in their homes and made house calls; few affiliated with hospitals, which were perceived as undesirable and unhealthy sites that served those without family to care for them. However, influenced by scientific developments in Europe, certain physicians in the United States attempted to modernize the field of medicine by emphasizing the importance of laboratory research, hospital-based health care, and the development of specializations. To institute new standards in the profession, these so-called regular doctors initiated a series of reforms through the American Medical Association (AMA) and the state.[16]

In this context of changing professional standards, Chung was relatively fortunate in her timing. Over the course of the late nineteenth and early twentieth centuries, the numbers of medical schools and students decreased as the AMA systematically reviewed the curriculum, faculty, facilities, and financial resources of each institution.[17] The changes, instituted under the banner of modern scientific reform, had a disproportionate impact on women and people of color. Most of the "unorthodox" schools, which taught more eclectic forms of medicine and admitted a more diverse student body, were recommended for closure. Even "regular" colleges, particularly women's and traditionally black schools, folded due to lack of resources to improve laboratory facilities and research programs. Had Chung applied a few years after 1911, she would not have gained admission to the USC medical school with just a high school education. Under pressure to match rising standards for professional training, USC instituted stricter entrance qualifications in 1914 and again in 1916.[18] She also was fortunate to complete her studies in 1916. In 1920, the school closed because of its financial inability to meet the requirements of a first-rate institution. Other individuals were not as lucky. The increasingly exclusive nature of the medical profession resulted in a 36 percent decline in male graduates and a 54 percent decrease in female graduates from 1904 to 1915.[19] Like Chung, the women who gained entry into the remaining coeducational institutions constituted a small percentage of their medical classes, with a national average of 5 percent.[20]

As at the high school level, a gender-mixed medical school did not necessarily mean an equal education for men and women. Some schools excluded women from learning about topics considered "unladylike," such as venereal disease. Others prevented female students from gaining clinical experience in male-dominated specializations, such as surgery. In addition to gender-biased school policies, the behavior of some male students tended to range from ostracism to harassment, making medical school all the more difficult for female students.

In the predominantly masculine environment of the USC College of Physicians and Surgeons, Chung broadened her experimentation with her gender persona. At the academy, she had appropriated a blend of Victorian and modern female attributes; in medical school, she expanded her range of behavior to facilitate assimilation into a male profession. During her sophomore year, when she was the only woman out of twenty-three students, school photographs reveal Chung practicing partial cross-dressing.[21] She retained her public identity as a woman, but she adopted a masculine style of dress. Pulling her hair back, she wore a dark suit with vest and tie, a choice of clothing that allowed her to blend in to the larger group of similarly attired male students. However, several subtle touches point to her femininity. The lapels of the men's jacket lapped left over right; Chung's lapped right over left. Her jacket was slightly longer than the men's, and it did not have the vee-shaped opening at the hem. Finally, she wore a skirt. Despite these touches, Chung's overall manly style in this photograph contrasts sharply with her look in previous photographs, which featured her in long dresses and feminine blouses with her hair carefully styled in a bun. Her position in the picture also suggests a different sense of her place in the group. Instead of standing on the edges of the group, perhaps an indication of her sense of herself as a marginal figure, Chung now appears in the middle of the front row.

A number of professional women adopted masculine dress to symbolize (and facilitate) their entry into traditionally male realms. Some women dressed in male clothing as a uniform or as a protective measure that would allow them to merge into the existing professional culture.[22] Chung, however, apparently enjoyed adopting masculine clothing and even a male name. During her early career, her favorite picture featured her in a similar dark suit. She sent autographed versions of the photo to her friends and identified herself as "Mike."

Chung succeeded in integrating into her class, at least partially. P. M. Suski, a male immigrant from Japan who entered the USC medical school one year after Chung, recalled that she was "a very bright and popular sophomore student."[23] During the year that she dressed in male clothing, she also served as an officer for the sophomore class as well as the general medical student body. In contrast to her preparatory school years, however, in which women assumed the highest ranking position of president, Margaret served in the traditionally female office of secretary.

Throughout, Chung maintained a sense of female solidarity. In 1914, the year she appeared in male clothing, Margaret helped found the USC chapter of Nu Sigma Phi, a medical sorority first organized at the University of Illinois in 1898.[24] Male USC students had four well-established medical fraternities. These organizations provided valuable social and career contacts, because the membership included faculty, alumni, and affiliates at other schools. In contrast, Nu Sigma Phi was the only organization available for female "fraternizing." As the only woman in her class, Chung no doubt welcomed the chance to share educational, professional, and personal experiences with both current and former students.

Chung also participated in the campus Young Women's Christian Association. Her speech to the YWCA in October of 1913 reflects the opportunities and the tensions in her medical school years. Speaking on the theme of "friendship," Chung stressed the importance of diversity: "We need the friendship of those whose interests and types of mind differ most from our own. The University offers a great opportunity for such friendship and students cannot afford to be exclusive."[25] This message about diversity delivered to a group of Christian women shows that Chung needed support from those like her.

"THE BITTERNESS OF RACIAL PREJUDICE"

The racial composition of Chung's classes throughout her education at USC mirrored the skewed gender ratio in the medical school. From the school photographs, it does not appear that she ever had any African American classmates. During her first year in the academy, she was one of three students of Chinese descent, including another woman, out of a total of ninety-two students. Her class also included one student of Japanese ancestry and one with a Spanish surname. In her subsequent years of attendance, the only nonwhite students had Chinese names. Their numbers ranged from two to four in classes of fifty to sixty students. Chung was the only Chinese American woman to graduate from the Preparatory Academy in 1911.[26] The number of students with Chinese ancestry decreased further during her medical school years. Despite her popularity, Chung, as the only nonwhite student in her class, became a target for discrimination. As she recalled, she "knew the bitterness of racial prejudice during the years when she was working her way through medical school."[27]

As with her strategies for gender integration, Chung experimented with her cultural identity to relate to the predominately white student body at USC. Born in the United States and raised by parents who had themselves been westernized by Presbyterian missionaries, she subscribed to mainstream American culture. She believed in the power of Western medicine, especially surgery, and expressed little interest in Chinese herbal medicine. She also avoided Chinese dress. While her baby pictures indicate that her parents occasionally outfitted her in traditional costumes, Chung adopted Western clothing for her schooling and her profession. As one of her mentors remarked, "She never wore Chinese clothes, but on all occasions appeared in a thin black tailored suit."[28] Through her attire, Margaret attempted to assimilate not only into the masculine world of professional medicine but also the American mainstream.

At the same time, Chung called on both her early experiences working in the ethnic service sector and her Chinese heritage as she made her way through her studies. She worked a number of jobs to pay for her medical education, recalling that "all the time that I was in Medical College I do not remember having three square meals a day."[29] To sustain herself, Chung resorted to some of the strategies she had used before she entered the USC academy. She used her entrepreneurial skills to sell "surgical instruments, rubber gloves, surgical aprons, and supplies" to other students.[30] She also returned to the Chinese service economy. One acquaintance saw her "reading a medical book propped on a shelf while doing dishes in a restaurant."[31] In addition, Chung discovered a new source of income that took advantage of her oratorical skills and her Chinese background: she earned money "by lecturing on China at churches and clubs."[32] Even though she never visited her ancestral country, she capitalized on the interest of school and community organizations in international affairs, cosmopolitan cultures, and missionary efforts in order to gain acceptance, recognition, and financial support for her education.

During Chung's years at USC, the school newspaper revealed a campus-wide interest in the political, cultural, and religious developments in Asia. International events at the turn of the century fueled the curiosity of USC students. In China, the overthrow of the last dynasty and the establishment of a republican form of government in 1911 sparked debate about the future of democracy there. The modernization movement in Japan and its victory in the Russo-Japanese War in 1905 also ignited discussion about the future alignment of world power. As an indication of the interest in international relations and cultures, students formed organizations such as the Japanese Student Association in 1910 and the Cosmopolitan Club in 1914. The Cosmopolitan Club invited "all students, American or foreign, men or women, who are interested in the furthering of international understanding and good will in the university."[33]

In addition, USC's long-standing religious mission also encouraged student interest in overseas affairs, especially in Asia and Latin America.

University publications explained, "Here on the Pacific Coast, close to another sister civilization, that of Latin America, and in immediate touch by water with the Great Orient, Californians have a unique position for doing honorable work in the world. . . . Particularly with our own institution . . . where religion has a definite place in the organization and in the curriculum, is there a call to send out representatives south and west to teaching and missionary posts."[34] Not coincidentally, there were sizable numbers of immigrants in Southern California from the two regions of the world that USC identified as targets for its missionary enterprise.

Speakers frequently visited the campus to discuss opportunities for teaching and medical work in Asia. The Rev. Ng Poon Chew, whose wife had resided at the Presbyterian Chinese Mission Home with Minnie Chung, addressed the student body in 1912 about the Chinese Revolution and China's relationship to the United States.[35] The YWCA, in particular, was quite active in sponsoring lecturers and workshops relating to the political changes in China and the need for female teachers and physicians to serve as missionaries there.[36]

The campus-wide interest in Asian politics and civilization provided opportunities for Chung to receive economic support for her education and to gain social recognition. Her family's cultural and religious background had instilled in her a concern about the moral and political future of China. The swell of student interest in international relations and cultures allowed Chung to transform her personal desire to become a medical missionary into a public platform. She most likely learned to adopt this role by observing the success of other students of Chinese ancestry. The year before she competed in the Interscholastic Oratorical Contest, a student from China, Ah Lok Tan, entered as the USC academy representative and won the event. According to the school annual, his speech, entitled "China's Call for Service," met with "long and enthusiastic applause [which] not only showed that he had won the hearts of his hearers but also heralded him the victor in advance."[37] His manner of delivery and his subject matter was so commendable that Ah Lok Tan, who had only resided in the U.S. for two years, was invited to speak at the Preparatory School Commencement in 1909.[38] His accomplishments likely encouraged Chung to focus her attention on developing oratorical topics relating to her ancestral country. During her first years at the academy, she exhibited an interest in Western literature. By her third year, she spoke on the topic of China's status within international politics. In fact, her award-winning speech at the Interscholastic

Oratorical Contest was entitled "China, the Future Leader of the Nations." Her outspoken interest in her ancestral country, especially in the role of women there, gained Chung a reputation as "a leader in her class in the College of Medicine and a strong advocate for the emancipation of Chinese women."[39]

Chung also used her connections with Chinese in the United States to further her professional goals. During and after her medical school years, she provided health-care services for Chinese Americans in Los Angeles. Although records relating to Chung's medical practice are not available, other sources suggest that she had patients of Chinese ancestry. She served as the attending physician for at least eight Chinese individuals, according to the files of the Evergreen Cemetery, where many Chinese Angelinos were buried.[40] Most of these people died in 1920, according to cemetery files, but one died in August of 1914, the summer before her junior year in medical school. Chung possibly treated the patient as part of her clinical training or without the supervision of her medical school. Because Western health-care facilities routinely refused to admit Chinese Americans, Chung may have offered medical advice on a more informal basis. Her services not only benefited her patients but also helped her gain medical experience.

The USC College of Physicians and Surgeons actually encouraged experimenting on racial minorities as part of the students' medical training. USC and other medical schools commonly operated public clinics to attract low-income patients in need of treatment. When the USC College of Physicians and Surgeons was located close to the Los Angeles Plaza, the school bulletin explained the benefits of the neighborhood for clinical practice: "This location is in the oldest portion of the city, founded more than a hundred years ago, and it is in this section of the city that the Mexican and foreign population is crowded. For these reasons, it has an admirable environment to draw from for clinical material."[41] The school's free clinic provided care to a daily average of sixty to one hundred nearby residents of Sonoratown, one of the centers of the Los Angeles Mexican American community. By the time Chung attended the USC medical school, it had moved to a different location, "a decidedly well-to-do neighborhood" but still relatively close to the San Pedro Chinatown. Despite the new locale, a similar philosophy regarding medical learning persisted. Juniors and seniors were allotted cases at the Los Angeles County Hospital, "where all manner of surgical and medical cases may be studied and observed." In addition, the school sponsored a Washington Street Clinic, "open to the needy poor," which enabled "the teacher and the student to carefully study each case in detail and note from time to time the effect of therapeutic measures." University publications assured their students that "material coming to this clinic is ample and of splendid quality."[42] In fact, the dean of the medical school, Charles W. Bryson, was a specialist in gynecology and known for treating Chinese prostitutes.[43] The provision of medical care to immigrant communities thus constituted a domestic version of the school's missionary goals. At the same time, the medical college objectified its intended beneficiaries as "cases" and "material."

AT A CROSSROADS

While Chung embraced Western science and medicine, she also viewed her education as fulfilling the higher religious purpose of uplifting the less fortunate. Following her graduation from the USC College of Physicians and Surgeons in 1916, she applied to serve as a medical missionary in China. Her goal of fulfilling a religious calling through the science of healing represented a culmination of her family upbringing and educational training. Her parents raised her as a Presbyterian and encouraged her vocational aspirations. She received her education at a religious institution that emphasized the need for female professionals in missionary work. Her desire to serve as a medical missionary may even have been heightened by the death of her mother. Even while Margaret was in medical school, she continued to care for her mother. Due to fears of contagion, she slept "in a tent in somebody's back yard with my mother who was very, very ill."[44] Minnie finally succumbed to her long bout with tuberculosis; she died on 14 July 1914, the summer between her daughter's sophomore and junior years in medical school.

Because of the importance that Margaret placed on becoming a medical missionary, the rejection of her application both surprised and troubled her. She declined to comment about this episode in her unpublished autobiography, but she spoke to a reporter in 1939 about her thwarted aspirations. In this account, Chung interpreted the rebuff as a result of her American birth and Chinese ancestry: "Three times her application came up before [missionary] administrative boards and three times it was turned down—not because of any lack in her qualifications, but because there was no provision in the rules and regulations governing funds to send American missionaries to China that covered a case of an American of Chinese descent."[45] The publications of the Presbyterian Occidental Board indirectly support Chung's claim of racial discrimination.

Of the forty-one missionaries sponsored in China from 1875 to 1920, none were of Chinese descent.[46] While the board frequently expressed the need for "native" helpers and published stories that featured the return of Chinese women to their ancestral homelands, the Presbyterian Church apparently did not support "native" missionaries in the same capacity as white missionaries.

The refusal of the Presbyterian missionary society to accept Chung as a medical missionary reveals the persistence of racial hierarchy, even among those who sought to uplift the Chinese. Although born in the United States and raised in areas with relatively small populations of Chinese, Chung had some exposure to the language and culture of her ancestral people. In fact, her background compared favorably with most white missionaries, who required linguistic and social training to function in China. However, Chung's Chinese ancestry would have placed her in an awkward position. Despite their goal of converting the "natives," the American missionary society in China was largely segregated.[47] Chinese Christians mainly participated as marginal figures, sometimes as domestic servants and sometimes as Bible women, who were paid small sums to proselytize. The few Chinese women who received their medical training in the United States were respected figures in the Chinese and white Christian communities. However, unlike Chung, they had been born and raised in China. They also had the ability to develop and utilize connections with Chinese political leaders and benefactors. As an American-born Chinese, Chung was both too American and too Chinese for the purposes of the white missionaries.

Chung's failed application to serve as a medical missionary filled her with professional and spiritual anxiety. Her goal of answering a religious calling through the science of healing had helped sustain her through the difficult years of obtaining an education. The gender and racial beliefs embedded in missionary ideology had assisted her during the years at USC. Entering the predominantly masculine and white world of medicine, she tried both to assimilate into the existing culture and to find support through women's organizations and her connections to China and Chinese Americans. However, the rejection of her application left her bereft of a professional as well as a spiritual calling. During this time, she stopped patronizing religious institutions. According to her youngest sister, Dorothy, Margaret "was never known to have gone to church after she graduated from medical school."[48]

Chung's graduating quote reflected her anxieties about the future. For the school annual, she selected the opening stanza of Henry

Wadsworth Longfellow's "Maidenhood" as her parting words: "Maiden! with meek, brown eyes, / In whose orbs a shadow lies / Like the dusk in evening skies." For a woman about to embark on a new career, Chung's selection reveals a surprising sense of foreboding.[49] The poem goes on to describe the tensions that a young woman faces as she approaches the crossroads of her childhood and her womanhood. The maiden in the poem stands reluctantly "Where the brook and river meet, / Womanhood and childhood fleet!"[50] She pauses with indecision about following the path to adulthood, which appears both as an attractive vision and as a dangerous trap. To face the hardships of life, the poem advocates the retention of innocence and purity:

> Bear through sorrow, wrong, and ruth,
> In thy heart the dew of youth,
> On thy lips the smile of truth.
>
> Oh, that dew, like balm, shall steal
> Into wounds that cannot heal,
> Even as sleep our eyes doth seal;
>
> And that smile, like sunshine, dart
> Into many a sunless heart,
> For a smile of God thou art.[51]

While acknowledging the difficulties of life, the poem conveys an optimistic message about the power of purity and idealism to sustain oneself and to heal others spiritually. Chung's selection of this poem demonstrates her self-awareness about the transition in her life as she graduated from medical school. The message of the poem also provides insight into her preferred strategy for facing the obstacles in her life. Even though her application to become a medical missionary had been rejected, she held fast to the goal of being a healer.

PART TWO

A Search for Belonging

CHAPTER 4

"A Noble Profession"

To me, the practice of medicine and surgery has always been a noble profession, a great responsibility and here I was, about to receive a diploma which would enable me to practice medicine and I knew so little! I made up my mind, then and there, before going to commencement exercises, that I would not open an office to practice medicine until I felt competent.

Margaret Chung, *"Autobiography"*

Margaret Chung had mixed emotions on commencement day in June of 1916. At twenty-six, she had succeeded in becoming a doctor. However, the denial of her request to serve as a medical missionary in China left her without a clear vocation. Over the next fifteen years, Chung would develop expertise in several medical specializations and cultivate varied clienteles in Chicago, Los Angeles, and San Francisco. Her eclectic practice and geographic mobility reflected her search for a professional and personal sense of belonging.

Chung initially faced limited career prospects. Like many medical school graduates, she felt inadequately prepared for an independent practice. However, by graduation, she still had not secured an internship, a position increasingly necessary to launch a career. As late as 1911, when she entered medical school, the USC bulletin explained that "internships and appointments in hospitals throughout the city and in surrounding towns" were readily available to their graduates; "in fact, in the past we have been unable to fill the positions open to appointments."[1] Just five years later, the number of graduates had outgrown the number of openings in the Los Angeles area. Twelve of Chung's classmates, including the student who received the highest exam scores, obtained internships at the Los Angeles County Hospital. Four others held hospital positions in California, while one served on the staff of a copper company in Mexico. Chung was one of six students without internships.[2] Instead, she accepted a position as a surgical nurse, not a physician, at the Santa Fe Railroad Hospital. The increased competition for internships reflected their growing importance.[3] As modern medicine promoted the development of specializations and hospital-based health care, graduates were increasingly expected to serve as unpaid interns before being appointed as paid residents in medical institutions. After gaining experience, establishing contacts, and earning the requisite resources, physicians could establish their own practices.

To secure a foothold into the medical profession, Chung left her family and native state of California. Her internship and residency in Chicago allowed her to develop an array of specializations, including surgery, gynecology, and psychiatry. Chung's career benefited from one of the most influential Progressive movements in the country. The label "Progressive" describes a wide range of reform efforts around the turn of the century.[4] One major strand of Progressivism addressed social problems that resulted from rapid industrial growth and massive immigration. To develop systematic solutions for economic exploitation and urbanization, reformers turned to scientific experts and the state.

In Chicago, the Progressive movement helped Chung to channel her missionary desires into secular reform. Her mentors, almost all of whom were women and/or Jewish, assisted the development of her career and her entry into their professional network. Although they traced their ancestry to Europe rather than Asia, they occupied a similar, though not identical, "outsider" status. Furthermore, they shared a passion for "civic medicine"—using their medical expertise to improve society.[5] Chung never attained the same "insider" status as her mentors. She also experienced difficulty balancing the ideal of uplifting the disadvantaged with the mandate of socially controlling her subjects through the authority of science and the state. She also chafed under the restrictiveness of life as an underpaid employee who resided at her place of work. Thus, although Chung profited professionally from her time in Chicago, she had largely negative memories of her internship and residency there.

A MIDWEST METROPOLIS

Chung's initial inability to obtain an internship reflected the persistence of gender and racial bias in the medical profession. Most hospitals in the late nineteenth and early twentieth centuries denied female and black doctors the opportunity for postgraduate training.[6] The only other woman in Chung's class, Agnes Scholl, had not secured an internship by graduation, either, even though she had won the Charles W. Bryson Prize, given to the senior with the highest scores in the gynecology and abdominal surgery final. Some of her male classmates were bound for hospitals specializing in the treatment of women, but Scholl did not receive an offer. She eventually became the first female intern at the Los Angeles County Hospital.[7] However, the County Hospital would not accept its first African and Asian American interns until the 1920s.

Chung finally obtained her internship at a hospital devoted to the care of female patients and the training of female physicians. She states simply in her autobiography that "Dr. Bertha Van Husen [sic] of the Mary Thompson Hospital in Chicago heard of me and offered me a job as an intern."[8] Van Hoosen, a prominent surgeon and advocate for women doctors, worked at an institution inspired by Victorian values of gender separatism. The hospital was initially established in 1865 to provide medical services for widows and orphans of the Civil War. It became one of many institutions created during the mid- to late-nineteenth century that focused on specialized care for women and children. The staff consisted entirely of female doctors, who not only cared for the sick but also trained female interns and nurses. Even as women increasingly attended coeducational medical schools during the early twentieth century, hospitals like the Mary Thompson offered much-needed opportunities for postgraduate training.[9]

Chung benefited especially from her mentor's commitment to assisting female physicians of Chinese ancestry. Van Hoosen had appointed the first Chinese woman intern at the Mary Thompson Hospital. Born in China, Li Yuin Tsao had received her training at the Woman's Medical College of Pennsylvania, the only remaining female medical school to survive the professional reforms during the early twentieth century.[10] Tsao was unable to obtain an internship following graduation, however. Van Hoosen explained,

> My first acquaintance with Chinese women physicians dates from the time that Dr. Mary McLean came to Chicago to get an internship in one of the hospitals for one of her protegees, Dr. Li Yuin Tsao.
> I wagered that she would not meet with success and told her, "When you fail, come back, and we will take Li Yuin at the Women's and Children's Hospital."
> Disappointed and resentful, she returned to accept my offer.

> Nevertheless, I began to regret my impulsive bravado and to dread the
> constant defense of a Chinese intern. I could almost hear such remarks as
> these: "I won't have a 'Chink' doctor me." "Don't let that foreigner come
> near me." "Why must we have a foreigner when we haven't enough posi-
> tions for our own women?"[11]

As it turned out, Tsao's medical and interpersonal skills encouraged Van
Hoosen to provide opportunities for other physicians of Chinese ancestry. In fact, the year before Chung arrived at the Mary Thompson,
another Chinese female physician was serving as an intern there.[12] Van
Hoosen most likely heard about Chung through a colleague, perhaps
one of Margaret's medical school faculty, mentors, or even sorority contacts. One of Van Hoosen's close friends served as a national trustee of
Nu Sigma Phi, the organization that Chung had founded at USC.[13]

Although female professional networks assisted Chung, her transition
to the Midwest proved difficult. Born and raised in Southern California,
she recalled being unprepared for the brisk winters of the Windy City:
"I landed in Chicago, on a cold, gloomy Thanksgiving day. . . . It had
snowed the day before, but a very black coal dust had settled over the
snow, and it was frozen hard, icy cold. All I had on was a thin suit and
a twelve dollar overcoat, which as you may guess provided very little
warmth."[14] Chung also had to learn to navigate a new urban environment. When she arrived in November 1916, Chicago was the second
largest city in the nation. It was growing at almost the same pace as Los
Angeles, but was roughly four times as large, with over 2 million
people.[15] As in L.A., Chicago's exponential growth resulted from a combination of rural-to-urban migration within the country as well as immigration from abroad.

As a single woman making her way in the large metropolis, Chung
shared similarities as well as important differences with the approximately thirty to forty thousand "women adrift" in Chicago.[16] At the
turn of the century, more women than men were moving into cities
because of the greater availability of female occupations, such as clerical
work, domestic service, and the needle trade.[17] Most women lived with
their families, but one out of five survived independently. Like her fellow
"sisters" adrift, Chung arrived alone, by train, with limited financial
resources. Unlike most of these women, who were immediately faced
with the difficult tasks of finding lodgings and work in an unfamiliar
environment, Chung held a professional position that provided room
and board. However, her status as an unpaid intern in some ways neu-
tralized her class standing as a medical professional. She lived at the

hospital and worked long hours for no wages. As she pointed out, the nurses, who ranked lower than doctors on the professional hierarchy, "received five dollars a month those days, but the interns received nothing."[18]

In Chicago, Chung had to adapt not only to a new work and living situation but also to a new racial and ethnic landscape. Unlike Southern California, where individuals of Mexican and Asian ancestry constituted sizable populations, the newcomers to the Windy City tended to be working-class immigrants from eastern and southern Europe and blacks from the American South.[19] Approximately two thousand Chinese, the same number as in Los Angeles, lived in Chicago. Some clustered around the old Chinatown in the downtown loop district, but there was a growing concentration on the South Side of Chicago, close to the burgeoning African American community.[20] In addition, a few international as well as American-born Asians attended the various academic institutions in Chicago. It is unclear how much contact Chung had with the Chinese communities in Chicago. A 1926 study of the population notes the presence of fourteen male doctors but makes no mention of the female physicians of Chinese ancestry who interned at the Mary Thompson Hospital.[21] Located on the West Side and close to the Hull House Settlement Project, the hospital was surrounded by Italian, Greek, Bohemian, Polish, Jewish, and native-born white residents. Even in the midst of these neighborhoods, scattered Chinese-operated laundries and restaurants catered to non-Chinese clientele.[22] Almost all immigrant men, they labored for long hours and had limited language skills to interact with their customers and neighbors. Chung, apparently the only Chinese American on the Mary Thompson Hospital staff for the year, experienced a similar sense of racial isolation. However, her formative years in Southern California had prepared her to function in "mainstream" and European "ethnic" America.

MATERNALIST MEDICINE

Chung's internship at the Mary Thompson Hospital was in many ways similar to her mother's upbringing at the San Francisco Presbyterian Chinese Mission Home. Both institutions attempted to train women to assist other women. The hospital and mission home also both focused on improving the lives of the immigrant poor. The Mary Thompson initially occupied a house with fourteen beds. By 1922, the hospital had expanded into a five-story brick building that accommodated 75 to 100

patients at a time. Chung worked with other medical personnel to care
for an estimated 1,800 patients per year. In addition, they treated 100
"charity" cases and also operated a free dispensary that treated 12,000
low-income individuals annually.[23] For four months of her internship,
Chung served as an "externe, visiting charity patients at their homes";
there, she "administer[ed] . . . medicines" and also taught "hygiene in
the everyday life and in the convalescence of the sick."[24] Like the missionaries at the Presbyterian Chinese Mission Home, Margaret's mentors used the idealized female role of motherhood to explain why
women physicians should exert a protective and nurturing influence
over their patients as well as their trainees. Margaret Culbertson, a
single woman dedicated to missionary reform, had become surrogate
mother for Minnie Chung. Likewise Bertha Van Hoosen, an unmarried
female doctor, referred to interns like Margaret Chung as her "surgical
daughters."[25]

The female community at the Mary Thompson also differed in
important ways from the Presbyterian Chinese Mission Home. Whereas
earlier reformers emphasized voluntarism and Christianity, Progressive-
era activists emphasized professionalism and interfaith cooperation.[26]
Van Hoosen exemplifies this new generation of female reformers. Born
in 1863 to a farming family in Stony Creek, Michigan, Van Hoosen
studied medicine at one of the best medical institutions and one of the
first coeducational schools in the country, the University of Michigan.
After obtaining postgraduate training at women's hospitals in Detroit
and Boston, she opened a practice in Chicago in 1892. While there, she
accomplished a number of firsts for women in the medical field: first
woman to be appointed under Civil Service as chief gynecologist at the
Cook County Hospital, first woman to be appointed as Professor and
Chair of Obstetrics in a coeducational medical school, and first woman
to present a paper at the International Congress of Medicine.[27] In addition to these personal accomplishments, she also advocated for better
medical care and opportunities for other women. In 1915, on the fiftieth
anniversary of the Mary Thompson Hospital, she helped found the
American Medical Women's Association (AMWA) to advance the professional interests of female physicians.

Van Hoosen's career exemplified Progressive strategies of using scientific expertise to improve society. For example, she gained recognition
during the early twentieth century for promoting a new medication,
referred to as "twilight sleep," to neutralize pain during childbirth.[28]
Hospitals provided the most effective setting for this delivery technique,

and thus it was associated with the general move away from home birthing under the guidance of female family members and midwives. In her eyes, only women with specialized training and access to medical institutions could offer the best health care.

In keeping with Van Hoosen's interest in promoting modern medical techniques, she trained her intern "daughters" in the highly prestigious and traditionally masculine field of surgery.[29] Chung's fascination with this particular branch of medicine began in her childhood. She explained: "My first love was surgery. . . . As a very young child, having no dolls or toys to play with, I would frequently take banana peels or cabbage stems and make believe I was operating upon them. Living on a farm or a ranch from time to time, I had to cook and prepare chickens, wild ducks, quail, or rabbit, and even while I was preparing the food I would make believe I was operating on the chicken or the rabbit."[30] Her preference for surgery coincided with its rising prominence at the turn of the century. Not only was surgery becoming safer, with new knowledge about sterilization and bacteriology, but the procedure epitomized the new scientific ethos of medical care. First, rather than a holistic approach to medical care, surgery emphasized the role of specialized physicians who could treat discrete illnesses and malfunctioning body parts. Second, surgery increasingly took place in hospitals, which provided the facilities, equipment, and personnel necessary for the procedures. Male-dominated hospitals denied women operating privileges; Van Hoosen and the Mary Thompson Hospital filled the void by undertaking the task of training female surgeons. Chung apparently displayed "a great aptitude for surgery," and Van Hoosen, "as well as others on the staff, gave her unaccustomed opportunities to operate."[31]

Van Hoosen's commitment to training Chung and other Chinese women physicians reflected the influence as well as transformation of female missionary efforts. When Van Hoosen appointed Tsao as her first Chinese intern, she explained that "at the Women and Children's Hospital we do not only profess Christianity, we practice it."[32] In other words, she viewed the acceptance of diverse individuals as an expression of Christian values. Not only did Van Hoosen train Asian women in the United States, she also traveled abroad to promote scientific exchange. Retracing the earlier movement of American missionaries overseas, Van Hoosen visited China, Japan, and India in the early 1920s to learn about medical practice in these countries and to offer instruction for Asian female physicians. She was particularly eager to reunite with Tsao and also meet Ida Kahn and Mary Stone, fellow graduates of the University of Michigan and two of the earliest and well-known Chinese medical missionaries.

With her international interests, Van Hoosen supported a secular version of religious medical missions. Shortly after the founding of the American Medical Women's Association, the organization began sponsoring health missions abroad to provide wartime, postwar, and emergency medical care. The female missionary movement had previously viewed science as a tool for spiritual conversion. Van Hoosen and other members of AMWA may have been motivated by Christian beliefs and used religious networks to assist their work, but they viewed the dissemination of scientific knowledge and the provision of medical care as their primary goals.

Chung benefited from the commitment of Van Hoosen and other female medical reformers to assist women who, by virtue of racial or ethnic background, were considered to be on the margins of society. All three of her primary mentors came from immigrant backgrounds and dedicated themselves to providing medical services and training for women, especially women in ethnic communities. Their willingness to help "outsiders" and "foreigners" partly stemmed from their personal backgrounds. Van Hoosen's father had emigrated from The Netherlands. May Michael, a Jewish pediatrician who vouched for Chung's "good moral and professional character" on her Illinois State Board of Health Application, had emigrated from England and devoted much of her practice and energies to Jewish service organizations in Chicago.[33] Rachelle Yarros, another female Jewish physician, eventually helped Chung obtain a medical residency. Born near Kiev, Russia, in 1869, Yarros had worked in a New York sweatshop before becoming a physician. In Chicago, she completed her residency at the Jewish hospital, the Michael Reese. Yarros eventually became affiliated with Hull House, a reform community in the heart of poor immigrant neighborhoods on the West Side of Chicago, and she became known for promoting sex education and birth control.[34]

The ethnic and religious backgrounds of Chung's mentors most likely fostered their ability to empathize with her status as a Chinese American. Nativist movements not only targeted immigrants from Asia but also those from Europe. As far back as the mid-nineteenth century, exclusionists argued that America should be reserved for the white Anglo-Saxon race. Whiteness, however, did not necessarily correlate with European ancestry. Along with individuals from Ireland, Italy, and parts of southern and eastern Europe, Jewish immigrants were commonly perceived as less than white.[35] They faced a variety of anti-Semitic restrictions and practices that determined where Jews could live, work, and attend school. Being ostracized oneself does not necessarily lead to compassion for other despised groups, of course. Some chose to reinforce discriminatory practices to gain mainstream acceptance, while others advocated racial equality.[36] Chung fortunately came into contact with female reformers who supported accessible health care and training. The Mary Thompson Hospital expressed their outlook in its mission statement that "no person shall be deprived of the benefit of this institution on account of nationality, race, or religious profession."[37]

THE LIMITS OF SISTERHOOD

Despite the Mary Thompson Hospital's ideal of creating a supportive professional environment for women of diverse backgrounds, Chung's memories of her internship largely dwell on the tensions within this female community. Instead of a nurturing workplace, she discovered social isolation and professional hierarchy. Her negative experiences reflect how women's institutions maintained and reinforced divisions between women to deflect emerging criticisms of gender-segregated communities in the early twentieth century.

Chung was struck by the impersonal and institutional character of the Mary Thompson Hospital on her arrival. When she got to Chicago on Thanksgiving in 1916, she discovered that "No one met me at the train. . . . The trees were leafless, the wind was cold, and the welcome in the hospital was hardly warmer. I was shown to my room—a little small cubicle with enough room in a little closet to hang up about four suits, an old iron bed which sagged unmercifully in the middle, one chair with the bottom out."[38] Facing financial difficulties that had almost forced closure in 1911, the Mary Thompson offered dining fare that was not much better than the accommodations. Chung recalled that "the meals were exceedingly meagre. For breakfast we had cold toast, coffee, and an egg; for lunch, meat, a vegetable, potatoes, bread and butter, coffee, and perhaps a dessert; for supper, cold toast again, and always, without exception, the same dish of stewed dried apricots and more coffee. . . . The few dollars which I had saved . . . were soon gone buying extra food to keep myself going."[39]

Despite these personal hardships, Chung recalled that the "work was exceedingly interesting," because the Mary Thompson provided numerous

opportunities to develop surgical skills.[40] However, she did not characterize her professional relationships in familial and nurturing terms.
Rather, she emphasized the hierarchical differences between the medical
personnel:

> The Staff Doctors of the Mary Thompson Hospital were very happy to turn
> over a great many of the clinic cases which were to be operated on free.
> Especially during the summer when it gets unbearably hot in Chicago, and
> of course in those days air conditioning was unheard of . . . and they had
> enough confidence in me to say to me, "Well, Dr. Chung, there's so many
> patients in the clinic to be operated on and when work is not too heavy here
> you can have the office send out postcards to these people and schedule a
> few operations each day for yourself, and you can clean up the list of opera-
> tive cases in the clinic." This was welcome news for me indeed, and by the
> time they came back in September I had cleaned out the whole clinic of all
> the operative cases which came to over six hundred cases.[41]

Chung acknowledges that the staff doctors had "confidence" in her.
However, she also suggests that they took advantage of her status as an
unpaid intern who could not afford to take a summer vacation.

Chung's critical attitude toward the Mary Thompson Hospital perhaps stemmed from the institution's efforts to monitor her private
behavior. Despite her initial sense of neglect, Chung apparently became
quite popular. In an unpublished draft of Van Hoosen's autobiography,
Chung's mentor described her as "a favorite with nurses and interns to
the degree that the hospital, for the first time, made a ruling that two
people must not sleep in a single bed."[42] The nature of Chung's relationships with these nurses and interns is not clear. Chung's own autobiography makes no mention of them. During the Victorian era, women
developed romantic friendships with one another that sometimes
included physical intimacy. In a society that presumed fundamental
gender differences, women tended to form their strongest emotional
bonds with other women. The passionate sensuality that characterized
some of these relationships appeared natural, not abnormal.

In preventing Chung from sharing her bed with other women, however, the Mary Thompson Hospital was in effect labeling her behavior
as socially unacceptable. The new policy responded to emerging ideas
about sexuality that critics used to stigmatize female institutions. As
women broke through gender barriers in the professional and political
arenas, their personal behavior drew increasing scrutiny. At the turn of
the century, a branch of medicine emerged that focused on "gender
inversion," the phenomenon of individuals who refuse their assigned

gender roles. Women who entered traditionally male professions or adopted masculine dress became suspected of harboring "mannish" sexual longings. In essence, this branch of study created new categories of identity, branding certain people as normal and others as deviant based on their behavior and desires. The new "sexology" research fueled criticisms of women's educational and professional training. In particular, female institutions such as the Mary Thompson faced charges of fostering lesbianism. In response, the hospital, along with other women's schools during the 1910s and 1920s, increasingly regulated female social and sexual behavior.[43]

Chung's mentors were not entirely unsympathetic toward her. Van Hoosen held Chung in high regard and kept in contact with her after her internship. In the published edition of Van Hoosen's autobiography, released shortly after World War II, she omitted the anecdote about her mentee's ability to attract bed partners. No doubt, she was attempting to shield both Chung and the Mary Thompson Hospital from public censure. The female community there provided valuable opportunities for Chung to continue her ascent up the professional ladder. However, as she gained scientific expertise, she was increasingly subjected to the scrutiny of modern medicine.

SAVING CHILDREN

In October 1917, as Chung neared the completion of her first year at the Mary Thompson Hospital, her father died unexpectedly in a car accident. According to her sister Dorothy, who was eight at the time, Chung Wong was driving his "first and only auto," when he became "caught between two Pasadena Red Cars . . . going opposite ways."[44] He lost his leg in the accident and died from loss of blood; he might have survived the accident, but the local hospital denied Chung Wong admission because he was Chinese.[45] Margaret could not afford to travel to California for the funeral. Instead, she sent a cable, inviting her siblings to join her in Chicago. Dorothy remembered that "soon after the funeral 'the Doctor' sent them a cable that told them she would bring them to Chicago. They all immediately quit school and it was some time before things were straightened out and back to school some of them went. Margaret could not afford proper winter clothes much less finance ten [sic] children. The children stayed in Los Angeles, the older ones worked and took care of the younger ones and Margaret sent a bit of money now and then."[46]

Lacking even a place for her six younger sisters and brothers to stay, Chung used her contacts among female medical reformers to seek a paid residency at the Illinois Juvenile Psychopathic Institute (JPI) in order to provide some financial assistance to her siblings in California. Her residency there exposed her to a new medical specialization and a new set of professional pressures. Her entry into psychiatry partly resulted from the professional obstacles that she continued to face. In April 1917, the United States entered World War I. As medical professionals left to fulfill their military duty, hospitals faced a personnel shortage.[47] Even under these conditions, Chung only obtained a position at a psychopathic hospital, a not particularly desirable posting. In the nineteenth century, the medical community generally held psychiatry in low regard. Practitioners primarily served as prison guards, detaining and isolating the mentally deranged in asylums. Despite the "low professional status" of institutional work, women doctors "were particularly happy to take such positions . . . Uncertain of the rewards of private practice, women were often attracted by the security of such appointments, and the opportunities they afforded to gain expertise."[48] Chung's career path in fact followed Van Hoosen's. Her mentor had interned at the Kalamazoo State Hospital for the Insane.

While the lack of attractive alternatives forced female physicians like Chung to accept institutional work, the changing field of psychiatry in the early twentieth century also offered an opportunity to use scientific expertise to improve society. Instead of detention and isolation, Progressive-era practitioners focused on research, education, and reform. For example, the Juvenile Psychopathic Institute, created in 1909, assisted the work of the Juvenile Court of Chicago by providing psychiatric evaluations for troubled youth and developing recommendations for their rehabilitation. The institute's mission, to understand and save children, may have appealed to Chung.[49] After all, Presbyterian missionaries in San Francisco had "rescued" her mother from a potential life of crime.

Rachelle Yarros assisted Chung in obtaining the residency through her connections with female reformers and Jewish physicians. Hull House activist Julia Lathrop, along with members of the Chicago Woman's Club, successfully lobbied for the creation of the first juvenile court in the country in 1899.[50] Seeking to exert a protective maternal influence over adolescents who ran afoul of the law, these female reformers explained that "children should not be treated as criminals, but as delinquent children needing wise direction, care and correction."[51]

Ten years after the founding of the juvenile court, Lathrop also played a crucial role in establishing the Juvenile Psychopathic Institute. With the support of philanthropist Ethel Sturges Dummer, Lathrop hired medical experts and social workers to study juvenile delinquency and encourage rehabilitation. The study was funded privately for five years before the institute officially became part of the state apparatus. Because the institute came under the purview of the newly founded Illinois Department of Public Welfare, Chung had to pass a civil service examination in order to qualify for residency.[52] Yarros, with her ties to the reformers who developed the vision for the Juvenile Psychopathic Institute, provided Chung's initial introduction.

Yarros's contacts with Jewish male physicians also assisted Chung's entry into this new field of specialization. In November 1917, Chung received a brief appointment as an assistant physician at the Kankakee State Hospital, where she took a course in psychiatry with the superintendent, Dr. H. Douglas Singer. Like May Michael, Singer was a Jewish immigrant from England.[53] When Chung joined the Juvenile Psychopathic Institute in December 1917, she worked under Herman Adler. Adler, the grandson of a prominent Talmudic scholar, had helped redefine the mission of psychiatry in the early twentieth century and had successfully obtained the newly created position of Illinois State Criminologist shortly before Chung's arrival.[54] Just as the initial low status of the specialization had facilitated the entry of women, so the emerging field provided opportunities for religious and racial minorities to advance their careers. In fact, "when psychology was viewed as a branch of medicine," the field "was understood to be potentially appropriate for Jews."[55] Chung recalled Adler and his wife with great fondness. They "did several nice things for her," according to Margaret's sister Dorothy, and even "noticed her inadequate winter clothing and bought her a coat." Dorothy remembered that Margaret "always had a soft spot for Jews" because of the Adlers' quasi-parental interest in her.[56]

Chung, however, did not enjoy the pressures associated with her new position. She worked and lived in two wards of Chicago's Cook County Hospital, which housed the Juvenile Psychopathic Institute. Unlike the Mary Thompson, where Chung worked with an all-female staff to help female patients, her JPI colleagues included male and female "psychiatrists, psychologists, psychoanalysts, [and] social service workers."[57] Men tended to occupy the primary positions of authority, as directors, judges, and physicians. Since male offenders came before the court in greater numbers than females, men even dominated the patient base.[58] Chung's responsibilities included training nurses from psychopathic hospitals throughout the state. However, she primarily assisted in "the examination, observation, and recommendation to the different judges as to the position of borderline cases, criminals who feigned insanity, and unusual court cases which the judges had difficulty in deciding what to do with the individual before them." Although the institute initially focused on juvenile cases, Adler advocated for an increased role in all court proceedings. As Chung recalled, "More frequently, we had adults rather than children." The large case load, an average of one hundred per month during her residency, overburdened the resources of the institute and allowed little time for research.[59] She found the work "very interesting" but also "nerve wracking for a young woman in her early twenties who would sometimes have to give a recommendation which might result in a man's getting a death sentence." Although Chung was then in her late, not early, twenties, the coercive aspect of her work as a court psychiatrist nevertheless disturbed her. Because the Juvenile Psychopathic Institute served as an extension of the legal system, researchers not only offered treatment but also assisted the court in meting out punishment. Overall, Chung found the experience "too depressing."[60]

Chung's anxiety over her responsibilities as a court psychiatrist partly stemmed from the inadequacy of the scientific tools at her disposal to understand criminality and abnormality. The field of psychiatry increasingly assumed cultural importance during the early twentieth century by offering explanations for social behavior. However, unlike most branches of medicine, psychiatry "lacked the critical capacity to inscribe itself on the body. Psychiatrists had few signs with which to identify disease; they had to be content to work with the ephemera commonly known as symptoms."[61] To buttress the scientific claims of their specialization, psychiatrists created categories of mental abilities and personality traits to classify and diagnose their patients. However, these classifications tended to reveal more about the subjective attitudes of the scientists and the nature of their interactions with the patients.

For example, the juvenile court and the JPI kept meticulous statistics on their subjects' "nationality" in the course of their study of correlations between criminality and insanity.[62] The concept of "nationality" did not refer to one's national citizenship, but rather to race and "racial stock." Separate listings existed for "American" and "colored," implying that "American" only referred to white individuals. American-born children of immigrants did not fall under the category of "American," either. Instead, researchers listed them under the nationality of their parents. This seemingly strange classification system revealed the influence of prevailing eugenics and nativist ideas that associated race and foreignness with mental defectiveness. The researchers, some of whom were immigrants and minorities themselves, increasingly emphasized environmental factors and individual personality to explain criminal behavior and psychological disorders. However, the statistics on and references to the patients' ancestry and race suggest that heredity lurked as a subtext for explaining mental deficiency.[63]

Chung's uneasiness with psychiatry perhaps also stemmed from the field's role in distinguishing deviant from normal forms of sexuality. The study of "sexology" emerged through research on "psychopathology." Physicians defined gender inversion and "sexual perversion" as mental disorders that required psychological and psychiatric treatment. In fact, cases involving cross-dressing and homosexuality appeared before the juvenile court and the Juvenile Psychopathic Institute during Chung's residency.[64]

Chung's internships and residency in Chicago introduced her to a variety of professional possibilities. At the Mary Thompson Hospital, she developed her surgical skills, a traditionally male specialization, in a female-staffed institution that catered to female patients. At the Juvenile Psychopathic Institute, she trained as a psychiatrist, focusing on traditionally "feminine" concerns such as emotional well-being, marital relations, and child rearing, while working under male experts and treating male patients.[65] Women reformers, seeking to assert a maternal influence over their communities, initiated both institutions. However, while the Mary Thompson remained a privately funded women's establishment, the Juvenile Psychopathic Institute became part of the state. The JPI demonstrated both women's success in shaping the state and the diminution of their status in gender-mixed settings.

The female and Jewish professional networks in Chicago helped Chung to establish her credentials.[66] However, dissatisfied with the nature of her work as well as the constraints on her life, she sought alternative opportunities. Following in the footsteps of her supervisor, Herman Adler, she requested indefinite leave from her civil service position in order to offer her skills to the military. During World War I, psychiatrists played an important role in conducting mental testing of soldiers and treating shell shock. However, the armed forces, despite the lobbying efforts of the American Medical Women's Association, refused to admit female physicians into its ranks.[67] Chung received her military leave from the JPI in November 1918, but the war ended the same month.[68] After two years away from her family and home state, she was ready to return to Southern California.

CHAPTER 5

"The Beginning of a New Era"

I loved everything about that Santa Fe Hospital! It was the
beginning of a new era for me! I loved the type of case we had
at the Hospital. . . . I loved the location . . . high on a hill,
overlooking Hollenbeck Park! I loved its sloping green lawns
and brilliant red poinsettas, proudly lifting their crimson
bloom to the very eaves of the building. . . . For the first time
in my life, I sat down to three square meals a day—and they
took a keen delight in filling my plate to overflowing—
especially with corned beef and cabbage, one of my favorite
foods!

Margaret Chung, *"Autobiography"*

I think that the men [my patients] were so anxious to see
what made the wheels go 'round in a woman doctor, much
less a Chinese one, that they didn't feel anything but curiosity
for the first few days.

Margaret Chung, *Los Angeles Times*, 1939

Hollywood has long been fascinated by Asia, Asians, and
Asian themes. Mysterious and exotic, Hollywood's Asia
promises adventure and forbidden pleasures.

Gina Marchetti, *Romance and the "Yellow Peril"*

Chung left Chicago during the dreary winter season and returned to a land
of sunshine, eager to start a new life. In February 1919, she applied for a
license to practice medicine in the state of California. Age twenty-nine at
the time and listed as five and a half feet, she appeared youthful and attractive in the accompanying photograph. Her eyes look straight into the
camera, and her expression conveys a sense of seriousness. As in her medical school pictures, she pulled her hair back, accentuating the roundness

of her face. She also wore androgynous clothing—a white blouse and a bow tie. A Chicago psychiatrist who worked with Herman Adler vouched for Chung's qualifications and character. He wrote, "I take pleasure in recommending her as being conscientious, reliable and industrious, and capable of fulfilling any position for which she might make application."[1]

During her three-year stay in Southern California, Chung achieved a sense of professional and personal fulfillment. She confirmed her love of surgery while she was a staff physician with the Los Angeles-based Santa Fe Railroad Hospital. She purchased her first home in the relatively wealthy community of Pasadena. She also cultivated a private practice that attracted entertainers and musicians from Hollywood, the emerging capital of the movie industry.

Chung's accomplishments appear anomalous in light of deepening social divisions during the late 1910s and early 1920s. World War I fanned nativist sentiments and racial antagonism. In 1917, 1921, and again in 1924, the U.S. Congress passed immigration exclusion laws that severely limited the entry of southern and eastern Europeans and almost completely barred Asians.[2] In Los Angeles, as in other cities that attracted large numbers of racially and ethnically diverse people, the practice of segregation expanded along with the creation of suburbs.

In the midst of these hardening boundaries, Chung discovered opportunities by capitalizing on her gender, class, and racial ancestry. While her medical training granted her professional and social clout, her identity as a Chinese woman imbued her with exotic difference. The modern celebrity and consumer culture, fostered by the Los Angeles movie industry, encouraged mainstream fascination with Asian culture and people, particularly with Asian women. Chung gained acceptance by non-Chinese and by men not due to their willingness to ignore her race and gender, or their ability to be color or gender blind. Rather, their consciousness of social difference fostered a desire to seek contact, knowledge, and entertainment from those unlike themselves.

A TRUE INTERNSHIP

Upon Chung's return to Southern California, she again joined the Santa Fe Hospital—where she'd served briefly as a surgical nurse before going to Chicago, this time as a staff physician.[3] Chung's experiences there solidified her medical specialization and revealed how her gender and racial identities could assist, not just hinder, her career. The Santa Fe

Hospital played such a formative role in shaping her career that she described her time there as a "true internship."

Working for a railroad hospital allowed Chung to continue in her role as a Progressive reformer from within the corporate structure. During its heyday, the Atchison, Topeka and Santa Fe Railroad spanned twelve thousand miles, winding its way throughout the Southwest, connecting Los Angeles to Chicago and Houston to San Francisco. The company employed tens of thousands of workers to build, maintain, and operate the railroad. The white-collar railroad workers, who tended to be white, native born, and only occasionally female, suffered few occupational hazards; however, the blue-collar laborers, men from predominantly immigrant backgrounds, experienced a high incidence of work-related injuries.[4]

In response to worker demands and public concern, the company adopted a corporate welfare strategy. While Progressive Hull House reformers like Alice Hamilton called for government legislation to institute workers' rights to health care and injury compensation, the Santa Fe Railroad Company sought a private alternative by creating a company medical plan.[5] In 1884, railroad executives called for the creation of the Atchison Railroad Employees' Association. Members contributed a monthly sum that provided the funds to build clinics and pay doctors. By 1916, the employees association had over fourteen thousand members and was operating seven hospitals throughout the Southwest. While some railroad stops had minimal health facilities, the Santa Fe Hospital in Los Angeles, situated on a hilltop overlooking Hollenbeck Park, was an impressive multileveled Hacienda-style building with one hundred beds. The hospital treated not only workers in the city but also those stationed as far away as Arizona who required more serious surgical and medical care.

Chung's appointment to the Santa Fe medical staff seemed fitting considering the history of Chinese involvement in building railroads throughout the American West. Her father may have worked for the Santa Fe during his early years in the United States. When Chung Wong fell ill with rheumatism when the family lived in Ventura County, Margaret hauled "freight to and from the Santa Fe Freight Depot" and even became acquainted with the railroad foreman, Frank Rosenfeld. His wife, Emma, also became Chung's Sunday school teacher. That Margaret should become a physician for the railroad twenty years later reveals an impressive degree of class mobility within one generation. Chung recalled that when Frank Rosenfeld came to the Santa Fe hospital for treatment, "he saw me there taking care of the Santa Fe patients, [and] he was as proud as though he had given birth to me."[6]

At the Santa Fe Railroad Hospital, Chung was mentored by physicians with backgrounds similar to those of her Chicago mentors. In fact, her Los Angeles supervisors had connections to Progressive doctors in the Midwest. She attributed her appointment to Dr. Adolph Tyroler, who was "the assistant chief surgeon of the Santa Fe at that time. . . . It was he, who gave me the job, and also he who 'god-damned' surgery into me."[7] Tyroler had graduated from the University of Michigan medical school, the alma mater of Bertha Van Hoosen. In addition, Tyroler, a Jew of Hungarian descent, was affiliated with the Jewish Hospital in Los Angeles. In fact, the Santa Fe Railroad Hospital was located in Boyle Heights, a community where one third of the city's Jewish population resided. And mentor George F. Thompson, who was affiliated with Cook County Hospital and who was a member of the American Railway Surgeons Association, sponsored Chung's application to the Chicago Medical Society.[8]

Chung affirmed her love for surgery at the Santa Fe. The traumatic nature of railroad injuries provided her with many opportunities to develop and practice her operative skills, especially in the field of plastic surgery. Her responsibilities contrasted dramatically with those of her previous specialization. As a psychiatrist, she treated indeterminate mental disorders that frequently required lengthy therapy with no guarantee of improvement. As a surgeon, she treated her patients' bodies and produced immediate results. Chung preferred this more direct, almost heroic, style of medical practice. She recalled that she liked "emergency work—I am at my best, when crowded and working under pressure. When they brought in a trainload of victims from a wreck in Kingman, Arizona, and we worked feverishly for 36 hours, I had a field holiday!" She thrived under the immediate pressures of working in the emergency ward and developed her skills at "good snappy surgery."[9]

Although the Santa Fe surgical ward was dominated by men of European ancestry, Chung recalled being "completely unconscious of any racial prejudice or sex resentment that might have existed on the part of the men."[10] She "loved everything about that Santa Fe Hospital! . . . Everyone at the hospital was kind and gracious to me, and there was no resentment on the part of the patients."[11] Ironically, the lack of hostility stemmed not from patients ignoring her racial and gender identities but rather from their fascination with her as an exotic: a Chinese female doctor.

She explained that the predominantly male and non-Chinese employees of the Santa Fe Railroad Company "were so anxious to see what made the wheels go 'round in a woman doctor, much less a Chinese one, that they didn't feel anything but curiosity for the first few days."[12]

Initially intrigued by Chung's racial and gender difference, her patients eventually expressed "enthusiasm for her differentness in administering to their needs." Her skill in removing steel filings from workers' eyes, a common injury in the machine shops, was attributed to the natural gentleness of a woman doctor. Her suggestion for increasing salt consumption to prevent heat exhaustion sounded like simple but effective advice that a mother would offer. In other words, Chung's patients perceived her as a good physician, not in spite of, but because of her sex. Their belief that a female physician would provide more gentle, maternal care resonated with Victorian ideas of womanhood. At the same time, Chung also may have attracted interest because of more modern notions of female sex appeal. One newspaper reporter described her as a "slim young Chinese woman." One worker suggested that "some of the men were deliberately getting hurt so that Dr. Chung could take care of them."[13]

Chung's racial status served as an asset in her professional interactions as well. On the one hand, her Chinese ancestry heightened her exoticism and sparked interest in her. Chung's comment about patient curiosity in her as "a woman doctor, much less a Chinese one" revealed that her ancestry increased her peculiarity in their eyes. On the other hand, this fascination with her cultural difference also coexisted with a sense of affinity, since many of her patients were immigrants and racial minorities. Margaret's sister Dorothy recalled that Mexican workers constituted a sizable portion of Chung's practice at the Santa Fe Railroad Hospital.[14] The institution was located just to the west of Belvedere, already well on its way to becoming the largest Mexican community in Los Angeles.[15]

Growing up with Mexican Americans and experiencing racial discrimination herself perhaps prepared Chung to treat her patients in a more humane manner. On at least one occasion, she substituted for the regular surgeons at the branch medical office in San Bernardino, located to the east of Los Angeles. The Santa Fe Railroad Company played an influential role in this small town, employing half of its total workforce.[16] The Santa Fe even created a barrio in San Bernardino through its practice of recruiting and then residentially segregating large numbers of workers of Mexican ancestry.[17] Chung became so popular with her patients there that "the entire shop personnel of 1132 men signed and submitted a petition to the main office asking that Dr. Chung be kept at the San Bernardino shops indefinitely." Their request for her medical skills signaled dissatisfaction with the care provided by the three regular male physicians. Rather than honor the request, the Los Angeles office sharply reprimanded her for "upsetting the status quo" and ordered her departure from San Bernardino.[18]

A HOME OF HER OWN

Despite the tensions at the Santa Fe, Chung remembered her time there as among the happiest in her life. Her sense of satisfaction stemmed from changes in her professional career as well as her personal well-being. When she first returned to Los Angeles, she rejoined her six younger siblings, then living in the San Pedro district. Her two brothers, Andrew and Virgil, then in their early twenties and late teens, respectively, followed in the footsteps of their father and worked as vegetable farmers and merchants at the Los Angeles City Produce Market. At the time, Chinese Americans constituted 40 percent of the produce wholesalers at the market.[19] Instead of using a horse and wagon like their father, Andrew and Virgil drove trucks to deliver goods. By 1920, Margaret had moved away from this working-class, multi-ethnic neighborhood. With the security and income afforded by her position as a staff physician, she was able to purchase a house in Pasadena, located to the northeast of Los Angeles. There she lived with her four sisters and a twenty-eight-year-old white nurse from Nebraska named Isabelle Shephard.[20] For the first time in Margaret's life, she had a home of her own.

Chung successfully moved in to a relatively wealthy and exclusive community just as a pattern of "land-use segregation" was intensifying in Los Angeles.[21] During the 1920s, the city became a metropolis. It "annexed 45 adjacent communities" and "added 80 square miles" as the population "more than double[d], from 577,000 to 1.24 million."[22] Most of the newcomers originated from the Midwest, the South, Mexico, and Japan, and they tended to settle with those of similar ethnic and class backgrounds. People of color predominantly lived "amidst commerce and industry in the small ghettos of central Los Angeles," while "white Americans" resided "in the suburbs sprawling north to Hollywood, east to Pasadena, south to Long Beach, and west to Santa Monica."[23]

In 1920, the affluent community of Pasadena did exhibit at least some racial and class diversity. Like other nonwhites who lived in the town, Chinese Americans tended to find work in wealthy residences as cooks, domestics, and gardeners.[24] Others operated businesses in the service and tourist industries, such as laundries, groceries, and Chinese curio and antique shops. Two physicians of Chinese ancestry, Margaret Chung and George Chee, lived in Pasadena. Also in his thirties, Chee practiced in downtown Los Angeles, not far from the Santa Fe Railroad Hospital.

Chee rented in a Pasadena neighborhood with working-class African, Mexican, and Japanese Americans; in contrast, Chung purchased a home in a white, middle-class community. Her neighbors consisted of families of midwestern origin. Almost all were native born, with a few descended from immigrants of northern and western European extraction. The male heads of households occupied white-collar positions, such as insurance and real estate agents. A few performed skilled blue-collar labor as machinists and glassworkers. The U.S. census indicates that almost none of the women held occupations. Not only were Chung and her sisters the only Chinese in the community, but Margaret had the highest professional standing of all her neighbors, male or female.

Given the increasing prevalence of racial segregation, it is not clear how Chung's neighbors responded to her or why someone chose to sell the home to her. A Christian minister lived next door and may have facilitated her entry into the community. A Chinese Methodist church was located a few blocks down the road. In addition, with a hospital on her street, Chung's presence may not have appeared too unusual. The fact that a white nurse lived in her home also suggests a certain degree of acceptance for interracial cohabitation.

The census lists Isabelle Shephard as a boarder in the Chung household, which was unusual in Chung's neighborhood. Generally, only working-class families rented rooms or beds in their homes to help make ends meet. Only one other residence housed a lodger, and that individual appeared to work there as a domestic. Perhaps Margaret needed the financial assistance to pay the mortgage. Perhaps she took advantage of her autonomy to create a home with another woman.

Chung's ability to achieve class mobility and racial integration helped to advance the status of her sisters. Almost all of them attempted to follow her lead into white-collar occupations. Coming of age after the medical profession contracted, however, they experienced difficulty duplicating Margaret's achievement. Anna, age twenty at the time of the 1920 census, along with Venus and Florence, ages seventeen and sixteen, eventually studied nursing.[25] Although that profession was

easier for women to enter, the difficulties that the Chung sisters encountered led them to pursue other occupations. Flo eventually served as
Margaret's receptionist and nurse, but Venus (or Vee) primarily worked
as a clerk. After developing tuberculosis, Anna left nursing school. As
the second eldest daughter, she bore much of the "mothering" responsibilities for her siblings and may have contracted the disease from
Minnie. She worked for the China Toggery, a clothing store for women
and children, and then obtained a position in a medical laboratory.[26]
Dorothy, only eleven at the time, attended school.

Although Margaret's sisters did not match her professional accom-
plishment, they made more progress than their brothers, who were
laborers. All the Chungs faced racial obstacles. However, a class difference emerged between brothers and sisters, illustrated by the location of
their respective homes in San Pedro and Pasadena. Andrew and Virgil
discovered fewer opportunities to move into managerial or professional
positions. Native-born men of northern and western European ancestry
filled 92 to 96 percent of these occupations during the 1920s.[27] Chung's
sisters gained white-collar jobs, but in low-level positions that were
reserved for women.

Even in the midst of racial segregation efforts, opportunities for
advancement existed. However, these niches did not necessarily indicate
a level playing field. Chung lived in a white, middle-class neighborhood
but not an upper-class community with those of similar professional
standing. The rest of the Chung sisters worked in low-paying but
respectable white-collar positions, while their brothers had greater
autonomy but less prestige because of their agricultural work.

A CELEBRITY PHYSICIAN

Several developments in Chung's personal life and professional career
helped her create a private practice and form a new circle of friends. She
received a regular salary from the Santa Fe for treating workers, but she
also could exact a fee from their family members and other patients.
The hospital subsidized her clinic by allowing Chung the free use of
office space, telephones, and secretaries. Working there introduced her
to a new pool of clients—musicians, actors, and entertainers, many of
whom were associated with the developing film industry in Hollywood.
Chung's interactions with her "star" patients reveal how the popular
culture of the 1920s influenced the lives of Chinese Americans and also
how people of Asian origin shaped the formation of modern identity.

In Los Angeles, Chung developed a reputation as a celebrity physician. Van Hoosen recalled that "the first news from her after she began practicing was that she had removed Mary Pickford's tonsils."[28] Chung's responsibilities at the Santa Fe Railroad Hospital brought her into contact with travelers who needed medical services. Musicians and actors on tour likely sought her assistance and then referred their friends and acquaintances to her. Chung's skills as a plastic surgeon, initially developed to treat work-related injuries at the railroad hospital, also helped attract clients from the entertainment world.[29] She became known for her deft finger work and the small size of her surgical scars, skills that Chung learned from Van Hoosen.

Chung's duties as a physician facilitated more personal relationships with her "star" patients. As their doctor, she inquired about their physical and mental well-being. The rapport she established facilitated social interactions outside of the office. She recalled that her patients included "some of the new people of the musical world like Charles Wakefield Cadman and Carrie Jacobs Bond who frequently came to my house and played some of their newest compositions."[30] Chung's invitations to her home for dinner and socializing were particularly welcome for those far away from home. As Dorothy recalled, "people on the road . . . don't get home cooked meals, so they loved it."[31]

Chung's interest in developing professional and personal relationships with celebrities reflects the rising influence of popular culture during the early twentieth century. Like most city dwellers, especially those from rural and immigrant backgrounds, Chung had a fascination with modern commercial culture. While her participation in the Willard Literary Society in the USC Preparatory Academy suggests that she aspired to achieve a Victorian sense of cultural respectability, Chung also enjoyed the bawdiness of cabaret shows during her medical school years.

The rise of the Los Angeles entertainment industry fostered Chung's interest in celebrities. In 1910, no film studios existed in Hollywood. By 1920, Hollywood "reigned as the center of the movie industry," accounting "for at least 80 percent of American production."[32] The rapid transformation occurred as entrepreneurs, many of them Jewish immigrants, relocated to the region to take advantage of the good weather and lower production costs in an anti-union town. Through the movie industry, Hollywood shaped the consuming habits and identities of Americans. The images and lives of movie stars portrayed in film and in print both entertained and instructed their audiences, creating a more nationally uniform sense of culture and self. Ironically, immigrants played an important role in shaping and consuming these idealized versions of American character, modernity, and urban life.[33]

Second-generation Chinese Americans like Chung and her sisters came of age as the Hollywood movie industry assumed national dominance. Although Chinese immigrants had been living in Southern California as far back as the mid-nineteenth century, few reproduced on American soil because of the scarcity of women. As late as 1910, only 147 Chinese women lived in Los Angeles. They resided in 61 households out of a total Chinese population of 2,602.[34] Due to the gender imbalance and the legal restrictions against interracial marriage, a second generation did not emerge until the 1920s and 1930s. Growing up with Hollywood almost in their backyards, Chinese Americans embraced the new mass culture. However, they faced both racial and community restrictions that impeded full participation.

Discrimination commonly prevented Chinese Americans from participating in "mainstream" forms of recreation. Even though the Chung sisters lived in a white neighborhood, Dorothy recalled that when she tried to swim in a public pool with her white classmates, "they wouldn't let me in because I was Chinese."[35] In response, Chinese Americans organized their own beauty pageants, jazz bands, sports clubs, and theatrical groups. Andrew and Virgil played on the Los Angeles Chinese baseball team from the late 1920s through the mid-1930s. They also competed in semiprofessional Chinese leagues against merchant teams throughout the Los Angeles area.[36] Their youngest sister, Dorothy, recalled attending games on Sundays to cheer for her brothers.

However, some Chinese American parents discouraged such Americanized forms of recreation. They feared the loss of Chinese culture in their children. For their daughters, in particular, they expressed concern about inappropriate gender behavior. The flapper lifestyle of carefree pleasure and sexual experimentation met with disapproval. The profession of acting, which became increasingly glamorous due to the popularity of movies, drew particular censure. Traditional Chinese society associated this line of work with prostitution and criminality.

Margaret Chung, as an orphan and the eldest sibling, had no obvious family pressures that would restrict her behavior. However, she witnessed the effects of parental disapproval among her second-generation cohorts. Chung became friends with Anna May Wong, one of the earliest Asian American actresses.[37] As pioneers in their respective professions and as single women who made unique choices in their personal lives, the two had much in common. Like Chung, Wong came from a working-class background. Born in 1905, she was raised in Los Angeles, where her family operated a laundry. Attracted by the glamour of the developing movie industry, Wong worked as an extra for several years before being offered a leading role in *Toll of the Sea* (1923), the first full-length Technicolor movie. Wong's family, especially her father, objected to her profession, especially since she tended to be scantily clad in her film roles. When she disregarded their advice to stop acting and rejected her father's plan for an arranged marriage, Wong became estranged from her family.[38]

Wong's separation from her family due to conflicts regarding sexuality and respectability in some ways mirrored Chung's distancing from the Chinese American community. Chung's status as a single woman limited her medical practice in that community. One acquaintance recalled that Chung "could get no practice in Los Angeles because she was unmarried . . . In Los Angeles an unmarried woman cannot converse with a group of married women."[39] She did treat some Chinese patients. In fact, from 1914 to 1922, she was the only physician of Chinese ancestry to appear in the records for Evergreen Cemetery, where both Minnie and Chung Wong were buried.[40] However, Margaret developed a predominantly non-Chinese clientele. Her decision to relocate away from the San Pedro area indicated a desire for professional as well as social separation from the Chinese American community there.

Facing a degree of social ostracism due to choices in her personal life, Chung rejected the traditional Chinese disdain toward popular culture. She even encouraged her youngest sister to pursue acting. Although three of the Chung sisters studied nursing, Margaret criticized the profession, explaining that "the nurse did all the dirty work and the doctor got all the credit."[41] Instead, Margaret supported Dorothy's aspirations to enter show business. Margaret even used contacts among entertainers to obtain her sister an entry-level job as a circus performer.

HOLLYWOOD ORIENTALISM

Ironically, while Margaret and other Chinese Americans asserted their Americanness through their enthusiasm for popular culture, "mainstream" Americans primarily accepted people of Asian ancestry due to perceptions of their exotic racial status. The Hollywood film industry played an influential role in cultivating this Orientalist image.[42] Following in a longer tradition of Western fantasies about the East, movies portrayed Asian people and their culture as the inferior yet desirable antithesis to the West.[43] Films allowed the audience to voyeuristically experience "forbidden pleasures," often embodied in the figure of the Asian female. For example, almost all of Anna May Wong's early roles featured her as a "Dragon Lady," an obviously foreign woman who is both evil and seductive. Wong and Chung both developed relationships with the same circle of actors and producers. Their Hollywood friends not only created the film industry but also formulated a particular cinematic depiction of Asia.

Margaret Chung's first celebrity patient, Mary Pickford, actually portrayed one of the first Asian women on screen. In 1915, she performed the tragic title role of *Madame Butterfly* in "yellowface." Using makeup to give the impression of being Asian, Pickford starred as a Japanese woman who kills herself due to the impossibility of her love for a white Western man.[44] Hollywood recycled this narrative about unfulfilled interracial romance multiple times. In fact, Anna May Wong's first full-length film, *Toll of the Sea,* retold the story, setting the plot in China instead of Japan. The repetitions and variations reveal a cinematic obsession with the desire to cross racial boundaries and the need to discipline these transgressive longings.

Pickford's associates also pursued these themes. In 1920, she formed United Artists with Charlie Chaplin, Douglas Fairbanks, and D.W. Griffith. Chung also developed professional and personal relationships with this circle of filmmakers. In fact, the Los Angeles manager of United Artists eventually introduced her to San Francisco, the city that would become Chung's home for the rest of her life. Anna May Wong also benefited from contacts with the studio. She gained national recognition after she starred with cofounder Douglas Fairbanks in the 1924 movie *The Thief of Baghdad.* She did not portray a romantic lead but instead appeared as a forbidden "other," a calculating yet beautiful Mongol slave girl. Another cofounder, D.W. Griffith, also elaborated on these fantasies of interracial sexuality. He is best known for making the first full-length feature film, *The Birth of a Nation* (1915). His negative depictions of African Americans, actually performed by white actors in blackface makeup, helped inspire the re-formation of the Ku Klux Klan. Griffith also created a number of movies on miscegenation between whites and people of Native American, Mexican, and Asian ancestry.[45]

These films mirrored modern experimentations in social and sexual behavior. During the Jazz Age of the 1920s, white, middle-class Americans entered New York's Harlem and Chicago's South Side to observe and participate in socially transgressive behavior.[46] In Los Angeles and in other parts of the country, they also became fascinated with the cultural exoticness of Asian people and culture. Such racial crossings continued to be considered scandalous, which enhanced the excitement of engaging in these practices. In California and in many other states, antimiscegenation laws existed to prevent marriages between whites and nonwhites. Hollywood even instituted the Hays Code in 1934, banning scenes that depicted the desirability of miscegenation. The tragic endings of interracial love stories provided one means of cautioning against forbidden love. The casting of white actors in Asian roles also helped lessen fears about interracial contact. Audiences could still engage in the fantasy of race mixture but feel assured that the actors truly were white.

The pervasive Orientalism of Hollywood filmmaking sparked mainstream interest in individuals of Asian ancestry, which perhaps explains why Chung gained entry into celebrity circles. In *On Gold Mountain*, a semifictional family history, Lisa See recalled that two relatives of mixed white and Chinese ancestry, Ming and Ray, were transformed from ostracized high school students to "playboys" in 1920s Los Angeles.[47] They attributed their sudden popularity to Rudolph Valentino. The "exotic sensuality" of Valentino, a by-product of his racial ambiguity, made Ming and Ray's "Eurasian blood" sexually appealing. "They looked for and found 'Beverly Hills People,' 'American Friends,' and 'Jewish People'. . . . They were asked to clubs and dances." The "new women" of the 1920s who reveled in experimentation "brazenly invited them out to dinner and to bed."[48]

The Asian craze also created economic opportunities for Chinese Americans. By the late 1930s, one in every fourteen Chinese in Los Angeles worked in movie studios. Most filled in as extras for films set in Asia. A few achieved more prominent billing, like Anna May Wong, but they did so through roles that did not emphasize their Americanness but rather their connections with a mythic Orient. In her work as a circus performer, Margaret's sister Dorothy was restricted to similar roles. For her first job with the L. G. Barnes Circus, she performed as Aladdin. Although Dorothy was neither South Asian nor a boy, she was channeled toward performing the role of an exotic other because of her Chinese ancestry.

Even Chinese Americans not directly involved in making movies benefited from the Hollywood fascination with Asia, as described by Lisa See in her *On Gold Mountain*. Like other Chinese Americans, See's family catered to the entertainment industry for their livelihoods. Beginning in the 1920s and continuing through the 1990s, their antique and curio shops rented out props and costumes for theatrical and movie companies. In the midst of the 1930s depression, they also opened a Chinese restaurant called Dragon's Den in Old Chinatown, a commercial and residential neighborhood located near the Central Plaza.[49] The creators of Dragon's Den strategically developed a marketing image for white customers and succeeded in attracting the bohemian, homosexual, and Hollywood contingents of L.A. "On any given night, Sidney Greenstreet and Peter Lorre could be found at a back table dining together. . . . Others—the men and women who created illusion in Hollywood—came as part of their work. There were directors, producers, cameramen, costume designers, set designers, and set decorators."[50] The popularity of Dragon's Den reveals the circularity and profitability of Hollywood Orientalism. The fascination with oriental objects and cultures, promoted by the movie industry, inspired the establishment of a restaurant that featured Orientalist decor. In turn, the individuals responsible for cinematic depictions of the Orient patronized Dragon's Den in order to obtain "authentic" ideas for their films. Influencing one another, moviemakers and restaurant entrepreneurs projected a mutually reinforcing fantasy of the Orient. Their respective patrons and even some of the creators did not necessarily recognize the image as a fantasy.

Even the movie industry attempted to capitalize on the physical, not just the visual, recreations of the Orient. In 1926, Sid Grauman built an ornate movie theater in the style of a gigantic Chinese pagoda with red and gold columns and picturesque dragons. Mary Pickford and Douglas Fairbanks inaugurated the building by being the first celebrities to leave their imprints in cement slabs on the nearby sidewalk. The success of the Chinese Theater, which became a Hollywood landmark, encouraged other commercial ventures. In the late 1930s, a white female developer funded the creation of China City. The district was dubbed "Chinese movie land," because it used film sets to recreate a Chinese village. Chinese American merchants played a pivotal role in offering the predominantly white tourists a commercialized and simulated experience of an imagined China. In fact, Dorothy, following in the footsteps of her father, operated a gift shop in China City with her husband, Jake. After consuming images of the Orient on screen, movie patrons craved the visceral experience of visiting the Orient.[51] China City, an economic venture that used its association with movies to attract tourists, represented a prototype for studio-sponsored theme parks.[52]

In one sense, Dorothy's interest in movies and involvement in the ethnic tourist industry would seem to be diametrically opposed to Margaret's profession of medicine. However, both sisters recognized that their status as Chinese American women created expectations for certain types of performances. While there is no evidence that Margaret purposely capitalized on her Asian identity to advance her career at this period in her life, she certainly developed an awareness of how her patients and the broader community perceived her "differentness." Margaret's affinity for entertainers provides insight into her personality as well as her strategy for negotiating social barriers. Just as an actor or actress has the ability to portray various identities to capture the interest of an audience, so Margaret recognized her patients' and friends' preconceptions regarding race and gender. In subsequent years, she would increasingly accentuate her "difference" and exoticness to gain professional, political, and personal opportunities.

CHAPTER 6

"The Ministering Angel of Chinatown"

A Chinese woman doctor, thoroughly Americanized, her
reception room in the office of a photographic studio in the
center of San Francisco's Chinatown, her clientele divided
equally among Chinese and Americans. Such is Dr. Margaret
Jessie Chung, a notable daughter of the West.

Gerald J. O'Gara, *Sunset Magazine*, 1924

In the early 1920s, Margaret Chung accepted the invitation of two
Hollywood patients to accompany them on a vacation to San Francisco.
She had just performed surgery on the manager of the United Artists
studio and his wife, and agreed to help them recuperate. During the trip,
she "fell in love with San Francisco at once."[1] The city, located on a
peninsula surrounded by the Pacific Ocean and the bay, held a distinctive
charm. Unlike the relatively flat, expansive terrain of Los Angeles,
San Francisco was a compact city, distinguished by over forty hilltops,
almost all of them with impressive views of the surrounding neighborhoods, sparkling water, and dramatic landscapes of the Marin
headlands and Berkeley foothills. The steepness of the San Francisco
hills initially made them undesirable places to reside, until the city
became the first in the country to install cable cars in 1873. By the
time of Chung's visit, one of the peaks, Nob Hill, had become home to
elite families and the site of luxurious hotels like the Fairmont and the
soon to be opened Mark Hopkins. The Golden Gate and Bay bridges
would not be constructed until the mid-1930s, so Bay Area residents
and tourists took the ferry to travel back and forth between San
Francisco and Marin County to the north and the cities of Oakland and
Berkeley to the east. In the summer, the cool temperatures generated a

86

billowing fog that added a sense of enchantment to the streets of San Francisco.

Chung was drawn to the allure of the city and the prospect of practicing medicine among the largest Chinese community in the United States. San Francisco, with over half a million people, was just slightly smaller than Los Angeles in the early 1920s. Its Chinese population, however, was more than three times the size of the Chinese community in Los Angeles, with just under eight thousand.[2] Furthermore, over seventeen hundred Chinese women lived in San Francisco—more than ten times the number in Los Angeles.[3] Because of racial segregation dating back to the mid-nineteenth century, the overwhelming majority of the Chinese in San Francisco resided in the area known as Chinatown, an approximately thirty-block area situated between the downtown financial district, the elite neighborhood of Nob Hill, and the Italian community of North Beach.[4]

The large concentration of Chinese in San Francisco would allow Chung to do something that had been difficult to accomplish in Los Angeles: to fulfill her original goal of serving as a medical missionary to people of Chinese ancestry. As she recalled, "At that time, there were no Chinese Doctors practicing American medicine and surgery in Chinatown, and I thought I saw a great future here."[5] Although her application to serve in China had been rejected and she increasingly cultivated patients outside her ethnic group, she still wanted to bring Western medicine to her "own" people, especially to other Chinese women. In 1922, despite her relative success in Southern California, she decided to relocate and establish a practice in San Francisco Chinatown. In her early- to mid-thirties at the time, she apparently made the move alone, without companions or family. With her sisters achieving greater independence, Margaret may have felt that the time was right to reevaluate her life goals.

Despite her hopes, Chung experienced a difficult transition when she moved to San Francisco's Chinatown. She entered a neighborhood in the midst of a cultural and generational transformation. The creation of the new Republic of China in 1911 and the coming of age of an American-born cohort of Chinese encouraged Chinatown leaders to "modernize" the community. Seeking to improve mainstream views of Chinese people, they endorsed American acculturation. They encouraged the use of Western medicine among those used to traditional herbal cures. They also encouraged the development of nuclear families, hoping to move beyond the stereotype of Chinatown as a "bachelor" society.[6]

Chung occupied an uncomfortable position in the midst of these civic reforms. She promoted "modern" medicine, especially surgery, but many Chinatown residents remained skeptical of Western health care. Many were also skeptical of Chung herself. Her status as a single, female physician who adopted masculine attire incited gossip and suspicion within a neighborhood interested in creating a more normative image of gender roles and kinship relationships. She encountered difficulty attracting members of her own ethnicity and sex. Instead, she drew "outsiders," akin to tourists, who were interested in sampling the exotic setting and services of Chinatown.

"MODERN" MEDICINE IN A "TRADITIONAL" COMMUNITY

To launch her career in San Francisco, Chung initially took a position as the house physician for the Hotel Wiltshire before establishing a private practice in San Francisco Chinatown. Her connections with Hollywood executives and celebrities may have helped Chung obtain this job. She resided at the hotel, which was located in the tourist area and shopping district of Union Square. From there, her office in Chinatown was within easy walking distance. Her clinic, in fact, was situated just down the hill from the Presbyterian Chinese Mission Home, an institution that remained active until 1939. Memories of her mother must have inspired Margaret. Elsa Gidlow, a bohemian poet who befriended her in the late 1920s, recalled that Chung "established her practice in San Francisco's Chinatown with a sort of missionary zeal to bring modern methods to that community."[7] Chung was the second doctor of Chinese descent to establish a Western-style clinic in San Francisco. She was the first American-born physician of Chinese descent, however, as well as the first woman.[8]

Despite her enthusiasm, Chung's practice got off to a wobbly start. She recalled that "for a solid month I sat in my offices without a single patient."[9] Her lack of clientele resulted from a combination of factors. As a newly arrived single woman, she lacked the family and social contacts that would help establish her in the close-knit community. Since the mid-nineteenth century, a variety of formal and informal mechanisms had developed to facilitate the incorporation of new residents, but these avenues primarily catered to men.[10] The most important neighborhood associations, which provided social services and promoted civic activism, excluded women. The male domination of institutions, while certainly not unique to Chinese Americans, also reflected the gender imbalance of the population. The gender ratio reached a national low of one woman for every twenty-seven men in 1890.[11] By 1920, women still constituted only one in five of the Chinese population in San Francisco. In response to their ban from male-led organizations, women created separate associations to facilitate their involvement in social, cultural, and political affairs.[12] However, Chung still needed connections to gain entry into these networks.

She had difficulties developing relationships in Chinatown, not only due her gender and lack of contacts, but also because of her limited Chinese language and social skills. Chung grew up in areas with much smaller numbers of Chinese Americans and had to learn how to function in a large, ethnic community. As she recalled: "My first few years in San Francisco were rather disheartening. I knew very few people socially, I lived alone in a hotel. I was afraid to go out and visit many Chinese people because of my limited Chinese. They thought me 'high-hat' because I didn't accept their invitations where, as a matter of fact, I was embarrassed because I couldn't understand their flowery Chinese."[13]

While Chung expressed a sense of humility about her inadequate Chinese language and social skills, she also demonstrated a patronizing attitude toward members of the segregated community. To perceive herself as bringing scientific enlightenment to Chinatown entailed a belief in the superior value of her offerings. Her recollections about her first visit to San Francisco reveal her social distance from the community. Traveling as a guest of her celebrity patients, Chung initially viewed Chinatown from a chauffeur-driven car. From this position of privilege, she "was shocked to see the conditions under which many of the Chinese people lived."[14] Chung's self-appointed role as a medical missionary reinforced her status as a community outsider.

Chinatown residents initially chose not to consult Chung, because they had access to alternative sources of health care. Chung explained, "At the time, Chinatown was divided into two classes—the older generation who still believed in Chinese herbs, and the younger, more modern generation who, if they required medical attention and wanted modern medicine and surgery would go to a white physician."[15] Chinatown residents who valued Western practices and culture also tended to internalize mainstream racial attitudes that ascribed superiority to whiteness. Even some Chinese who favored traditional methods of healing "preferred American [i.e., white] women doctors to minister to their women during childbirth."[16] Like Chung, these female physicians came from a maternalist medical tradition and offered their scientific expertise for the women and children in Chinatown. Unlike Chung, they automatically were accorded more prestige due to their race. They also faced less social pressure to follow Chinese protocol.[17]

While Chung faced competition from white physicians, she encountered the greatest resistance among critics of Western medicine. In the 1920s, less than a handful of "regular" physicians of Chinese descent practiced in Chinatown. During the same time, the neighborhood supported thirty-seven herbal stores.[18] Traditional Chinese doctors, who arrived in the United States with the earliest immigrants, tended not to charge for their diagnoses but instead made their profits through selling herbs.[19] Chinese medicine was also diametrically opposed to Chung's preferred specialization of surgery. Patients remained fully clothed during examinations, which consisted of observation, conversation, and pulse detection. Accustomed to this form of health care, Chinatown residents were particularly skeptical of Western hospitals, because these institutions were associated with operations. Joseph Lum, who would become the superintendent of the Chinese Hospital in San Francisco, explained that "in those days . . . they [the Chinese American community] did not trust American doctors, and they thought the hospital was a place where you came to die."[20] While critics of these attitudes argued that hospital deaths primarily resulted from the reluctance of Chinese patients to enter the hospital "until it is too late," the patients explained the cause of death as a result of "being 'cut-open' . . . and to [other] totally unheard of remedies."[21] Advocates of Western health care criticized these fears as evidence of the "backwardness" or "superstitious" nature of traditional Chinese. However, many non-Chinese Americans shared these views of hospitals as unsanitary death traps, a description that accurately described these institutions during much of the nineteenth century.

In addition, some Chinatown residents resented the role that Western medicine played in reinforcing racial discrimination. Public health reform movements from the mid-nineteenth to the mid-twentieth centuries assisted wider political efforts to exclude and segregate Chinese.[22] Immigration officials instituted racially selective and humiliating medical examinations to target individuals considered undesirable for the American nation. These screening measures continued after entry as well. Health officials and anti-Chinese forces depicted the Chinese as the physical embodiment and the source of dangerous and infectious diseases, such as bubonic plague, leprosy, and syphilis. In essence, the Chinese served as "medical scapegoats."[23]

Ironically, even while Chinese Americans were being accused as diseased, governmental and medical regulations made it difficult for them to seek health care. Hospitals routinely denied admission to Chinese patients. At the same time, the San Francisco Board of Supervisors repeatedly prevented Chinese Americans from building their own hospital, a solution commonly adopted by immigrant and religious minorities.[24] The community finally received permission to establish a dispensary in 1900, but only after they promised to include Western-trained physicians on the staff. The American Medical Association deemed Chinese herbalists "irregular" and would not grant them medical licenses. Well into the twentieth century, they faced charges of criminal practice and were fined for diagnosing ailments and dispensing medicine.[25] Public health officials even barred Chinese herbal doctors from signing death certificates, requiring instead the authority of a licensed physician.[26] This regulation may explain why Chung's name appeared on the death certificates of Chinese in Los Angeles.

SPECIALIZING IN FEMALE CARE

Given the layers of gender, racial, and cultural conflicts in Chinatown, it is not surprising that Chung met with community reluctance to patronize her new practice. After six weeks of inactivity, when, she wrote, she "had almost reached the end of my rope," she suddenly benefited from a historical accident. In her autobiography, she recalled receiving an urgent call from a Chinatown restaurant:

> I walked in and found a young Chinese woman who was seriously ill, practically in shock. Calling an ambulance I rushed her to the hospital. They say that fools rush in where angels fear to tread. . . . I did not realize how my professional reputation and my future livelihood depended upon that case. It hung like a slender thread. . . . God was good to me, for she was an exceedingly poor risk . . . and if she had died my name would have been "mud" and I might just as well have folded my little tent and gone elsewhere.[27]

Her patient turned out to be a well-respected businesswoman who frequently served as a translator for other Chinese women during their visits to doctors. Chung recalled that "in less than twenty-four hours, the news had gotten around. Business picked up considerably following that successful operation."[28]

As this case indicates, a Chinese American female network launched Chung's career in Chinatown. Women in the community assisted each other in gaining access to medical treatment; as women, they shared the responsibility of ensuring the health of their families, particularly their children.[29] During the 1920s, Chinatown witnessed a baby boom. The maturation of the second generation, combined with an improving gender ratio, resulted in Chinese women giving birth "at a rate 90 to nearly 250 percent higher than women in the city overall."[30] When these women consulted health-care providers, they preferred midwives and female doctors. Margaret's sister Dorothy suggested that Margaret played an important role in Chinatown because women there "were too shy to let a man examine them."[31] They also likely believed that women would provide better quality care for mothers and children.

The population explosion assisted Chung in developing a professional niche. She volunteered her time at a local school, conducting physical exams and giving educational talks to the 178 children enrolled.[32] She also helped found the Chinese Hospital in 1925. After years of planning, the Chinatown community finally succeeded in establishing a five-story, fifty-five-bed institution.[33] Following the standards of the California medical board, all the physicians held medical licenses. The hospital grudgingly accommodated more traditional medical approaches, explaining that "we Chinese have used herbs for many thousands of years. Since this is in the blood, we cannot but retain it."[34] While Chinese patients could request herbs and foods to assist their recovery, all such treatments were subject to the approval of the licensed physicians. The hospital maintained a cultural hierarchy between Western and Chinese medicine, but the institution did challenge the racial hierarchy in some ways. Each department was headed by one of the four Chinese American Western-trained physicians in the community. They, in turn, presided over the remaining thirty-two white doctors on the hospital's staff. Significantly, although Chung had trained in a variety of surgical procedures, she was not listed under that division. Instead, as the only female among the four Chinese American doctors, Chung led the Gynecology, Obstetrics, and Pediatrics unit.[35]

The kinds of assistance that Chinese American women provided Chung reveal that their influence extended beyond female networks. By 1927, she became known as the only physician for "the entire 'Four Families'—Lowe, Quan, Jung, and Chew."[36] This family association included members with the last name Chung, a variation on Jung. Women could not join these organizations, which were among the most important in the community. At best, they became auxiliary members based on their kinship ties to men. Margaret's new reputation as a family association doctor indicates that female patients helped establish her in male-dominated arenas.

THE BURDENS OF COMMUNITY SERVICE

Although Chung achieved some recognition and acceptance among Chinese in San Francisco, she felt uneasy about her professional position. By the late 1920s, she sought opportunities to "give up her practice in Chinatown entirely" and promised her "remaining Chinese patients" to a newly licensed Chinese American male physician.[37] Despite her desires to serve her own people, Chung continued to encounter suspicions regarding her professional skills and her personal life.

The medical community in Chinatown during the 1920s and 1930s was rife with jealousy. The competitiveness simmered as increasing numbers of Chinese American doctors established clinics in the neighborhood. Like other professionals of color, many of whom faced insurmountable racial barriers in mainstream society, they turned to segregated neighborhoods to establish their careers.[38] As members of the professional and social elite, Chinatown physicians tended to socialize with one another. Frequent contact could produce close friendships, but this "limited society" also had the potential to transform "the friendliest feelings . . . into the bitterest criticism of a colleague in private conversation with patients or friends."[39] The tendency of clients to quickly switch physicians if immediate improvements did not occur also exacerbated the tensions between professional colleagues. As one doctor complained: "They expect one to be [a] miracle worker. Even God could not do the things they wish us to perform for them. Then they blame us for their own shortcomings. They never come to us until it is practically too late. They will doctor themselves with herbs and when this practice fails to help them, they will plead for us to help them. Quite often, all we can do is to help them ease their dying pains."[40]

Chung was not immune to this world of gossip, innuendo, and criticism. In 1927, the Hip Hop Association of San Jose sent a handwritten letter to the California State Board of Medical Examiners requesting that Chung be stripped of her medical license.[41] The organization charged her with selling cocaine in federal prisons with a Chinese accomplice identified as her husband. In response, the board queried the American Medical Association about Chung's practice and marital status.

The AMA's response briefly listed her credentials, and the California board subsequently took no action about the complaint. The episode is revealing on a number of levels. The letter writer assumed a fictitious identity to present false charges against Chung. The Hip Hop Association did not exist.[42] However, whoever wrote the letter realized that the medical board had the power to grant and revoke medical licenses. Furthermore, the writer understood the type of charges that might damage Chung's reputation. Accusing her of selling narcotics, clearly an illegal act, would evoke popular perceptions of Chinese as opium smokers and dealers. Condemning Chung for lying about her marital status, not necessarily a criminal or professional matter, would impugn her character by implying personal impropriety. It is unlikely that another Chinatown physician wrote the letter, which contained multiple grammatical errors. However, the letter indicates that a community member or someone who wanted to assume the guise of the Chinese sought to besmirch Chung's public and private reputation.[43]

Chung also received criticism from more respectable circles. James Hall, one of the four Chinese American physicians who founded the Chinese Hospital, increasingly criticized his Chinese American colleagues as he assumed greater leadership in the institution. He accused them of being self-interested, unwilling to volunteer their services to the hospital's free clinic. There was some resistance among Chinese American physicians to provide low-cost or free health care. During the Great Depression, the doctors affiliated with the hospital would vote to close the clinic. The pressure to provide low-cost and free health care for impoverished communities existed not only for Chinese Americans but other professionals of color and women physicians.[44] These demands for personal and financial sacrifice, while potentially rewarding for those committed to community service, also represented a continuous financial drain, especially for those seeking a professional livelihood in the competitive market of Chinatown. The Chinese American physicians Hall criticized might have conducted "charity" work on their own, or they might have disliked Hall's administration of the clinic. They might have decided that providing free medical care was not worthwhile given the lack of loyalty among some Chinatown patients. Bessie Jeong, who began practicing in the San Francisco Bay Area in the 1930s, recalled that she treated Chinese patients, but many "did not pay their bills."[45]

Hall also specifically criticized the quality of Chung's surgery. Chung took pride in the efficiency of her procedures, but Hall complained that he had to "follow up on many of her tonsilectomies" due to her inattention.[46] He hinted that she was "not ethical" and had been barred from practicing in many hospitals. These allegations are difficult to verify because Chung had a dedicated following among both white and Chinese patients and developed affiliations with a number of medical institutions in San Francisco. By 1929, Chung had achieved enough prominence to be listed in the *Who's Who in California*.[47] Even as her Chinatown clientele declined, some Chinese Americans continued to seek her out for medical treatment, especially for surgical procedures. Hall's charges perhaps reflected changing medical standards as well as professional rivalries. Hall, who took pride in having graduated from Stanford University in the early 1920s, criticized the medical education that Chung had received at the University of Southern California in the 1910s. And, he was head of the surgical staff at the Chinese Hospital, a position that Chung may have wanted given her interest and training.

In addition to these criticisms from Hall, Chung also faced competition from other Chinese American female doctors who entered the Chinatown market. The relatively cool reception that Chung received in the early twenties contrasts with the community's warm acceptance of Dr. Rose Goong Wong, when she began her practice in 1927. A graduate of the Philadelphia Woman's Medical College, Wong played a central role in transforming community attitudes toward Western medicine, hospitals, and childbirth. Like other Americans during the early twentieth century, expectant Chinese parents preferred giving birth at home. Wong, who specialized in obstetrics and gynecology, made house calls but also coaxed parents to use the services of the Chinese Hospital. "The popularity of Wong's reassuring bedside manner" contributed to a dramatic increase in hospital deliveries "from only 20 percent of all Chinese births in 1929 to 56 percent in 1939."[48] A history of the Chinese Hospital characterized Wong as a widely respected community resource, leaving behind a "legacy of twenty-four hour devotion to her patients in which fatigue never dulled her joy." Chung, by contrast, was described as catering less to the Chinese community, with a "huge non-Chinese following."[49]

The difference in community reception of Chung and Wong stemmed from a variety of factors. First, Wong's medical expertise and approach to health care proved more suitable for a community focused on reproduction yet distrustful of Western medicine. Chung had been trained in gynecology and obstetrics, but she identified herself as a surgeon, a field dominated by men and a field especially mistrusted by many Chinese.

In contrast, Wong viewed herself as a specialist in women's health. Furthermore, she willingly provided free and low-cost medical care, possibly as a means to develop her practice. Described as a "dynamic, business-minded physician[,] she was nonetheless kind, understanding, and did not press her less fortunate patients for debts. She was among the first to provide free postnatal care for mother and newborn."[50]

Differences in the two women's personal backgrounds may also have played a role. Whereas Wong grew up in San Francisco Chinatown and attended the nearby University of California, Berkeley, as an undergraduate, Chung, like many of the first wave of Western-trained physicians who moved to Chinatown, came from outside of San Francisco. Wong's familiarity with Chinatown may have fostered a greater sense of commitment to its residents.

The two women's marital status and personal reputation also probably influenced their reception in the community. Both Wong and Chung practiced cross-dressing, adopting male professional attire to indicate their status as medical doctors.[51] However, while they transcended established gender roles in their professional career and identity presentation, Wong followed a more traditional path in her personal life. She married and eventually had a family. Chung remained single, a status that became increasingly anomalous in the nuclear-family-centered community.

Chung's standing as an unmarried woman, coupled with her practice of cross-dressing, led Chinese in San Francisco to question her sexual propriety. Some community members conflated her personal history with her mother's, describing Chung as a former prostitute rescued "from a life of white slavery by a social worker."[52] A more common charge against Chung centered on her sexual orientation. When physician Bessie Jeong was asked decades later whether she and Chung shared a sense of camaraderie, she exclaimed defensively: "Oh, no! Margaret and I were as different as [pause] She was a homo, a lesbian."[53] The rumors regarding Chung even surfaced in a 1940 report by the Federal Bureau of Investigation. The agent noted that the doctors in Chinatown "will not say anything about [Chung] but raises his [sic] eyebrows when she is mentioned. There are rumors that she is a lesbian."[54]

Competition from other Chinese American female physicians, in combination with the rumors about Chung's sexuality, resulted in a loss of Chinatown clients, especially female patients. Speculations about Chung as a former prostitute and as a lesbian marked her as a transgressor against sexual norms. In essence, she represented a liability for a community seeking to demonstrate their normality through a celebration of nuclear families.

SELF-ORIENTALISM AND MEDICAL TOURISM

While Chung sparked controversy within Chinatown, she discovered that the exotic mixture of her personality and her Asian ancestry attracted white patients, particularly male ones. Surprisingly, other Chinese American physicians also developed a similar client base, because they faced comparable professional and social pressures from within Chinatown.[55] The phenomenon of white men seeking medical care from a Chinese American woman appears to invert established racial and gender hierarchies. However, Chung's patients traversed social boundaries not because of their desire to ignore her identity as a Chinese American woman but rather to partake of her social difference. Just as middle-class white tourists visited racial communities during the 1920s for purposes of leisure, so Chung's patients practiced a form of medical tourism. They sought medical assistance from someone on the margins. The close-knit Chinatown neighborhood had more daily interactions with Chung and consequently more ability to regulate her professional and social interactions. In contrast, members of the mainstream society, because of their geographic or cultural distance from her, could view her through their preconceptions.

Chung regularly came into contact with tourists through her responsibilities at the Hotel Wiltshire, and she led them to her Chinatown office. As in her interactions with Santa Fe Railroad Hospital patients, Chung discovered that her "otherness" proved an asset. Just as her Los Angeles clients projected their ideas onto her, so she actively cultivated an Orientalist image to attract San Francisco patients. Capitalizing on the desire among travelers and even local residents for exotic yet safe cultural experiences, Chung in effect staged her medical clinic as a tourist site. The woman who always dressed in Western clothing decorated her Chinatown office with "furnishings in Oriental artistry."[56] Both residents and visitors noted the significance of this decision. Writer Pardee Lowe, who recorded his observations about Chinatown life in a series of research notes, repeatedly commented on Chung's decision to decorate her office in an "electively Chinese" style. While Chung maintained "100% Western" medical equipment, her office was "thoroughly Chinese."[57] This commingling of the West and the East reflected Chung's cultural identity. Moreover, it reflected her predilection for popular culture, her savvy reading of the potential market for authentic Oriental experiences, and her delight in performance. Chung shared a reception room with a photography studio, a setup that automatically linked her practice with the tourists who wanted their pictures taken in Chinatown. Her clinic was a natural complement to the studio, a staged backdrop that would attract patrons curious about the authentic Chinese experience. Her plan worked effectively. When Bertha Van Hoosen visited her former intern in the 1930s, she remarked that the "very beautiful Chinese furnishings took my fancy."[58] Pardee Lowe also commented that "her office has become one of the main sights in Chinatown."[59] Chung, dressed in Western clothing and practicing Western medicine, provided a safe yet culturally distinctive experience for non-Chinese patients.

Other Chinese Americans also adopted Chung's strategy of self-Orientalization.[60] That is, they created of a particular cultural image to fulfill people's fantasies about Asia. For example, the few second-generation women who found work outside of Chinatown usually appeared as "exotic showpieces"; they were required to "wear oriental costumes" to add "atmosphere" for "teahouses, restaurants, stores, and nightclubs."[61] Similarly, some Chinese herbalists, intent on impressing their non-Chinese clientele, resorted to dressing in "Chinese robes and round Mandarin hats" to prove the cultural "authenticity" of their medical cures.[62] In fact, during the 1920s and 1930s Chinatown as a community debated how to encourage "Chinafication" of their neighborhood to attract tourists.[63]

These self-Orientalist practices attracted non-Chinese patients who purposely sought medical care from someone of a different cultural background. Traditional herbal physicians actually developed a reputation among both Chinese and non-Chinese patients for treating "embarrassing" ailments such as venereal disease and infertility. White patients also felt more comfortable approaching non-white but Western-trained doctors to remedy socially disreputable ailments. Bessie Jeong recalled that a relative of a movie producer once approached her for narcotics. Native American physician Charles Eastman recounted the temptations of financially remunerative requests. He was "persistently solicited for illegal practice, and this by persons who were not only intelligent, but apparently of good social standing."[64]

Chung's perceived status as an outsider not just in terms of race and culture but also gender and sexuality helped to attract patients. For example, she became the physician for Elsa Gidlow, a self-identified lesbian, and Gidlow's female lover, Tommy. Gidlow suspected that Chung "might be a sister lesbian" and felt comfortable revealing that she and Tommy lived together.[65] Because of this assumed bond, as well as their mutual status as independent women, Gidlow also requested assistance regarding her unmarried pregnant sister. Although abortion was illegal, motherhood was "financially impossible" and "unthinkable":

> Abortion was the only solution. I had no idea how one went about getting one and was horrified at what I heard about that violent recourse. . . . Finally, I asked Margaret Chung for advice. She told me what I already knew, that she could not risk such an operation. But she was warmly sympathetic. She had young sisters and would feel as I did. She said, "I'll help you." She wrote a name and an address. "This man is a competent medical doctor and surgeon. He will do a clean, safe job. I'll telephone and tell him he is not to charge you over $50." There are no words to express [my] gratitude for such compassion.[66]

In addition to providing the abortion referral, Chung also agreed to sterilize another of Gidlow's sisters. Chung apparently also offered medical options for other women to control their fertility. In 1950, a letter to the Board of Medical Examiners reported "rather ugly rumors in circulation about the abortion activities of Dr. Cecil A. Saunders [a fellow graduate of USC] and his relationship in business with Dr. Margaret Chung."[67] James Hall's comment about the unethical nature of Chung's practice may have referred to these rumors.

Chung, like other female doctors, no doubt provided access to birth control for Chinese American women as well.[68] In fact a non-Chinese physician operated a birth control clinic in Chinatown.[69] Some residents monitored the size of their families, since uncontrolled reproduction indicated an inability to practice American norms regarding the appropriate size of the nuclear family. Pardee Lowe commented that "birth control [was] practiced by 2nd & 3rd generations, particularly 3rd for higher standards of living"; the most common strategies used included "late marriage," "contraception," and "abortion."[70] The decline in reproduction during the Great Depression further indicates the practice of birth control.[71] Chung's willingness to help women regulate their fertility likely stemmed from her mother's experiences as well as her training in Chicago. Minnie's numerous pregnancies had aggravated her tubercular symptoms. Recognizing the sufferings of working-class immigrant women, Rachelle Yarros, one of Chung's Chicago mentors, led the effort by Hull House reformers to promote birth control. In San Francisco Chinatown, despite the community desire to monitor reproduction, Chung's efforts might have contributed to her marginalization. Facilitating access to birth control and illegal abortions put her at odds with the strong pro-natalist movement in Chinatown.

Although Chung developed a significant clientele among white women, the majority of her patients were white men. In addition to tourists and others seeking remedies for potentially embarrassing illnesses, she cultivated a patient base among police officers. At the time, the Hall of Justice bordered Chinatown. In fact, a special "Chinatown Squad" was created to deter tong wars and other illegal activities in the community.[72] Merchants and professionals like Chung welcomed these cleanup efforts, which helped to promote tourism. However, other Chinese Americans routinely complained of the harassment and humiliation that they experienced at the hands of the police, who did not necessarily distinguish between law-abiding residents and criminals.[73] The Irish working class, historically one of the most virulently anti-Chinese groups, dominated the police force, which likely exacerbated tensions with the Chinatown community.

Chung's family history and work experience help explain her interest in attracting police officers as clients. While they represented a racially oppressive state presence in Chinatown, they also intervened in correcting gender abuse. The police served as allies for white female reformers and accompanied missionary rescue efforts, which continued through the 1930s. In contrast to Chung's lack of cultural skills in interacting with a large Chinese American community, she had ample experience with men of various ethnicities. Her position at the Juvenile Psychopathic Institute in Chicago had brought her into almost daily contact with law enforcement. Also, she treated a large Irish clientele among her patients at the Santa Fe Railroad Hospital. Except for her internship at the Mary Thompson Hospital and her initial years in Chinatown, Chung mostly worked in ethnically diverse male environments. Her training thus facilitated her rapport with male colleagues, friends, and clients, especially those from outside of the Chinese community.

Just as Chung used the blending of her cultural identities to attract white patients, so her mixture of gender identities elicited the interest of male clients. Along with her masculine dress, she also adopted "male" professional mannerisms. Her relatives, friends, and patients characterized her in stereotypically "masculine" terms; she was "bossy," "brusque," and straightforward. A San Francisco tour book containing an entry on Chung in the chapter on Chinatown described her as possessing "a gruff voice, a hearty manner," and affecting "masculine styles."[74]

Despite her male gender persona, many of her patients as well as acquaintances insisted on portraying her in traditionally feminine ways. For example, a 1924 *Sunset Magazine* article featured Chung as "The Ministering Angel of Chinatown." The phrase evoked Victorian ideas that characterized women as inherently nurturing and pure. The writer from *Sunset,* an Irish male, acknowledged Chung's masculine clothes and specialization in surgery. "Professionally mannish are the silk shirt-waist, soft collar and bow tie that Dr. Chung wears, but a woman's tenderness and a mother's love she has showered on a growing family."[75] The passage demonstrates his desire to assert a fundamentally maternal nature underneath Chung's masculine exterior.

Just as Chung's femaleness allowed male patients to project their need for female nurturance, so her Chinese ancestry allowed white patients to fulfill their fantasies about cultural difference. The article also describes Chung as "a Chinese woman doctor, thoroughly Americanized . . . [fighting] against the oriental ideal of homebound womanhood, against oriental distrust of everything Western, against the ignorance of sick persons who would die with herbs rather than live with modern medicine."[76] In celebrating Chung's ability to traverse cultural and gender boundaries, the writer also asserts a fundamental dichotomy between "oriental" values and "everything Western." He characterizes the East as stubbornly clinging to ignorance and patriarchy. In contrast, America represents rationality, freedom, and modernity.

The article captures the mainstream fascination with Chung's in-between status as Western and Oriental, male and female, modern and traditional. Individuals who considered themselves cosmopolitan found her appealing because Chung successfully demonstrated the ability to cross multiple boundaries. She also could provide discreet remedies for their experiments in social transgression. At the same time, her admirers insisted that she embody essential gender and racial differences to gain assurance that fixed distinctions would remain.

Chung's efforts to establish her medical career in San Francisco Chinatown reveal the shifting racial, gender, and sexual boundaries in the ethnic neighborhood as well as the broader society. Her weariness of Chinese Americans and her popularity among white Americans cannot be explained simplistically by characterizing the former as more close-minded and the latter as more liberal. Rather, her experiences demonstrate that the transition to a modern society did not eliminate, but rather reconfigured, social hierarchies and distinctions. In the process of "modernizing" their community, Chinese Americans accepted some elements of Western medicine and female professionalization. At the same time, they also expressed suspicion and rejection of those outside of established kinship networks and emerging heteronormative families. Chung's white patients also navigated shifting social values; for them, Chung's exoticism marked both their cultural adventurousness and their need to reinforce the boundaries between white and nonwhite, male and female. Described as "oriental" and "Americanized," "mannish" and "motherly," she fulfilled mainstream desires to cross but not to erase social boundaries of the early twentieth century.

CHAPTER 7

A Sister Lesbian?

By this time, Margaret Chung became Tommy's and my
doctor and our friend. She was Chinese, but American-born
and educated, western in her general medical practice and in
surgery at which she excelled. . . . Her office was a couple of
blocks down the steep Sacramento Street hill where we lived.
As I walked home from work, I would see her sleek blue
sportscar. She was a striking woman in her late thirties,
smartly dressed in a dark tailored suit with felt hat and
flat-heeled shoes. . . .

   With my increasing interest in Chinese people, their
philosophy and literature (and suspecting she might be a
sister lesbian) I was immediately attracted.

Elsa Gidlow, *Elsa: I Come with My Songs,* 1986
(Courtesy of Celeste West and Booklegger Publishing)

By the late 1920s, Margaret Chung had achieved a degree of professional stability and social status in San Francisco. Her entry in the
1928–1929 edition of *Who's Who in California* indicates that she had a
private practice in Chinatown and served on the executive staff at the
Chinese Hospital. In addition, she continued as a resident surgeon at
the Hotel Wiltshire. Reflecting her class status and ability to cross racial
boundaries, Chung participated in "mainstream" women's professional
and civic organizations, such as the San Francisco Medical Women's
Club and the San Francisco Women's City Club.[1] Like other entries in
this genre, the brief biography conveyed Chung's respectability in the
public realm. During this same period, however, rumors circulated
about her masculine attire, marital status, and sexual orientation.
No doubt recognizing the power of these speculations, Chung shielded
her personal life and regulated her behavior to minimize public
censure.

Given the difficulties of unearthing information about romantic desires and relationships, it is fortunate that one of Chung's admirers was a writer.[2] When she and Elsa Gidlow first met in the late 1920s, Gidlow was a struggling poet about ten years younger than Chung, who was then in her late thirties. In 1923, Gidlow, a Canadian who originated from Great Britain, published *On a Gold Thread,* considered the first collection of explicitly lesbian poetry in North America. Turn-of-the-century sexologists formulated the category of "lesbian" to identify "deviant" and "mannish" women. Creating lesbian-themed literary works allowed individuals like Gidlow to offer their own portrayals, often more sympathetic ones, of same-sex desire and relationships. Some writings, like British author Radclyffe Hall's 1928 novel *The Well of Loneliness,* reached a large international audience despite being banned in England for depicting lesbian love. Gidlow's volume, however, sold poorly. In 1926, she moved to San Francisco and worked as an editor for a health journal to meet expenses. She lived with her female lover, Tommy, just on the border of Nob Hill and Chinatown. At the time, no cohesive, visible lesbian community existed, which was not surprising given the stigma attached to this new identity. Instead, Gidlow and Tommy relied on personal networks to recognize and socialize with lesbians.

Gidlow's observations of Chung, although filtered through the writer's projections and desires, offer a unique glimpse into the intimate world of the physician. Chinese American women of that era generally married and did so within their ethnic group. In contrast, Chung elected to remain single, expressed homoerotic desires, and developed romantic relationships with white women and men. At once transgressive and yet longing for respectability, she explored both heterosexuality and homosexuality.

Chung's physical location on the border of Chinatown facilitated her efforts to create a liminal or in-between personal space. The Chinese district in San Francisco is regarded widely as a racially bounded neighborhood. However, Chinatown and its surrounding communities, particularly the Italian neighborhood of North Beach, also functioned as "interzones," "areas of cultural, sexual, and social interchange."[3] Individuals interested in personal and artistic experimentation created a bohemian subculture that crossed racial and ethnic borders. The exoticness associated with "foreign" cultures and the marginalization of these communities fascinated individuals who viewed themselves as outsiders. This alternative network allowed Chung to explore unconventional desires and relationships and offered some protection from public criticism.

A MANNISH WOMAN

Gidlow was not alone in perceiving Chung as a possible lesbian due to her masculine persona. The prevailing social attitudes and emerging medical literature linked female cross-dressers with "sexual perversion." The connections between gender presentation and sexual orientation were more complex, however.[4] Chung consciously adopted an obviously Western and masculine style of dressing. As former mentor Bertha Van Hoosen recalled: "When on the street, [Chung wore] a black sailor hat. This costume would have been very inconspicuous had she not always carried a short sport cane."[5] Chung did not mind attracting attention to her traditionally male accessories, because they visibly demonstrated her successful entry into the world of white, professional men.

Chung's desire to achieve the status of elite men could be traced to childhood memories and perceptions of her inadequate femininity. She described herself as "a homely little child."[6] While working on a farm pitting apricots in Ventura County, she noticed that attractive girls received better treatment from boys: "There were always some pretty teenage girls around whom the boys liked. The boys would give them the large ripe apricots which they could simply run a knife through and slip the pit out; whereas they would give me the small green ones. . . . Needless to say, I did not make very much money pitting apricots."[7]

Instead of emphasizing her femininity to gain favors from men, Chung learned to participate in traditionally masculine activities as an equal companion. In medical school, she not only adopted male dress, but also supplemented her income by gambling with "the boys": "When I was too broke to pay the carfare to and from the County Hospital and the Medical School I would borrow a penny or two from some of the boys, shoot craps with them until I won about thirty-five or forty cents which would be enough to buy a half a pie, a sandwich, and assure me of carfare for the next day."[8] Reflecting Chung's limited economic resources at the time, she engaged in working-class forms of masculine camaraderie. In addition to gambling, she also was fond of drinking and swearing.

Chung's eventual professional success allowed her to assume elite male privileges. For example, she owned a series of expensive cars. In

California, the state with the highest percentage of female car owners, only one in five motorists was a women.[9] In San Francisco Chinatown, "only 4 percent of the . . . families . . . had cars, and few women knew how to drive."[10] And, just as Chung's habit of sporting a cane attracted attention, so did her ownership of cars. Elsa Gidlow noticed Chung's "sleek blue sportscar," and Bertha Van Hoosen recalled that her former mentee purchased a "spiffy red auto" soon after establishing a practice in San Francisco.[11] Edmund Jung, a physician who grew up in Chinatown, remembered that all the young boys in the community admired Chung's Cord. The car had the reputation of being "the most innovative, most modern, and most luxurious" car available at the time. Not only did the Cord have a distinctive appearance, it also had a "super charged V-8 engine."[12] As Chung advanced in social status, she employed a chauffeur and moved from driver to passenger. When Van Hoosen visited San Francisco in the late 1930s, she was escorted in Chung's Cadillac limousine.[13]

Chung's attempts to transcend class, gender, and racial boundaries resonated with the goals of other second-generation Chinese Americans. For example, Bessie Jeong echoed Chung's desire to participate as an equal in an elite white and masculine world. In fact, Jeong's personal history echoed elements from the lives of both Margaret and Margaret's mother. Born in San Francisco Chinatown, across from the Chinese Hospital, Jeong ran away from home at the age of fifteen, when her father decided to return to China. Fearing that he would arrange a marriage for her, Jeong turned to the Presbyterian Chinese Mission Home, the same institution that had assisted Ah Yane. Seeking to become a medical missionary, Jeong became the first Chinese American woman to graduate from Stanford University and eventually attended the Woman's Medical College in Philadelphia. Jeong explained that her desire to study biology and medicine stemmed from an early childhood interest in "boys' games," which were much more challenging to her than "girls' games." Medicine, to her, was a "man's game," and she believed she had a "man's mind."[14] Like Chung, Jeong accepted existing gender divisions, which associated certain abilities and privileges with men, even as she sought to transcend those boundaries.

However, Jeong distinguished between women who sought opportunities in traditionally male professions and women like Chung, who extended their challenge to include dress and behavior. While in medical school, Jeong observed that two sororities existed: in "one of them, the girls smoked and drank a little. They wore those gloves and wore suits and acted mannish. They'd sit down and put their legs this way. They were the mannish type. The men don't like them and the girls don't like them. The other group was more socially acceptable—real girls."[15] Jeong's comment reveals her effort to classify certain challenges to gender privilege as "normal" and others as "abnormal."[16] She could desire to enter the "man's game" of medicine but still consider herself a "real girl." However, Jeong clearly regarded Chung as the "mannish type," describing her as a "homo, a lesbian," who "went for her nurses."[17] Chung's ability to transcend gender and class barriers could be admired, but her success in acquiring male mannerisms and privileges also elicited unfavorable perceptions of her sexuality.

HOMOEROTIC DESIRE

Chung's views of her own sexuality are difficult to gauge, given the lack of sources from her perspective. Gidlow's accounts suggest that Chung engaged in a flirtatious and romantic friendship with her. However, Chung had reservations about expressing her desires publicly, especially in the Chinatown community, or acting upon them. Conscious of other people's censure, Chung resisted efforts to classify her as deviant or abnormal.

Gidlow, who had a non-monogamous relationship with Tommy, courted Chung. The writer invited the doctor to her apartment for dinner and regularly visited Chung in her office, sometimes bringing her flowers. Gidlow even wrote poetry about Chung and gave her a copy of *Teasedale's Anthology of Women's Love Lyrics*.[18] According to Gidlow, Chung understood the nature of these advances. Gidlow recalled one particular house call that Chung made: "Observing Tommy's and my domestic scene, [she] smiled a knowing smile."[19] One turning point in their relationship occurred when Gidlow departed for Europe to attempt a writing career. Chung invited Gidlow to a speakeasy in North Beach, the Italian community bordering Chinatown, for a farewell luncheon. Drinking bootleg liquor, Gidlow wrote in her journal, helped Chung reveal more about herself.[20] The growing intimacy of their relationship was sealed two days later by an exchange of good-bye presents and a kiss. Gidlow reflected: "I believe she was really sorry to see me go and heaven knows she is one of the few I part from with a pang. She gave me a pint bottle of bourbon, Government sealed, 160 proof and—what I value many times more, a spontaneous kiss on the mouth. I had never dared to hope she would kiss me."[21]

Chung made no apparent attempt to contact Gidlow while the writer lived in Europe. However, when Gidlow returned to San Francisco the following year and became dangerously ill, Chung finally expressed her growing feelings. Gidlow wrote poems about Chung while under her care at the Chinese Hospital. One composition so moved Chung that she kissed Gidlow again.[22] In and out of consciousness following an operation, Gidlow recalled two conversations she had with Chung: "I took her hand and would not let it go. How long she stayed I do not know, nor whether it was there or while still on the operating table that I heard myself say: 'Do you love me?' Her answer seemed to come after a long time: 'yes—if it will make you feel better.'"[23] Hours later, Gidlow and Chung conversed again:

> The door opened and M. came in 'I have been thinking about you all afternoon', I heard myself say. Then I begged her to stay with me for a little while and she said she would. . . . Was it then that M said: "You gave me hell this morning for operating on you; and then you asked me if I loved you. There were people around too," I felt a vague concern for her. Had I put her in an awkward position? "Was I very indescrete?" [sic] I asked her? "No, no," she assured me. . . . For a while—I remember it as a long while—my mind was a blank, yet I was aware, with the curious comfort, of Ms presence and thought of her constantly. Suddenly I asked: "Do you love me?" This time she said "Yes" immediately and quietly.[24]

Chung apparently never acted on her declaration of love. After Gidlow's recovery, Chung avoided contact with her. Gidlow wrote, "M. denies herself to me almost completely."[25] A few months after the operation, Gidlow's journal reported Chung's engagement to a wealthy man: "M is going to get married. It is bald, but it is a man and it has half a million— another sacrifice to the twin gods, manners and respectability."[26]

The interactions between the two women reveal that Chung felt romantic attraction toward Gidlow but also ambivalence about pursuing a relationship with her. The meals, gifts, and kisses that they exchanged demonstrated the eroticism underlying their professional rapport as doctor and patient. Perhaps Chung's reluctance about Gidlow stemmed from the presence of Tommy. Certainly, Chung's concern about public perceptions played a role in her considerations. She hesitated to declare love for another woman in front of other people. In fact, she attempted to express her sentiments as an extension of her responsibilities as a physician. Chung's engagement to a wealthy and respectable man, soon after an unqualified and private declaration of love, demonstrates her desire to retreat from an explicitly lesbian relationship.

BOHEMIAN CROSSINGS

Chung's decision to distance herself from Gidlow reflects her efforts to negotiate sexual norms in overlapping racial and cultural communities. Her vigilance regarding her personal reputation dovetailed with her efforts to gain professional recognition in Chinatown. That the intimate conversations between Gidlow and Chung took place at the Chinese Hospital is significant. As a relative newcomer to the community, Chung had to guard her image, especially because her initial efforts to establish herself met with mixed results. While homophobia existed in the broader American society as well, Chung very likely felt more vulnerable about her status in the close-knit Chinatown neighborhood. Consequently, she searched for alternative physical and social spaces to develop relationships that would be seen as transgressive by the Chinese American community.

The interactions between Gidlow and Chung took place in Nob Hill, Chinatown, and North Beach. Chung's geographical mobility was rather unusual, in light of Chinese American complaints of racial harassment and even violence outside of the Chinatown confines.[27] Chung's occupation facilitated these racial border crossings. She encouraged non-Chinese patients to enter Chinatown. Gidlow, who had limited resources, discovered that a private room in the Chinese Hospital was less expensive than in "American Hospitals."[28] Chung's professional status and responsibilities also allowed her to leave Chinatown. She visited patients in their homes. Also, as a physician for the Hotel Wiltshire, she developed professional and personal relationships with the white guests. Chung also likely became familiar with popular eating and entertainment establishments that catered to tourists. It is noteworthy that she introduced Gidlow to the speakeasy in North Beach. As the writer recalled, it was Chung who rang the doorbell at a nondescript and "dumpy house." The physician gained admission for them after a "soiled Italian . . . peered out" and then welcomed Chung "reverently."[29] The host's manner of greeting indicates his familiarity with her. Perhaps Chung frequently patronized the speakeasy. Perhaps she offered emergency medical care for the establishment, just as she had provided similar services for Chinese restaurants. Chung's profession allowed her to partially invert traditional "slumming" practices. Instead of middle-class white individuals visiting more economically disadvantaged and racially marginalized communities, Chung, as a Chinese American physician, could enter an Italian working-class neighborhood to seek amusement.

Chung's ability to cross into North Beach also stemmed from the marginal racial status of Italians. Like the Irish and the Jews, Italians, who arrived in large numbers at the turn of the century, were not readily accepted as "white."[30] Gidlow referred to North Beach as "Dagoetown," a racially derogatory term in common usage at the time.[31] While Italians did not face the same degree of legislative or political restrictions as Asians, they experienced economic discrimination and social segregation. Over the course of the first half of the twentieth century, the mainstream perception of Italian immigrants and their offspring evolved from nonwhite "Dagoes" to white ethnics. However, Italian Americans continued to be viewed as socially disreputable, especially due to their perceived association with organized crime. Like Chinatown, North Beach became a tourist site in part because of its reputation for seediness. During prohibition, mob-sponsored speakeasies in the community offered bootleg liquor to their patrons.

North Beach attracted individuals, like Chung, who wanted to pursue unconventional lifestyles, not just scandalous pastimes. During the early decades of the twentieth century, the area became a bohemian hub, with many cafes and art salons. This sense of cultural experimentation appealed to Chung. During the farewell luncheon with Gidlow, she expressed a desire to visit Paris, the destination of choice for aspiring writers and artists. Chung never traveled to Europe, but she did move into North Beach in the mid-1930s, becoming one of the first Chinese Americans to successfully integrate the neighborhood. She resided in a modern apartment on Telegraph Hill, where her immediate neighbors included authors, painters, and architects.[32]

This mecca for cultural exploration also fostered sexual experimentation. Gidlow described the Italian speakeasy that she and Chung visited as a "queer place." The use of the term "queer" may simply refer to the strangeness of the establishment. However, the fact that Chung chose the speakeasy for a private luncheon with Gidlow suggests that she felt more comfortable developing their relationship in that space. In fact, the illegal speakeasies in North Beach and the legitimate bars that opened following the repeal of Prohibition fostered the development of San Francisco's "queer subcultures."[33] Individuals who identified as homosexuals or who were interested in exploring non-normative possibilities frequented these establishments. They served as transgressive sites where individuals of diverse backgrounds and interests could encounter one another. The culture of organized crime during the Prohibition era even influenced the argot of homosexual communities: "'Straight' referred primarily to law-abiding citizens before the 1930s," but it also became a term to refer to heterosexuals; in addition, "criminals, rather than gays, were said to be 'in the life.'"[34] In the 1930s, a circuit of North Beach bars became known as "gay bohemian nightspots," which were particularly popular with the "literary crowd."[35] Gidlow and her friends occasionally patronized businesses that catered to lesbians, such as Mona's and the Black Cat. Some establishments, like Finocchio's, continued to appeal to a "mixed" clientele of "straights" and those "in the life" by titillating them with performances of male and female impersonators.

The neighboring community of Chinatown, with its low rents and exotic cultural allures, also attracted the interest of bohemians and homosexuals. Gidlow recalled that some of her white friends "lived in a loft above a Chinese laundry on Jackson Street," where they composed music and experimented with instruments and sounds. Musicians such as Lou Harrison and John Cage used the Chinatown setting as inspiration, "combining brake drums and buffalo bells with a dozen other exotic instruments from Orient and Occident to produce sounds never heard in Western composition."[36] As in North Beach, the milieu of cultural experimentation in Chinatown encouraged transgressive sexual exploration as well. Gidlow and Tommy ate in inexpensive Chinatown restaurants and met their first San Francisco acquaintances who identified as lesbian and gay while walking through the community during a New Years parade. The overlapping artistic and sexual subcultures included Chinese Americans other than Margaret Chung. One Chinatown resident, who grew up during the 1930s and 1940s, recalled that "there were many white homosexuals in North Beach 'who had a thing for Asian and Black boys.'"[37]

ORIENTALIST DESIRE

The cross-group interactions that occurred in Chinatown and North Beach do not mean there was social equality; rather, the dynamics reveal asymmetrical forms of power. Even though Chung had the financial resources and professional status to move outside of Chinatown, she still contended with mainstream perceptions of her Chinese ancestry. Western fantasies about the Orient fueled white interest in Asian people, explaining why Gidlow became attracted to Chung and also why many white homosexuals "had a thing" for Asian boys. However, these projections tended to define Chung as an exotic outsider, regardless of her efforts to craft her own identity.

Although Chung embraced Western science and culture, she evoked the mysteriousness of the Orient for Gidlow. In the writer's poem, "For a Gifted Lady, Often Masked," Gidlow claimed to see past the professional persona of Chung: "Matter-of-fact manner,/Brusque speech,/Expert hands—These are not *you*."[38] Instead, Gidlow posited the doctor's real identity as evocative of an ancient and foreign civilization: "Your soul is a cool tuberose/Drowsy with perfume,/Languorous, dreaming. . . . Its fragrance wafts me/To far-off times and lands." Gidlow's description of Chung reveals the pervasiveness of Orientalism. Like most Westerners, the poet perceived the Orient as the "contrasting image" of the West. Instead of representing science and modernity, Chung inspired Gidlow's fantasies about Asia as "a place of romance, exotic beings, [and] haunting memories."[39] Gidlow even imagined Chung in the stereotypical role of a wise and inscrutable sage, remarking that "there is no one to whom I can talk. . . . I want someone neutral, and someone with a special sort of maturity and wisdom. M seems to me the one person. . . . More, far more than I want to possess M physically, I want to understand her; but she eludes me continually."[40]

As in her professional career, Chung understood white fantasies about her Chinese identity. In some ways, she resisted Gidlow's perceptions of her. Chung described herself to Gidlow as a Westerner, explaining that "I am Chinese, yes, but I am a new soul."[41] In contrast, she described Gidlow as an "old soul," therefore having a greater affinity with the "Orient." In this exchange, Chung suggests that Gidlow's fascination with her stemmed primarily from the writer's interest in Orientalist difference and less from the physician's actual identity. However, Chung's use of dichotomous categories of "new" and "old" also reinforced the juxtaposition of between the Occident and the Orient. As Gidlow points out to Chung, if the physician sought to deny cultural differences between the West and the East, why "speak of 'old souls', 'new souls'?"[42] Even as Chung distanced herself from Gidlow, she continued to ponder the dilemma of how to both benefit from and challenge Orientalist thinking.

PROSPECTS OF MARRIAGE

Chung's decision to marry did not relieve her anxieties about how to achieve both social acceptance and personal freedom. While she was reluctant to pursue an explicitly lesbian relationship with a white woman, she also felt ambivalent about the prospect of marriage.

Although a substantial number of educated, professional women during this time chose to remain single, Chinese American women "still considered marriage and motherhood as their destiny."[43] The gender imbalance in their community, the exclusion of immigrants, and the ban on interracial marriage compelled them to marry other Chinese. Despite these social pressures, Chung initially contemplated an interracial marriage and then rejected marriage altogether.

Although Chung did not discuss her engagement, others testified that she had intended to marry at one point in her life. Gidlow remarked on the vast amount of wealth and the scarcity of hair of Chung's fiancé, but she made no comment about his race. From other sources, it appears that Chung's intended marriage partner was white. Her sister-in-law, Lucile Chung, remembered that Margaret was engaged to an "American" doctor.[44] Lucile used the term "American" to refer to a "white" individual, a common linguistic practice that conflated race and nationality. Pardee Lowe believed that Margaret Chung actually married an "American" and included a note about her and her siblings, two of whom eventually married white partners, in his file on interracial marriage.[45] Chung did not shy away from interracial relationships, an interest manifested in her professional and homoerotic relationships. Although California had an anti-miscegenation law, determined couples could travel to other states or out of the country for the marriage ceremony. Occasionally, local officials also overlooked state laws.[46]

Chung's Chinese American friends and family explained her choice in marriage partner as a combination of class, age, and legal considerations. Few eligible candidates existed within the Chinatown community because of the scarcity of educated professionals. Chung's age also eliminated potential marriage partners. She was at least a decade older than most of the second-generation Chinese Americans, who came of age in the 1920s and 1930s. Immigrant men tended to be working-class "bachelors," many of whom had wives in China, or merchants with families. Furthermore, due to the 1922 Cable Act, American-born women who married immigrants ineligible for citizenship would lose their U.S. citizenship.[47]

Instead of choosing a marriage partner who would detract from her social status, Chung selected a white and wealthy man to bolster her position. She apparently viewed marriage as a means to improve or at least secure class standing, a view not uncommon in both Chinese and middle-class American society. Lucile Lai, who married Andrew Chung in 1928, recalled that Margaret strongly opposed their marriage. Although Andrew, like his father, could be considered working-class, Margaret

wanted him to marry someone who was more educated and acculturated. Lai actually came from a fairly well-off family and had attended
school in China. However, she lacked an American college education
and spoke mainly Chinese. Consequently, Margaret believed Lucile
would "never amount to anything."[48] Similar status considerations may
have influenced Margaret's eventual decision not to marry. According
to Lucile, Chung requested her fiancé's assistance to fund her sisters'
education and eventually declined to marry him because he refused to
do so. She might have interpreted his refusal as a portent of his behavior as her husband.

Chung ultimately preferred to remain single rather than entangle herself with a marriage partner who did not meet her expectations. Although
few Chinese American women chose this path, some professional women
served as role models for Chung. She undoubtedly heard stories from her
mother of the dedicated missionaries who rescued Chinese women from
servitude. Although the mission home reformers promoted companionate
marriage for their charges, many of the women, including Chung's surrogate grandmother, Margaret Culbertson, chose to remain single to devote
their lives to missionary careers.[49] In addition, Chung's medical colleagues and mentors, including her surgical mother, Bertha Van Hoosen,
were members of the first generation of female physicians, a significant
percentage of whom never married or had children.[50]

Even in San Francisco Chinatown, Chung was not completely alone
in her decision to reject marriage. Significantly, rumors of lesbianism
surrounded the single Chinese American professional women: a lawyer,
a banker, a teacher, and a physician.[51] In a note about homosexuality in
Chinatown, Pardee Lowe commented that these acts were "noticeable
only in a few isolated cases. Or attributable in a few isolated cases, particularly among the native born Chinese girl who is employed in the
professions and has never found a suitable suitor to marry because to do
so meant either a loss of prestige or income."[52] The speculations reflected
an array of communal anxieties regarding women who transgressed
their assigned roles. Women who achieved greater professional success
than their male counterparts were perceived as lacking in suitable marriage partners and therefore vulnerable to lesbianism. Left unstated was
the possibility that the women's economic independence allowed them
to pursue romantic and even sexual fulfillment outside of marriage and
heterosexuality. The charges of lesbianism may not reflect the actual
practices, desires, or self-perceptions of these women. Chung herself
criticized the rumors as a "malicious effort to affect her practice."[53]

However, her professional status certainly facilitated her ability to develop relationships with individuals interested in transcending gender, sexual, and cultural norms.

Chung's decisions regarding her personal life reflected both romantic interest in other women and a desire for respectability. Given Gidlow's relationship with Tommy and her Orientalist proclivities, she was perhaps not an ideal companion for Chung. Nevertheless, Chung's expressions of love for the writer and then her subsequent retreat from Gidlow suggest that Chung had difficulty reconciling a lesbian identity with her professional and social goals.[54] Her simultaneous rejection of marriage, however, also indicates her desire to seek an alternative to heterosexuality.

Although Chung developed her community of friends mainly with white Americans, she was not the only Chinese American living an unconventional private life.[55] In addition to the Asian men who were pursued by North Beach homosexuals, "there were also many spinsters and unmarried sisters in the [Chinatown] families."[56] At least one wife and mother, and probably many more, formed romantic and sexual relationships with other women. In a poem entitled "chinatown talking story," writer Kitty Tsui described her grandmother, a Chinese opera singer who first traveled to the United States in 1922:

> my grandfather had four wives
> and pursued many women
> during his life.
> the chinese press loved
> to write of his affairs.
>
> my grandmother,
> a woman with three daughters,
> left her husband
> to survive on her own.
> she lived with another actress,
> a companion and a friend.[57]

Even as Chung chose spinsterhood, she would continue to search for fulfilling emotional and romantic relationships through alternative forms of family.

PART THREE

Orientalized Motherhood

CHAPTER 8

Becoming Mom Chung

Then, one fine day, into my office came the first of my Beloved
Sons, and suddenly a new and wonderful life was opened to me.

Margaret Chung, *"Autobiography"*

For Margaret Chung, 1931 was a momentous year. Then in her early
forties, she regarded her life accomplishments with mixed feelings. After
nearly a decade in San Francisco, she still had not attained a sense of fulfillment. Chung claims that she "had been too busy in a struggle for a
mere existence to laugh or to have fun."[1] She actually engaged in a relatively active social life. However, her comment reflects a lack of satisfaction, perhaps regarding her status in Chinatown and her personal
life. Despite her goal of serving her ancestral people, Chung increasingly
focused her professional and personal attention on non-Chinese
Americans. In addition, her attraction to and discomfort with both lesbianism and marriage also revealed some confusion about her private
desires. The creation of a fresh identity offered a solution to her quan-
daries and endowed her existence with a renewed sense of purpose.

Chung's life changed as the indirect result of global geopolitical
conflicts. In 1931, Japan invaded Manchuria and then followed with a
strike on Shanghai. The advancing forces initially met with little
resistance. At the time, Chiang Kai-shek, head of the Chinese Nationalist
government, insisted on targeting Mao Zedong and his Communist
supporters. However, a Japanese full-scale offensive in 1937 eventually
forced a temporary halt to the civil war. The Nationalists and the
Communists united to fight the Sino-Japanese War (1937–1945). The
assault on China invigorated a patriotic movement among Chinese in
the United States as they mobilized to support their ancestral nation.

Japanese aggression also altered the American public's perceptions of the Chinese.[2] Previously deemed alien and diseased, Chinese people increasingly became viewed as sympathetic and even heroic. The growing support for China escalated after the attack on Pearl Harbor on 7 December 1941 and the U.S. entry into World War II. The domestic repercussions of these international conflicts catapulted Chung into the public limelight. She met the need for a symbol of U.S.-China unity and in the process gained recognition from both mainstream Americans and her own ethnic community.

AN "OLD MAID" AND HER "FAIR-HAIRED BASTARDS"

Following Japan's initial attack in 1931, Steven G. Bancroft, an ensign in the U.S. Navy Reserves, approached Chung for assistance to gain a commission in the Chinese military. Reflecting the growing pro-China and anti-Japan sentiments, he wanted to "bomb Tokyo out into the middle of the Pacific."[3] It is not clear why Bancroft thought Chung would be able to help him. Mainstream Americans generally had little contact with Chinese in the United States. Perhaps Chung's professional success among white patients brought her to his attention. In any case, she had no influence with the Chinese military.

Unable to fulfill his request, yet impressed by his political fervor, Chung invited Bancroft and his six housemates to have dinner with her. They enjoyed each other's company so much that they became dedicated friends. Bancroft and his friends, all of them unemployed pilots, recent graduates from the University of California, Berkeley, and former college football players, ate dinner with Chung "almost every night for many happy months." They also went camping and hunting together. Her generosity and support became the subject of one after-dinner discussion; Chung recalled: "Red [Frank Fulgham Gill] spoke up and said, 'Gee, you are as understanding as a mother, and we are going to adopt you; but, hell, you are an old maid, and you haven't got a father for us.' Feeling facetious that night, I cracked back at them, 'Well, that makes you a lot of fair-haired bastards, doesn't it?' And quick as a flash, they pounced on that idea and said, 'Swell! We'll call ourselves your fair-haired bastards from now on, and we'll spread your fame into every corner of the world!'"[4]

Chung's surrogate family grew steadily as she and her original seven sons recruited other members through their personal contacts and as their unusual kinship network garnered public attention. The number of her children had reached over five hundred by the start of the Sino-Japanese War in 1937. Throughout the 1930s, but especially after 1937, articles about Mom Chung and her adopted children appeared regularly in local and state media. After the attack on Pearl Harbor, Chung increasingly gained national and even international recognition. She was featured in newspapers throughout the country and in publications with widespread circulations, such as *National Geographic, Life,* and *Christian Science Monitor.* As a result of this publicity, Chung's family had swelled to approximately fifteen hundred members by the end of World War II.

Chung assigned her "children" to one of three "branches," giving each a number to identify the order of his or her entry. The oldest, largest, and most publicized group consisted of pilots who called themselves the "Fair-Haired Bastards." In order to qualify for adoption, these nine hundred members, almost all of them men, had to demonstrate a willingness to dedicate themselves to, and possibly sacrifice their lives for, a higher purpose.[5] In Chung's words, each of her sons was "a good guy, who can fly, who's not afraid to die, a courageous man who is loyal, tolerant, a 'square' man who contributes to the progress and glory of aviation, who makes the world a better place because he lives."[6] Chung characterized the "Fair-Haired Bastards" as the "Phi Beta Kappa of Aviation" for attracting the "Who's Who" among pilots.[7]

Recognizing the growing support for China among larger sectors of the American public, even prior to the U.S. entry into the war, Chung expanded her kinship network. Those who were "good bastard material" but did not fly became known as "Kiwis," named after the flightless bird. Chung's approximately three hundred Kiwis included entertainers, politicians, and other military personnel. Because men dominated aviation, the relatively small numbers of "daughters" that Chung adopted tended to enter this branch of the family. Chung herself became Kiwi number 1, although she eventually learned to pilot a plane.

Chung established the final branch of her family in the spring of 1943. At the request of a naval lieutenant who had read about her adopted network, she created the "Golden Dolphins" specifically for submariners. The requirements for this group, which grew to almost the same size as the Kiwis, reflected U.S. engagement in the war at the time. Those admitted as Golden Dolphins had to have sunk "five enemy ships" or "at least 100,000 tons."[8] Chung founded this new division to recognize the unique qualities of submariners. While her pilot sons exhibited a sense of "confidence and self-assurance that sometimes may

almost become cockiness," submariners demonstrated a sense of inter-
dependence and "a very democratic spirit."[9]

Chung's surrogate family raises a number of questions. What motivated Chung and her sons to form fictive kinship relationships? Why
did Chung, a single professional woman of Chinese ancestry, want to
serve as a maternal figure to white men? Why did individuals in the
American military, entertainment world, and political circles seek membership in her family? And, why did Mom Chung and her adopted children capture popular attention during the 1930s and 1940s? What
propagandistic function did they serve during the Sino-Japanese War
and World War II?

The origins of the Fair-Haired Bastards, which Chung repeatedly
retold to other adopted children and to the press, provide insight into
their motivations for establishing the family. Like other friendships, the
relationship between Chung and her initial sons and subsequent children fulfilled their needs for companionship and support. As members
of her family expressed in letters and interviews, Chung's "sons"
became deeply devoted to one another. It may be that the marriages of
Chung's brothers and sisters in the 1920s and 1930s created a void in
her life that she sought to fill by forming an alternative family of her
own.[10] However, the particular configuration of her consciously constructed kinship network requires further exploration. For Chung,
becoming a mother to all-American sons and daughters allowed her to
fulfill a normative gender and cultural role. Motherhood not only
brought Chung recognition but also protected her from public censure,
even as she stretched the boundaries of socially acceptable behavior. For
her children, incorporation of Mom Chung into their family symbolically represented the expansion of the U.S. national family during the
international conflicts of the 1930s and eventually World War II. At the
same time, Chung's image in the popular media, the composition of her
kinship network, and the different responsibilities assigned to its members reveal that wartime inclusion simultaneously maintained certain
social barriers and hierarchies.

"MOM, SHE'S A GREAT GUY"

In forming a surrogate family that crossed racial boundaries, Chung
recreated—with variation—her mother's and her own adoptions. White
female Presbyterian reformers had adopted Chung's mother into their
missionary family. Chung's mentor, Bertha Van Hoosen, had adopted

surgical daughters of varying racial backgrounds and nationalities. With Chung's new family, she reprised but also inverted the roles of these religious and professional forms of maternalism. First, she reversed the racial hierarchy by assuming the more authoritative role of parent over her white children. Rather than being a nonwhite daughter, she became a nonwhite mother. Rather than being adopted, she did the adopting. In a second inversion, she formed her family primarily with men rather than exclusively with women. Instead of seeking out an all-female environment, Chung constructed an adopted family by nurturing young men, for the most part. In so doing, she created an alternative social possibility for herself, a woman who had gone against the grain by rejecting marriage and biological reproduction. Previously perceived as a traditional female nurturer, despite her male dress and professional style, she consciously adopted a socially expected and accepted role for women. Ironically, by becoming Mom Chung, she could engage more freely in masculine forms of behavior.

For Chung, her sons epitomized the ideal qualities of manliness. She described her first group of sons as "All-American football heroes" and "the most glorious specimens of real American manhood."[11] Chung's conception of manhood encompassed physical as well as personality attributes. Her original sons were "big, strong, [and] husky," averaging "well over 200 pounds each." They also exhibited a fun sense of recklessness and daring. To Chung, "they were as full of mischief as young colts." By becoming their mom, she could join in their fraternity-like camaraderie. Reminiscent of Chung's tomboy days and medical training in Southern California, she enjoyed traditionally male pastimes, such as sports, camping, and hunting, with her sons.

Chung's fascination with airplanes, like her enthusiasm for automobiles, reflected her desire to participate in modern manly pursuits. During the interwar years, aviation captured the popular imagination.[12] With the World War I flying aces and the 1927 trans-Atlantic solo flight of Charles Lindbergh, flying became associated with freedom, excitement, romance, and masculinity. Amelia Earhart, whom Chung claimed as one of her few bastard daughters, proved that modern women could match male accomplishments after her trip across the Atlantic in 1928.[13]

Like Chung, Earhart lived in Southern California during the late 1910s and early 1920s and described the region as "particularly active in air matters."[14] In fact, the first Chinese American woman to earn a pilot's license, Katherine Cheung, resided in Los Angeles.[15] The San

Francisco Bay Area became similarly "air-minded." The city airport, originally located at Crissey Field, was dedicated in 1919, and the first transcontinental airmail flight landed there the following year.[16] By the late 1920s, the region boasted at least six airports, which facilitated the development of military and commercial aviation.[17] In 1935, the *China Clipper* established regular airmail flight to Asia from the Bay Area. That same year, Earhart landed in Oakland following her record solo flight from Hawaii. The Bay Area served as the base for another of Earhart's widely publicized adventures, the 1937 attempt across the Pacific Ocean during which she disappeared.

Despite the iconic status of Amelia Earhart in the American imagination, flying, even more than driving, was an exclusive class and gender privilege.[18] To obtain flight instruction, let alone purchase a plane, required a heavy expenditure of capital. The military provided training and opportunities for men to fly planes. Commercial aviation also preferred male pilots. Female aviators needed wealth or sponsorships to support their interest.[19]

Chung, who took flight lessons and flew on trips, sought to participate in this male-dominated world of aviation. As a middle-aged woman who became increasingly heavy, she did not embody the image of the youthful, athletic aviatrix.[20] However, she could live vicariously through the exploits of her pilot sons. Members of her flying family recalled the pleasure of sitting at the bar in her home and exchanging stories, or as one son expressed it, enjoying "hanger flying."[21] Captain John F. McGinty, son number 149, reflected, "The best part about your bar, Mom, is the people that you meet there. It is strictly a place for good fellowship, something that must be kept alive in this world."[22] Chung's ability to facilitate and share this sense of masculine platonic companionship led her fictive sons to attest, "Mom, she's a great guy!"[23]

Wearing the protective mantle of motherhood, Chung could live her life without the censure that would otherwise have shadowed her: a single woman of Chinese ancestry in her early forties fraternizing regularly with white and usually much younger men. In fact, surrogate motherhood allowed Chung to avoid matrimony yet still enjoy male companionship. In contrast to marriage, in which a woman expresses love and commitment to one man, her voluntary maternal status allowed her to select as many sons as she desired to befriend. One reporter commented that the adoption ritual resembled a "wedding-like procedure."[24] Chung usually held the adoption ceremony on Sunday evenings after dinner. She opened these occasions with a prayer and then proceeded to give a speech about the history of the family before announcing the qualifications and accomplishments of the inductees for that occasion. She gave her sons silver rings, engraved with their assigned numbers, to symbolize the bond between them. The bestowing of rings, reminiscent of wedding vows, also connoted other forms of love and loyalty, such as fraternal allegiance or religious devotion, that complement, rival, and occasionally replace marriage. Chung established family ties, not through matrimony and biological motherhood, but through adoption. By becoming a surrogate mother, Chung evoked the emotional power of family to naturalize her communion with her sons yet also alleviate the need for conjugality. In fact, the acceptability and the humor in the phrase "Fair-Haired Bastards," which raised the specters of miscegenation and illegitimacy, stemmed from the impossibility of biological connection between Chung and her sons.

In the absence of a legitimate father figure, implied by the term "bastards," Chung assumed the role of both mother and father in relation to her "children." She performed the female tasks of cooking and "nursing" for her sons. At the same time, her professional success in relation to her unemployed sons also meant that she played the traditional masculine role of bread winner. Her recollection of her relationship to H. Joseph Chase, son number 3, who eventually became a Pan American pilot, demonstrates her dual gender roles:

> When Joe was out in Haiti he contracted malaria and black water fever. . . .
> He said, "Well, I'm going out to see Mom, she will fix me up." So he took
> the first plane out and I took care of him and nursed him back to health.
> Frequently, I would find him standing over my bed at three or four o'clock
> in the morning and hear him plaintively say, "Mommie, I'm hungry." So
> I would get up and heat some thick vegetable soup which all the boys liked,
> broil him a couple of filet mignons which I kept in readiness for him, fry
> him some mashed potato patties, fix him a couple of vegetables, or fry some
> rice with ham and green onions and eggs. Then we would sit up and talk
> until about seven in the morning. I would tuck him into bed again, and
> I would go off to the hospital and start work.[25]

While Chung praised the masculinity of her sons, she also infantilized them to highlight their need for her as both a surrogate mother and father.

Chung's original sons accepted her efforts to care for them partly because of their unemployed status. With the United States in the midst of the Great Depression, Bancroft and his housemates had difficulty finding work. Their reliance on her to provide dinner "almost every night for many happy months" revealed the impact of the widespread financial crisis on their lives. Her sons were in such desperate straits that their diet consisted of "nothing but eggs for breakfast, lunch and dinner," because "the egg man is the only guy who has given us any credit in the last six weeks."[26] The direness of their situation likely motivated her sons to seek employment in the Chinese military, where they could use their piloting skills to fight the Japanese and sustain themselves.

It is unclear how the financial crash affected Chung's medical practice. On average, the net income of physicians in California dropped "from approximately $6,700 in 1929 to $3,600 in 1933."[27] It is possible that Chung's economic niche protected her from the worst of the depression, since her social life and personal appearance became increasingly glamorous during this time period. Her clients from the entertainment world, who continued to patronize her despite her relocation to San Francisco, thrived during the 1930s as Americans flocked to movie theaters to gain some emotional relief from their economic distress. Those who suffered financially but still required medical attention no doubt found the lower cost of health care in Chinatown more affordable. Families concerned about extra mouths to feed likely requested Chung's assistance regarding birth control. Members of the police force, as government employees, had some protection from the vagaries of the economy and also the clout to advocate for medical care programs through their union. Though the national Social Security program declined to include health insurance, "local hospitals and social agencies began to charge welfare departments for services previously rendered free."[28] Even Chinatown residents gained increased access to health services during the depression as federal relief extended "free medical care at a local clinic."[29]

Even if Chung's income fell by half during the depression, she still occupied a more secure position than her unemployed sons. Chung's status as their mother made her generosity acceptable. She emphasized that "feeding them [her sons] was *not* an act of charity. It was the most selfish thing I've ever done because it was more fun than I had ever known in all my life."[30] Furthermore, Chung's sons reciprocated her affection through their efforts to care for her physical and emotional well-being. She remembered:

> We all loved to eat, and when we didn't have anything to eat we would sit around and talk about fine foods. One evening I said that I wished I had some frog legs sautéd in butter, sprinkled with fine herbs, and cooked with white wine. A couple of days later, Steve walked into my office with a

package of the most beautiful frog legs I had ever seen. He was an Ensign in the United States Naval Reserve and was supposed to fly a certain number of hours each week to keep up his rating. So he had taken up a Hell-diver and gone up to Livermore where he had caught the frogs in one of the sloughs! . . . {He didn't have any money then, but he was anything but a moocher.} He was extremely thoughtful.[31]

Though unconventional in many respects, Chung's kinship network resembled Chinese American arrangements to some degree. Due to the imbalance in gender ratios, only a small minority of the Chinese in the United States historically lived in nuclear family units. Instead, the predominantly male immigrants formed households with extended members of their ancestral network. Some even claimed fictive kinship connections in order to facilitate entry into the country, obtain jobs, and foster companionship. During the depression, these connections became even more necessary. Even male heads of nuclear families participated in extended networks through the surname societies. In essence, Chung created her own family association. Her decision to adopt a male lineage actually followed Chinese cultural dictates that encouraged women to achieve honor by raising sons. Rather than biologically reproducing Chinese men, she mothered surrogate white ones who could fight on behalf of China.

NATURE VERSUS NURTURE

Chung's decision to adopt white children stemmed in part from her conflicted relationship with people of her own ethnicity and her greater affinity with mainstream Americans. Although the Sino-Japanese conflicts of the 1930s fostered solidarity among Chinese, Chung initially encountered difficulties finding a niche within the growing nationalist movements in China and Chinatown. Despite her marginal standing, white Americans insisted on perceiving her as a leader among Chinese in San Francisco, and by extension, a representative of her ancestral country. This misperception allowed Chung to search beyond her ethnic group, essentially to adopt outside of her bloodline, in order to advocate for China. By associating with "All-American" types, such as sports champions, flying aces, military heroes, political leaders, and entertainers who portrayed these roles in popular culture, she gained a platform among the mainstream public.

Adoption served as both mechanism and metaphor for Chung's efforts to build an interracial coalition. The adopted nature of her

family deemphasized the significance of blood or racial lineage in deter-
mining national allegiance. Her white children demonstrated that non-
Chinese could dedicate themselves to the welfare of China. Chung's
status as their mother proved that people of Chinese ancestry could be
all-American as well. However, her efforts do not signify the primacy of
environmental factors, such as culture and politics, over genetics. The
political symbolism of her family was based on the racial identities of its
members. Chung chose almost all white individuals, particularly men,
because they unambiguously represented the central constituents of the
American polity. Both her children and the media focused on Chung's
Chinese ancestry in order to portray her as symbol of China. Just as
Chung sought entry into male spheres by assuming a traditionally
female role, so she promoted interracial and international unity by
affirming the association between race and nationality.

Throughout the late nineteenth and the first half of the twentieth centuries, overseas Chinese closely followed the political turmoil in
China.[32] Their interest partly stemmed from domestic considerations.
White Americans historically perceived Asian immigrants as members
of their native homelands and not their "adopted" country. Mainstream
Americans even viewed the U.S.-born offspring of Asian descent as
having stronger blood ties to their ancestral land than to the nation in
which they lived. Perceived as aliens, Chinese in the United States recognized that their status depended on the international position of
China: a strong, stable China could command respect and negotiate for
better treatment for its people abroad.

The Sino-Japanese conflicts and the Great Depression fueled these
nationalist sentiments, even among those born in the United States. The
second generation came of age in the midst of an economic recession,
which further constricted their opportunities for employment. At the
same time, they learned about the plight of China and the country's
need for educational, technical, and military expertise. Consequently,
an estimated 20 percent of the American-born Chinese went to China in
the 1930s to find work and establish families.[33]

Chung wanted to be among this group. As military conflict broke out
in Asia, she offered her services to China. Attempting to fulfill her original desire to serve as a medical missionary for her ancestral country, she
applied at least twice to the National Government of the Republic of
China, once in 1933 and again in 1937. Both times, Chinese authorities
discouraged her from leaving the United States. In 1933, Dr. J.H. Liu,
chief of the Chinese National Health Administration, wrote to the

Chinese Consulate General in San Francisco to dissuade her from coming to China: "While the spirit of Miss Margaret Chung is commendable I do not advise her to leave a lucrative practice when the need in North China is really not urgent. It is in any case impossible for her to receive a salary. So unless she can afford to come as a real volunteer I should advise against her coming."[34] When Chung applied again in 1937, the Chinese government could not reasonably use the explanation that the situation in China was not "really urgent." Instead, Chung's American citizenship was hinted as a possible obstacle. In a newspaper article discussing Chung's offer of medical service in war-torn China, the writer suggested that "the Chinese government is anxious not to involve Americans in the present conflict."[35] Just as Chung's missionary application was rejected because she was an American of Chinese ancestry, so the Chinese government used her U.S. citizenship to discourage her involvement.

This explanation, however, does not square with China's attempts to gain official and unofficial assistance from the United States and their acceptance of other Americans of Chinese descent. The government's reluctance toward Chung likely stemmed from gender bias. As early as the 1910s, the recently created Republic of China, contending with external and internal threats to its sovereignty, became interested in training and recruiting Chinese Americans with aviation skills. In 1917, the Chinese Nationalist Party popularized the slogan "National Salvation through Aviation" and established flying schools in the United States.[36] Japan's attack on China in the 1930s further fueled these efforts. Chinese throughout the United States formed flying clubs with two such organizations in San Francisco alone. These institutions and groups eventually trained between 150 and 200 people who went on to serve in the Chinese Air Force. Women participated in these efforts as well. In addition to Katherine Cheung and Margaret Chung, other Chinese women in the United States learned to fly. At least two women volunteered their services to China. However, the Chinese Air Force refused the female aviators, accepting instead the eleven male pilots who accompanied them.[37] Although the government official espoused the need for "new women" for a modern China, resistance to female participation in traditionally male realms persisted. Discouraged from serving in China, Chung chose to focus her energies on supporting the war effort from within the United States.

As a middle-aged single woman with a questionable sexual reputation, however, Chung was not positioned favorably to participate in

Chinatown's community efforts. Chinese American women played significant roles in war relief efforts. They promoted a boycott of Japanese products in the United States, raised funds for humanitarian aid in China, and disseminated information about the Sino-Japanese war.[38]

In contrast to most Chinese American women who became active within San Francisco Chinatown, Chung lacked familial connections to serve as social and political resources. Seven women's China relief organizations existed in the community during the international conflicts of the 1930s and 1940s. Each group differed in terms of the membership's "nativity, class, age, and cultural and political orientation."[39] In addition to these factors, a woman's family connections also influenced her decision to join a particular organization. For example, the New Life Association, officially affiliated with the first lady of China, Madame Chiang Kai-shek, tended to attract immigrant women who were "married to businessmen, ministers, or community leaders."[40] Similarly, the Fidelis Coteri attracted elite "matrons . . . who met regularly at expensive restaurants 'for the sake of friendship and to promote good family life.'"[41] Chung did not fit in easily with the wives and biological mothers of middle-class and elite Chinatown families.

As an American-born, single woman, Chung more likely would have joined the Chinese YWCA or the Square and Circle Club, a community service organization of business and professional women. However, her age may have a represented barrier to her involvement. By the 1930s, she was in her forties, while most of the second generation tended to be in their twenties and thirties. The Square and Circle Club granted her an honorary membership, but she did not regularly participate in their activities.[42] Chung's reluctance may have stemmed from negative perceptions of her sexuality.

In contrast, her white children and the mainstream media embraced her. In exchange for her generosity and emotional support, Chung not only participated in masculine camaraderie but also gained access to white America. Her family of white men helped her to culturally "pass" as an American. The description of her sons as "Fair-Haired" highlighted their whiteness. Furthermore, the characterizations of her sons as "the most glorious specimens of real American manhood" and "all-American football heroes" emphasized their "Americanness," their identification with and participation in mainstream culture. Like other parents, Chung shared in the glory of her children's accomplishments; her sons' achievements reflected her commitment to American values.

Since she was not the biological parent, her contributions to her sons were not genetic (i.e., racial). Instead, as the surrogate mother, she influenced via "nurture," not nature. In essence, her role as a surrogate mother deemphasized her racial identity and highlighted her cultural identity as an American.[43]

As Chung's initial sons rebounded from the poverty of the Great Depression and as her family increasingly attracted well-known and successful members, her surrogate kinship ties distanced her from negative images of Chinese Americans. A *New York Post* account of Chung demonstrates how her sons' social status supported her claims to cultural acceptance: "Last night she was interrupted to be told a Mr. Lee was calling. Some wit mentioned that it was a member of the famous laundry family. 'No,' said Dr. Chung. 'I know who it is—Son No. 348, Robert Lee, Vice-President of the John Manville Corp.'"[44] By emphasizing her close connection with a white male corporation vice-president, Chung disassociated herself from the servile status of Chinese people.

Chung not only gained social acceptance through affiliation with white men. She also adopted masculine behavior to achieve respect among mainstream Americans. In an interview to researcher Pardee Lowe, Chung explained: "Before they get a chance to step on me, I sock them in the jaw. If they try to put something over on me, I hit them then twice as much. I use to be ladylike and deferential but I found it didn't pay. Everywhere I was stepped on. Now I treat them rough, they lapped it up. Since then I have changed. They regard me with respect."[45] It is not clear whether Chung actually engaged in the physical behavior that she described, or whether she used this descriptive language figuratively to characterize what she regarded as being less "ladylike" and more assertive. However, she perceived that her engagement in masculine combativeness generated positive results among people who had previously "stepped" on her. Lowe's commentary to Chung's interview revealed that he regarded her as representative of a group of Chinese Americans who "aspire towards American friendships," especially among those with "prestige & wealth." "On the one hand they boast of their altruistic American friends and on the other they are bitter in their denunciations of the social [in]equality visited upon them."[46]

Chung took many opportunities to stress her Americanness, even choosing to distance herself from the label of "Chinese American." One newspaper reporter recalled that "no one refers to Dr. Chung as Chinese, although that is her ancestry. She was born in San Francisco [*sic*] and got perfectly furious once because she was called 'a great Chinese-American.'"[47] Those who knew Chung agreed with writer Gertrude Atherton's characterization of her: "The fluid in her body may be Chinese but her brain cells are American."[48]

Chung's Chinese ancestry, however, was not eclipsed but repeatedly invoked to promote internationalism among Americans. Although friends emphasized her "Americanness," they also consistently noted her Chineseness, a heritage that became a political asset during the Sino-Japanese War and World War II. Newspapers also frequently referred to Chung as a voice for China and Chinatown. One article in the mainstream press clearly exaggerated her status by suggesting that "the countless residents of the Golden Gate's Chinatown . . . worship[ped] her."[49] Chung embraced this role as a figurehead for her ancestral people. Earlier in her life, at USC, she had gained experience as a public speaker on topics relating to her ancestral country. She utilized these skills again during the 1930s and 1940s, speaking to women's organizations, university audiences, and on radio broadcasts such as "What China Is Fighting For" and "China's View of the Present." Although she never visited China, she adopted the role of national spokesperson for white American audiences.

Ironically, her success among "mainstream" Americans bolstered her standing in San Francisco Chinatown. Given her conflicted relationship with her ethnic community, she rarely participated in neighborhood functions. Her status as a marginal social figure can be detected in the coverage of the *Chinese Digest,* a Chinatown-based English language newspaper published by and primarily for second-generation Chinese Americans. From 1936 to 1939, the publication highlighted the political and cultural activities of Chinese in San Francisco, the United States, and the world. In contrast to respected community leaders, Chung appeared infrequently in the newspaper's social columns, which featured fashion shows, sporting events, dances, and banquets. When she did appear in the *Digest,* she was usually accompanied by a high-status white friend. In 1936, Jim Musick, a well-known pilot, served as her escort to a dance. The *Chinese Digest* reported that "Dr. Margaret Chung looked charming, and guess who was also there, and we believe, at Dr. Chung's invitation? Good 'old' Jim Musick, skipper of the good ship "China Clipper" on her maiden voyage to Manila."[50] The doctor's affiliation with a white celebrity known for his involvement in promoting trans-Pacific transportation helped to legitimate her social position within San Francisco Chinatown.

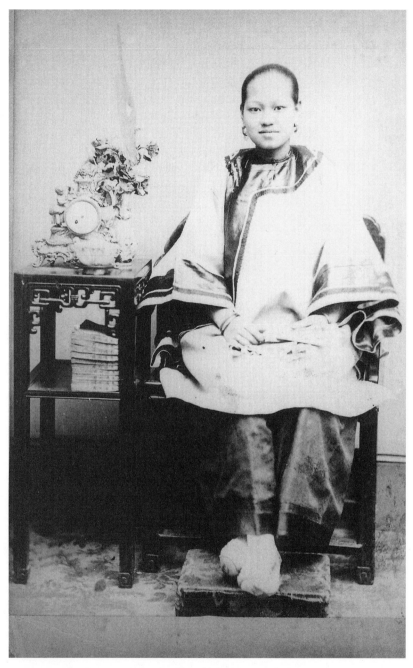

Figure 1. Ah Yane, Margaret's mother. Photograph by William Shew, San Francisco, California. California Historical Society, FN-31714.

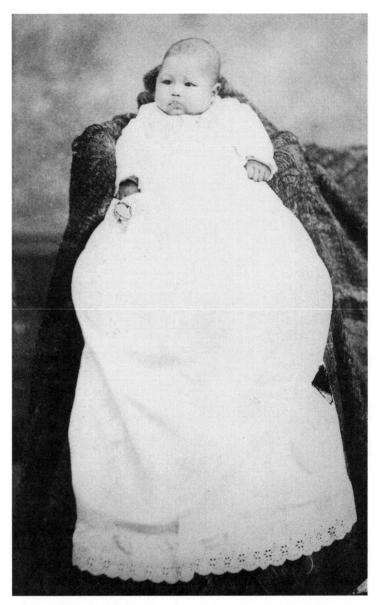

Figure 2. Baby Margaret, 1890. Photograph by Cook's, Santa Barbara. California Historical Society, FN-31715.

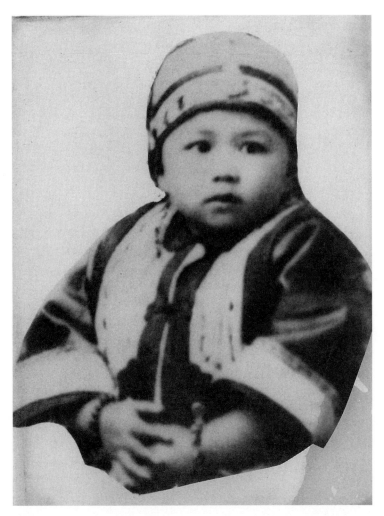

Figure 3. Baby Margaret in Chinese costume. Chinese American Museum Collection at El Pueblo de Los Angeles Historical Monument, Dorothy Siu Collection.

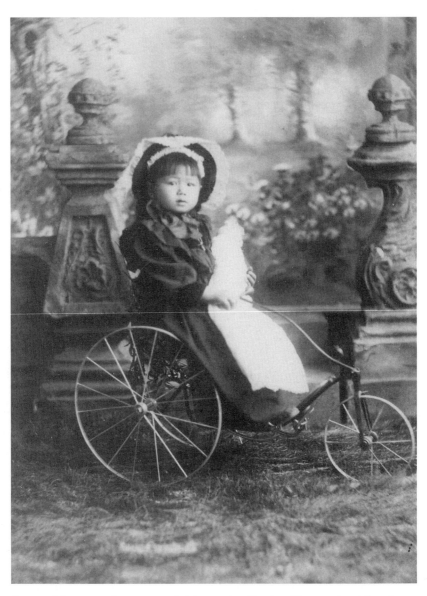

Figure 4. Margaret at three years and eight months old, 1893. Photographer: Edwards, Santa Barbara, California. Chinese American Museum Collection at El Pueblo de Los Angeles Historical Monument, Dorothy Siu Collection.

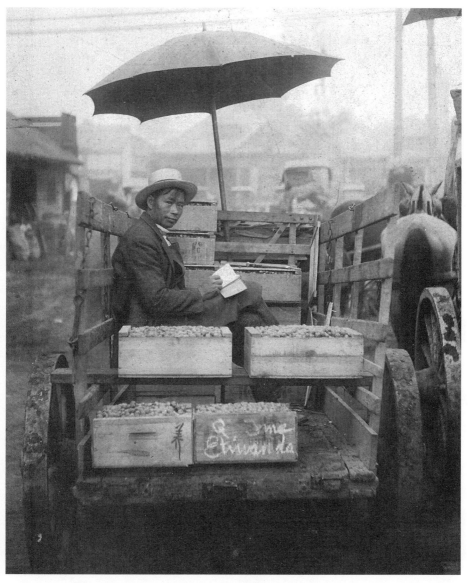

Figure 5. Chung Wong, Margaret's father. Photograph by Western Foto Co., Los Angeles. Siu Family Collection.

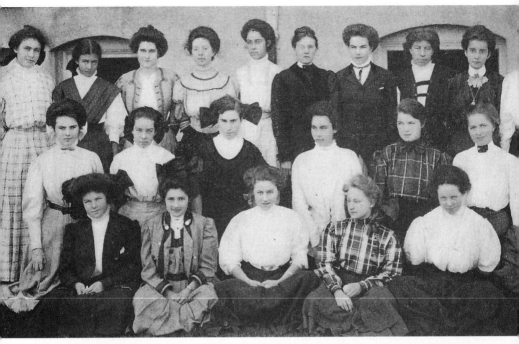

Figure 6. The University of Southern California's Willard Literary Society (*El Rodeo*, 1910). Margaret Chung in back row, far right. Courtesy of University of Southern California, on behalf of the USC University Archives.

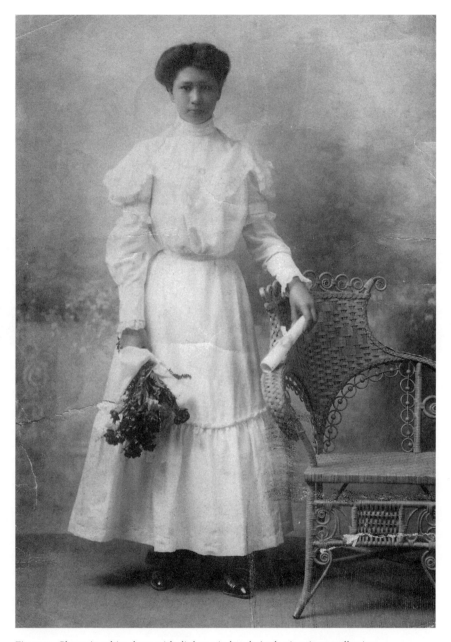

Figure 7. Chung in white dress with diploma in hand. Author's private collection.

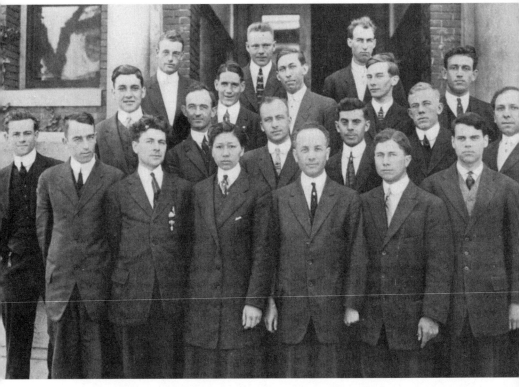

Figure 8. The Sophomore Class of the USC College of Physicians and Surgeons (*El Rodeo*, 1915). Margaret Chung in front row center. Courtesy of University of Southern California, on behalf of the USC University Archives.

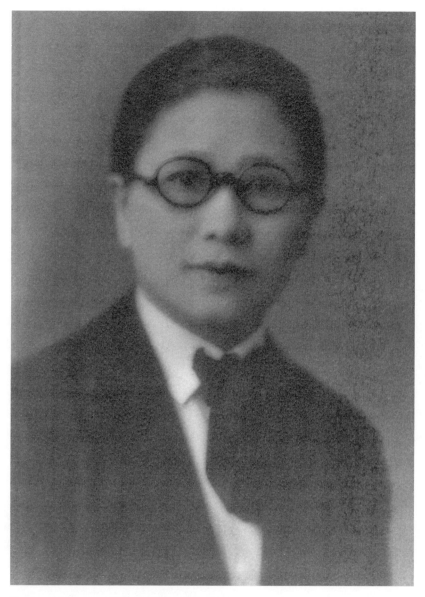

Figure 9. Margaret as "Mike." Siu family collection.

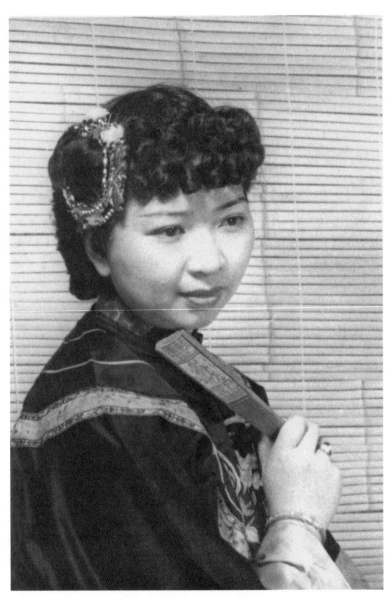

Figure 10. Dorothy Siu in Chinese costume, January 1941. Siu Family Collection.

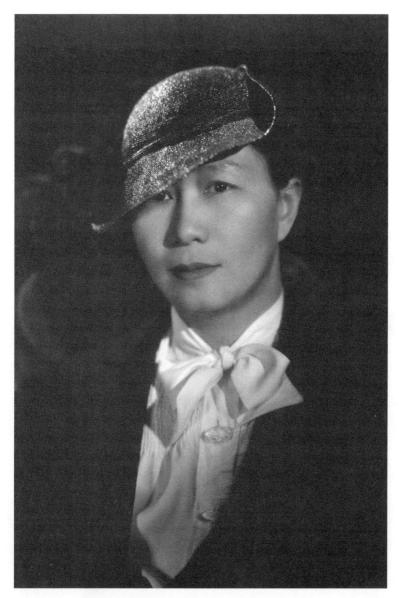

Figure 11. Chung, smartly dressed. Author's private collection.

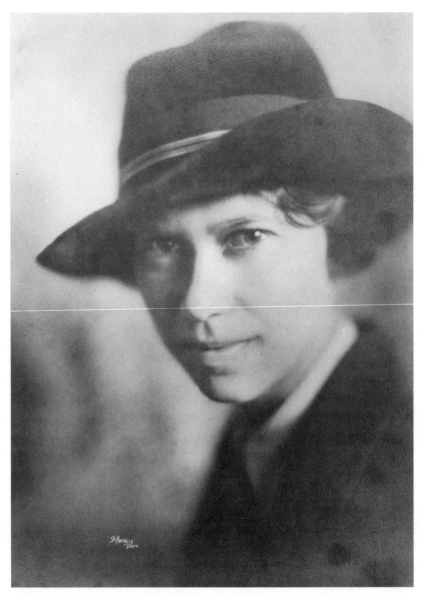

Figure 12. Elsa Gidlow, age twenty-seven. Courtesy Gay, Lesbian, Bisexual, Transgender Historical Society, Elsa Gidlow Collection.

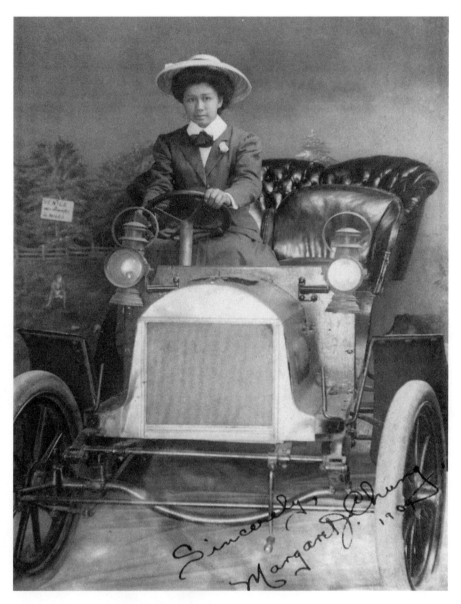

Figure 13. Chung in the driver's seat, 1909. Original caption reads: "Want a Ride?"
Credit: Security Pacific Collection, Shades of L.A. Archives, Los Angeles Public Library.

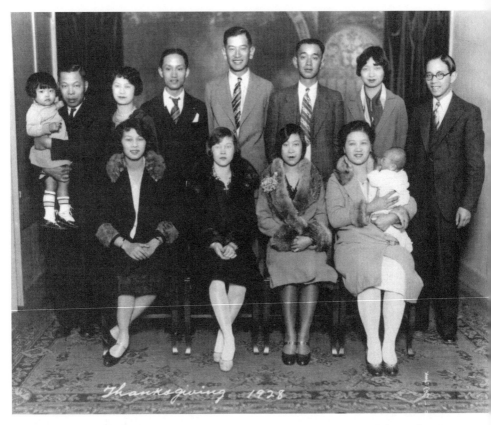

Figure 14. The Chung siblings and their families, Thanksgiving 1928. Front row (left to right): Anna, Margie (Virgil's wife), Lucile (Andrew's wife), Flo, and Rodney. Back Row: Shirley, Bill Yip (Anna's husband), Vee, Ernie Tsang (Vee's husband), Andrew, Virg, Dorothy, and Henry Low (Flo's husband). Margaret not pictured. Siu Family Collection.

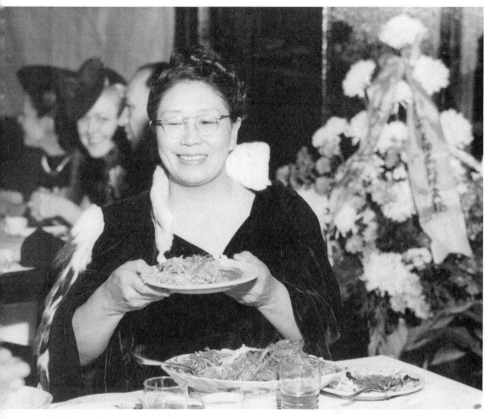

Figure 15. A meal out with Mom Chung. Author's private collection.

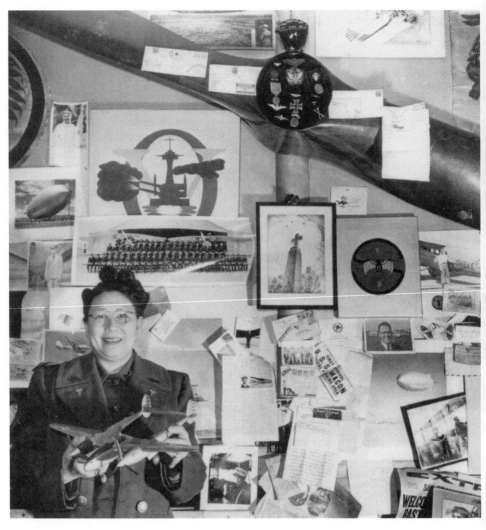

Figure 16. Mom Chung's War Memorabilia Room. Source: Doheny Memorial Library, University of Southern California, Regional Historical Collection. Credit: AP/World Wide Photos.

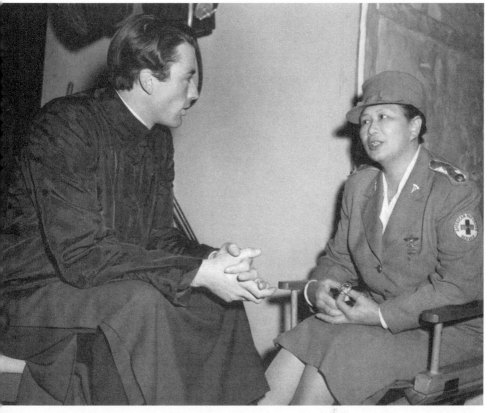

Figure 17. Chung with Gregory Peck on the set of *The Keys of the Kingdom* (1944). Siu Family Collection.

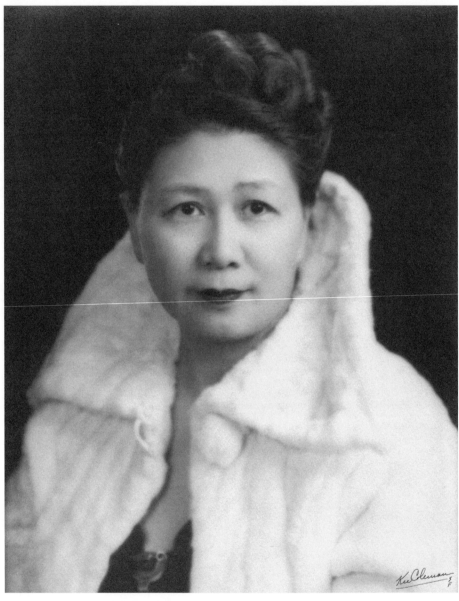

Figure 18. "Mom" Chung in ermine; this was her favorite photograph. Author's private collection.

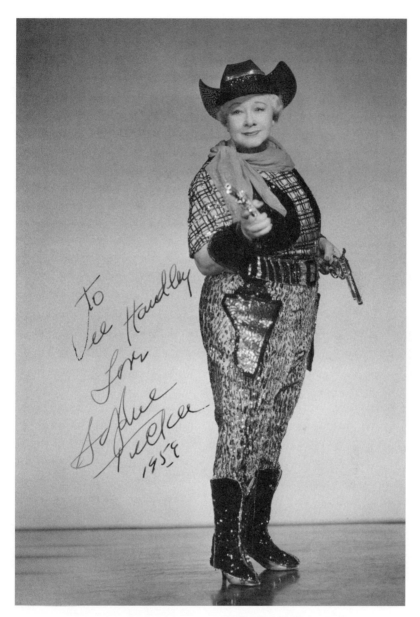

Figure 19. Sophie Tucker performing "Pistol Packin' Mama." Photographer: Maurice Seymour. Courtesy of Ronald Seymour. Author's private collection.

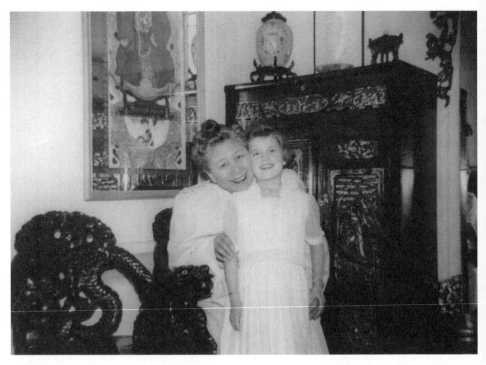

Figure 20. Mom Chung with Kiwi Mickey Hamilton, September 1949. Taken at Chung's home during a party for the cast of *Kiss Me Kate*. Photographer: Lynn Bingham. Private collection of Betsy Bingham Davis.

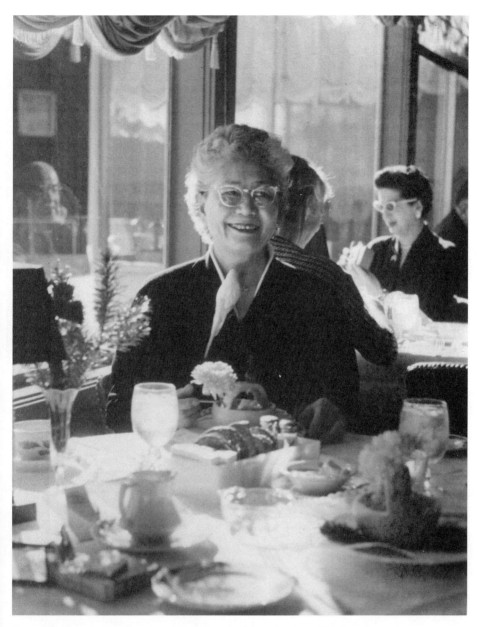

Figure 21. Chung with pet parakeet, Sweetheart. Private collection of Rodney Low.

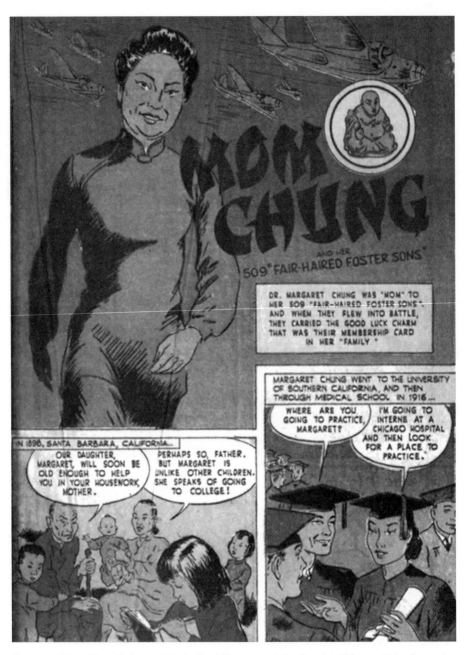

Figure 22. Mom Chung is featured in the *Real Heroes* comic book series (February/March 1943).

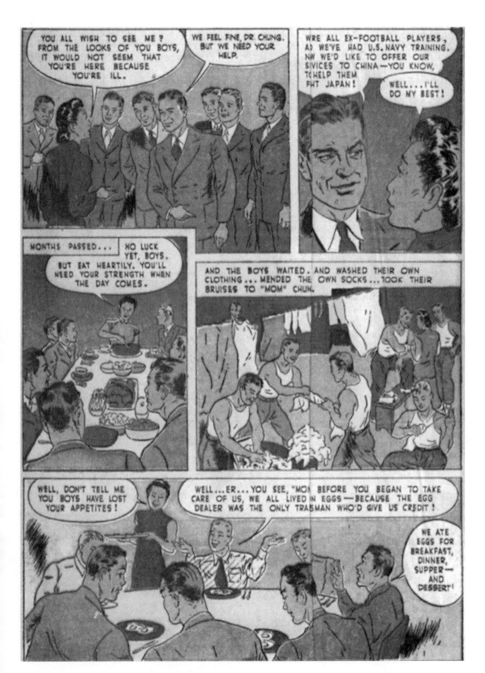

Figure 23. The *Real Heroes* story portrays a young and slender Mom Chung with her "fair-haired foster sons."

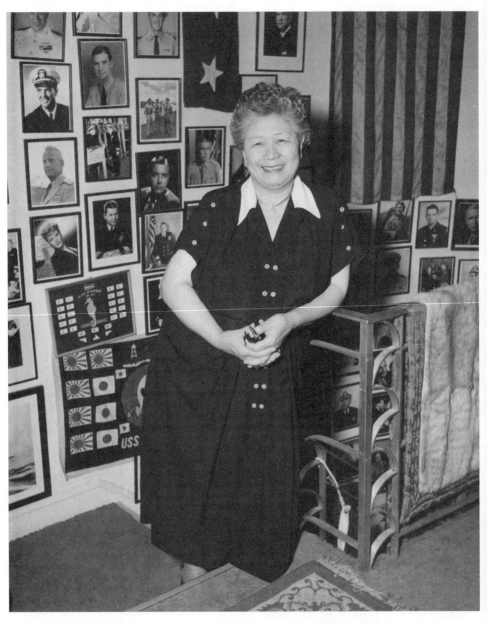

Figure 24. Mom Chung at home, 29 July 1952. Photographer: S/Sgt. Higgins, 8th Army Central Photo Lab. U.S. Army photograph.

Chung's relationships with white Americans also became a political and commercial asset for the Chinese American community. During the 1930s, the community engaged in a dual effort to "save" their ancestral homeland from external aggression and their own neighborhood from the economic downturn of the Great Depression. "Selling China" as a nation in need of humanitarian and military aid from the United States coincided with an effort to sell Chinatown as a tourist experience. Both goals relied on generating mainstream interest in China and Chinese culture.

Chung used her contacts with influential white Americans to sponsor a series of events to promote these humanitarian and commercial campaigns. For example, she co-founded the Rice Bowl Parties, elaborate festivals held in over seven hundred cities during the late 1930s and late 1940s. San Francisco alone hosted three such celebrations, which featured parades, cultural performances, carnival concession stands, and fashion shows. Each Rice Bowl Party attracted hundreds of thousands of attendants, who not only contributed a combined total of $235,000 of aid to China but also spent freely in Chinatown restaurants, stores, and bars.[51]

Chung facilitated the partnership between the other two cofounders of the festival.[52] B.S. Fong represented the male merchant class that dominated the Chinatown establishment. In addition to his role as the president of the most important community organization, the Chinese Six Companies, Fong also served as the chairman for the Chinese War Relief Association, an organization that coordinated fund-raising efforts among three hundred communities throughout North and South America. Paul C. Smith, editor of the *San Francisco Chronicle,* could be considered Fong's counterpart among the broader American community. Responsible for the main newspaper in the San Francisco Bay Area, Smith helped mold public opinion about diverse social, cultural, and political issues. Smith was a close friend and neighbor of Chung's in North Beach. In addition, he also was one of her adopted sons. With her skills as a cultural broker between mainstream and Chinese San Francisco, Chung became, in the words of a Chinatown resident, one of "the big bosses . . . [who] knew all the Caucasians."[53]

While Chung became valuable to Chinese Americans because she facilitated access to the resources of mainstream America, she became an asset to the U.S. government because of her ability to represent China. Although she could not initially fulfill Steve Bancroft's request for a commission in the Chinese military, the publicity about her growing family of military aviators led American officials to contact her. According to Chung, Major James Marshall McHugh, an assistant naval attaché at the American Embassy in China, asked her to recruit two hundred pilots to assist the Chinese war effort prior to official U.S. involvement in the war in Asia. She recalled his words in her autobiography:

> We do not dare send out the regular men from the aircorps of the Army, Navy, and Marines, for Japan would use that immediately as an incident. If you are willing, you could do a great service to America and China by getting two hundred of your aviators and sending them out to the Orient a few at a time. The pay will be $650.00 a month gold, and the round trip passage. Here is the address of the people who will arrange for their transportation and their salaries. But of course, if the Japanese hear about this and try to make an incident of it, we will simply shrug our shoulders and say, "Well, what the hell! We know nothing about it. She's a Chinese woman with her own private army of aviators, and we know nothing about it. After all, you have been attacking the land of her forefathers for several years."[54]

McHugh's recruitment instructions reveal how Chung's identity as an American of Chinese ancestry could be used in contradictory ways. On the one hand, he recognized her dual national commitments by asking if she "could do a great service to America and China." On the other hand, he warned that if her involvement was exposed, then the U.S. government would deny her American status and emphasize her identity as a "Chinese woman" whose ancestral land was under attack by the Japanese. The government's willingness to negate Chinese American claims to America and to underscore their political allegiance to China was consistent with racial conceptions of Asians in the United States as perpetual aliens. The same logic eventually justified the internment of approximately 120,000 Japanese Americans during World War II. Regardless of citizenship, cultural identity, political beliefs, or personal actions, all individuals of Japanese ancestry were suspected of harboring loyalties to Japan. Ironically, the American government strategically manipulated these same perceptions of the inalienability of racial ties to ask for Chung's assistance to serve both the United States and China.

Chung's status as both a dual-nationalist and a perpetual alien reveals an additional reason for her passion for aviation. On the one hand, the act of flying allowed for the possibility of transcending geographical, and hence social and national, boundaries. Chung explained the appeal of flight in a passage regarding her pilot sons: "They fly so far into the heavens they are not 'earth-bound'. Flying in the clean stratosphere, daring in and out of fleecy clouds into the blue of the sky, they get a different perspective on life—they see and realize how pettiness and meanness have no place in their firmament."[55] The act of flying also served as a metaphor for her surrogate family. The ability to rise above everyday barriers and to perceive the society around in a different light—these were the goals of her fictive kinship network. On the other hand, while flight allowed the possibility of transcendence, air power also represented a means to wage warfare and protect geopolitical boundaries. Even the blue skies of heaven could be partitioned to mirror the "pettiness and meanness" of the realms underneath. In creating an ideal world, Chung and her family worked within certain constraints that reflected their beliefs as well as the larger society's values. Consequently, the tools with which they used to transport them into a higher sphere inevitably returned them to the ground.

Chung's surrogate maternal identity allowed for transformative possibilities within existing social constraints. She had lived on the margins for much of her life, and her new adopted kinship network endowed her liminality with personal and public significance. Her Chinese ancestry and perceived maternal qualities became assets for fostering an interracial and international family. The cultural authority that she gained through association with her sons reveals the reciprocal but unequal nature of the adoption process. As the adopting parent, Chung helped mold the identities and outlooks of her surrogate sons, and through them the values of the broader American society. At the same time, her sons, as the central members of American society, adopted Chung, granting her legitimacy and recognition by fulfilling their expectations of gender and racial roles. The contradictory nature of her surrogate family provided the basis for their popularization during World War II, when Mom Chung and her Fair-Haired Bastards captured both the promise and the anxieties associated with wartime transformation.

CHAPTER 9

A Model Family at War

Just before Hong Kong fell, two hurried tight-lipped
American flyers settled next to each other at a bar. They said
brusque "Hellos." Then one grinned at the tiny jade Buddha
tie-pie on the other.

"Got one, too," he said. He dug his forefinger inside his
collar, pulled out a gold chain and on it hung a jade brother
to the first Buddha.

"How's Mom?" they both exclaimed.

Sigrid Arne, *Boston Daily Globe,* 1942
(Reprinted with permission of the Associated Press)

I have just left you, but that is only physical. I guess I'm now
one of hundreds of boys who can never leave you. Your love
of America and desire to see our Nation strong through the
courage and sacrifice of the people have deeply impressed me.

I want to thank you from the bottom of my heart for the
perfectly swell way you treated me today. Meeting such fine
people, eating like a King, and mainly, being around where
you were in constant evidence every moment was a pleasure
I couldn't believe would ever be mine. . . .
I don't ever expect to repay you for what you have done.
But I want you to know I will be a strong, more diligent
fighting man for you. . . . If I get into the fighting in the
islands and I get a crack at the monkey boys I'll get them
for you and what you stand for.

"Son" Chuck to Margaret Chung, 6 February 1944

The nation's official entry into World War II fundamentally changed
people's lives. Nearly 16.5 million citizens and residents, more than
10 percent of the American population, left their homes and families to
serve in the armed forces. Three to four hundred thousand never

returned and seven hundred thousand more sustained injuries. The need for servicemen provided unique opportunities for those traditionally marginalized by American society. Nonwhite men, including Japanese Americans whose families remained in internment camps, tended to enlist in greater proportions, because military service offered benefits and recognition reserved for honored members of the American citizenry.[1] Women of all colors also demanded the right to protect their country. Approximately 350,000 would serve in the newly created female units of the armed forces. Many more, an estimated 6 million, joined the 12 million women already in the workforce to fight the war from the home front.

The scale of wartime changes created unprecedented opportunities to transform the racial and gender contours of American society. At the same time, there was resistance to required alterations to daily life and to social changes that threatened traditional roles.[2] Because a "total war" required the mobilization of privately owned resources and intrusion into personal lives, American participation in the Allied cause entailed an interpenetration of public and private interests.[3] Whether a woman chose to work and even how she fed her family no longer appeared as personal domestic decisions but rather as issues of pressing national concern. Soldiers fighting for the Allied cause were reminded that they not only defended their country and the values that America represented but also the safety and well-being of their families.

The wartime emphasis on personalizing the political and politicizing the personal was responsible in large part for the celebrity status of Margaret Chung and her surrogate family. What began as a private arrangement that expressed the political sentiments and served the emotional and economic needs of a relatively small group of people became a propagandistic vehicle to promote the war cause. Chung and her expanding kinship network received national and even international attention because they created a model family that stood for patriotic service. Chung and her children demonstrated how women and men, whites and nonwhites, could work together toward victory.

At the same time, Chung relied on traditional conceptions of gender roles and race relations to advocate for the recognition and inclusion of women and individuals of Chinese ancestry in the Allied family. She demonstrated the value of women's contributions to the war effort by highlighting their roles in maintaining the domestic comforts of white military men. She also included Chinese people in the political intimacy of the Allied family by reinforcing Orientalist perceptions of Asian culture and racial hostility toward people of Japanese ancestry. Chung received recognition during World War II largely because her strategies resonated with the broader persistence and even heightened importance of social hierarchy in the wartime context. Her persona as a war mother demonstrated how other Americans could reconcile the demands for greater inclusion and the desires for social stability.

A NEW PLACE LIKE HOME

Margaret Chung's primary claim to fame during World War II centered on her maternal support for her military "children." Although newspaper articles mentioned her professional status as a physician, her responsibilities as a surrogate mother inevitably garnered greater attention. She fulfilled traditional gender expectations of physically and emotionally nurturing her sons, almost all of whom were separated from their biological and conjugal families. While other women provided similar services, Chung's Chinese ancestry marked her as an anomaly. By reinforcing traditional conceptions of female domesticity, she racially expanded her children's vision of family and nation. In personalizing the political experience of war and politicizing the personal offerings of domesticity, Chung also familiarized the exotic and exoticized the familiar. Her home, both literally and figuratively, offered comforting nostalgia and fascinating difference.

The military emphasis in Chung's adopted family reflected the strategic position of the San Francisco Bay Area as a "home base" for the war effort.[4] The region hosted one of three main navy stations in California. Along with San Diego and Long Beach–San Pedro, San Francisco-Alameda served as a training, send-off, and receiving base for naval aviators and submariners, two of the main branches of Chung's surrogate network. In addition, California as a whole and the Bay Area in particular represented a primary location for the burgeoning defense industry. The Kaiser shipyard in the East Bay employed close to one hundred thousand workers by 1944 and boasted the highest productivity in the country during the war. Bay Area factories and plants, which received over $4 billion in war supply contracts, stimulated the region's economy and created opportunities for women, Chinese Americans, and other previously excluded groups.[5] The expanding economy, characterized as a "Second Gold Rush," helped attract nearly half a million Bay Area newcomers; "everyone, it seemed, had come from somewhere else."[6]

In the midst of this dynamic and transient world, Chung's abode in San Francisco represented "home base" for her adopted family. Especially for her sons in the military, a highly mobile group, Chung's residence served as a place to prepare for and recover from the hardships of the war. As one reporter pointed out, "She really is a 'mom' in a practical way. She goes over them when they light in San Francisco between assignments, suggests sleep, gives them medicine, plans fun, feeds them, [and] hears their stories."[7]

Chung's most frequent and memorable performances of her maternal identity centered on her weekly Sunday night dinners, each attended throughout the war by seventy-five to a hundred family members and their guests. A 1949 literary tour book of San Francisco referred to these gatherings as examples of San Francisco's "saloniéres," assemblies of the "artistic, musical and literary world."[8] Chung drew upon her network of bohemian and celebrity friends to add glamour to family gatherings. However, she primarily sought to foster a traditional sense of home and domesticity for her itinerant children.

Her selection of Sunday supper as the event to showcase her hospitality evoked the connotations of a special family meal. For these weekly buffets, Chung reinforced her maternal identity by cooking the food while "robed in a gingham apron," a costume selection that contrasted sharply with her former masculine professional suits.[9] The menu also tended to replicate dishes consumed by "typical" American families, such as barbecue spare ribs, Caesar salad, and chocolate cake. Despite the large numbers of guests and the expansive size of her adopted family, Chung sought to emphasize the personal nature of her offerings. She made special efforts to fulfill the requests of her children. Tex, son number 632, recalled, "I'll never forget my joy and surprise at just saying I'd like red beans and finding the best ones I'd ever tasted right before me."[10] Her thoughtfulness compared favorably with institutional military fare. As son number 640, nicknamed "Rascal," wrote to Chung, "Every time we get a dish of spam or peas we say something dedicatory to you & your cooking."[11] Chung's famous weekly parties alleviated some of the loneliness and alienation of those who were separated from their own families because of the war. As one of her sons wrote, "Many thanks, Mom, for everything you did for us those weeks. The pleasant experience of meeting your friends and inhaling tons of garlic seasoned food at the house was warming to the soul."[12] Like other mothers, Chung expressed her love through the provision of food; by physically nurturing her family, she also spiritually rejuvenated them.

Chung's sons so valued her residence as a "home" that they contributed financially to the purchase of her first house in San Francisco. Sometime between 1942 and 1943, Chung moved from her apartment in North Beach into a three-story but modestly proportioned house in a white, middle-class neighborhood. Situated on Masonic Avenue in the Western Division neighborhood, her new home was some distance from her practice in Chinatown. Her relocation preceded the difficult postwar suburbanization efforts of Chinese Americans but paralleled the movement of European immigrant groups out of ethnic ghettoes before and during the war. Chung's professional status, combined with her well-publicized support for white American patriots, no doubt assisted her efforts to circumvent racial covenants in the restricted wartime housing market. Her sons, some of whom had enjoyed her hospitality for over a decade, solicited contributions among one another to assist Chung with the down payment. In exchange for serving as a surrogate mother for her white sons, she gained not only a symbolic but an actual geographical niche in "mainstream" America.

Chung's children not only enjoyed the comforting sense of familiarity when they visited her home. They also experienced the thrill of the exotic, and many of them wanted her to introduce them to her ancestral culture. One of her out-of-town friends, a white journalist, recalled, "Dr. Chung and I always go to eat at a Chinese restaurant—which represents for her a sacrifice on the altar of friendship. She doesn't like Chinese food and I do. And she usually eats with American knife and fork while I use chopsticks."[13] Although Chung described corned beef and cabbage as her favorite meal, she strategically introduced certain types of Chinese fare in an otherwise typically "American" menu for her Sunday night dinners. She combined "Chinese" and "American" ingredients—soy sauce and ginger as well as ketchup, mustard, and honey—to prepare her signature dish of BBQ ribs.[14] In addition, she offered fried rice as an accompaniment to the main meat course, which usually consisted of ribs, but also steaks and turkey for special occasions.

The pairing of meat and rice at Chung's parties held political significance. Historically, anti-immigrant rhetoric focused on the allegedly strange eating habits of the Chinese to justify racial discrimination. Charges that the Chinese enjoyed eating rats, dogs, and even other people supported perceptions of their subhuman nature.[15] Even the American Federation of Labor evoked the powerful cultural connotations surrounding food to argue for Asian immigration exclusion. In 1902, Samuel Gompers coauthored a tract entitled "Meat versus Rice: American Manhood against Asiatic Coolieism—Which Shall Survive?"[16]

By World War II, with the Sino-U.S. alliance, American men and women were encouraged to regard the Chinese as worthy allies instead of a despised group. In fact, the 1882 Chinese Exclusion Act, which prevented entry of laborers and denied naturalized citizenship for immigrants, was repealed in 1943 as a gesture of wartime friendship. Chung assisted this campaign to emphasize the mutuality of U.S. and Chinese people. Fried rice, as opposed to some esoteric delicacies that might repel her predominantly white guests, constituted a rather "safe" introduction to Chinese fare. In catering to her family's interest in "Oriental" food, she reminded them of the compatibility of "meat and rice"—that is, American and Chinese culture.

The cultural diversity of Chung's menu, along with her maternal identity, helped expand her sons' conception of family. As Fair-Haired Bastard number 4, "Red" Gill, explained after receiving a letter from Chung: "What a wonderful day this has been, how good God is to me! A letter from you is like an October day in San Francisco with chop suey, like the thrill of the kickoff at 'Big Game' time."[17] Gill's nostalgic memories of his Bay Area home included Chinese food as well as the cross-bay college football rivalry between Stanford and Berkeley; both chop suey and football served as reminders of what it means to be a San Franciscan and by extension an American. Tellingly, Gill's invocation of chop suey reveals how Chung's sons frequently misperceived Americanized versions of Chinese culture as authentic. She encouraged such Orientalist perceptions by giving jade and ivory Buddhas as good luck charms to her sons. These trinkets commonly served as tourist souvenirs without promoting in-depth cross-cultural understanding of religious beliefs and practices. However, like fried rice and chop suey, the palatability of these cultural emblems allowed Chung's sons to expand the imagined home and nation that they were engaged in defending.

FIGHTING THE WAR ON TWO FRONTS

Chung not only fed and entertained her sons during their visits on the home front, but also eased the process of adjustment for those fighting on the warfront. Like biological mothers, she played an important role in facilitating communication between family members and sustaining the emotional bonds of kinship. Some of her sons only met her once, while others visited only infrequently due to the demands of the wartime schedule. However, many of her sons wrote to Chung to thank her for her hospitality and to sustain their emotional and political bonds. Their expressions of gratitude highlighted the racial reversal of Chung's family compared with her mother's earlier adoption. Ah Yane, like other Chinese "slave girls," offered letters of thanks and obligation as a form of repayment for her "rescue" by white Presbyterian female reformers.[18] During World War II, Chung's white sons articulated their appreciation for their surrogate Chinese mother, who sustained them both physically and emotionally.

Chung spent much of her time writing letters and sending care packages. She explained in an interview, "Certainly I write them [her sons] back. . . . Everyone of them, although I am only able to answer 14 letters a day. I would like to write each one of them more often but I still have my practice to keep me busy a great deal of the time."[19] She became such a famous correspondent that letters addressed simply to "Dr. or Mom Chung, San Francisco, U.S.A.," would arrive at their intended destination. In addition to her daily letter writing, she gathered large numbers of her friends and adopted family members to wrap and send Christmas presents to every one of her sons. A typical care package contained toilet paper, a bottle of scotch, a "big delicious box of Blums confections . . . gum enough for a squadron, oodles of noodle soup, toothpaste, shaving cream, razor blade, cigs., coffee candy . . . , fruit cake, and sardines."[20] In the war front context, these simple household items represented valuable luxuries and commodities. Perhaps more importantly, the gifts affirmed a sense of communion between soldiers on the war front and their loved ones and supporters on the home front. One son, writing from Australia, explained, "Unfortunately most of the men out here feel like they are forgotten back home. . . . The fighting is just about the toughest there is and the boys can stand that but what really gets them is the feeling of being neglected."[21] Another pleaded, "Please drop me a line, dear Mom—for a letter is a priceless reward—when we get back, from a few days of toil. Don't fail me Mom—because news from one at home, from one you hold close to your heart is enough to keep one going."[22]

Chung's sons also developed valuable fraternal relationships with one another that assisted their wartime adjustment. While some were good friends before they were adopted, others became companions through their mutual association with Mom Chung. Outside of her presence, they identified one another through the little Buddhas, silver rings, and leather wallets that she gave to them as well as through the stories that they told about her and other members of the family. One Kiwi and one Bastard cowrote a letter to Chung about their chance meeting in South America; Elmer Awl exclaimed: "Never in a thousand years, could you guess with whom I am having a drink to-night. I remember well your claim to having so many 'bastardios' and at last I have met up with one of them—#413 and now a *Full* Colonel and Naval Attaché at Bogota, Columbia. . . . We are having one for you and wish you were here to join us."[23] Another son wrote about an unplanned encounter at a restaurant: "I find myself 'selling you' to everyone & work myself into an amazing enthusiasm. Last night while in Reno I was talking about you at a restaurant—when suddenly a waiter who shouldn't have been listening to our conversation leaned over my shoulder & asked 'Are you illegitimate too?' For a moment I was ready to hit him, and then it dawns on me that he had heard our conversation & and in deference to ladies present was unwilling to call me a bastard."[24]

These fraternal connections facilitated an immediate emotional bond between strangers; they also provided potential career contacts. War correspondent Bill Baldwin used his status as a Kiwi to send in the first story about the U.S. strikes on Formosa. Following the attacks, which were led by one of Chung's sons, Admiral William F. Halsey Jr., Baldwin learned that the military carrier that he was on would continue to the Philippines to cover General MacArthur's landing. Because that story was assigned to two other journalists, Baldwin worried that his report would lose its relevance. He decided to request "permission of the Captain of our Carrier to send a visual message to Admiral Halsey. I had never met him—still haven't, but in the message, I said . . . 'Mom Chung sends her best wishes. I am endeavoring to get my radio story back to Pearl Harbor for release before General MacArthur lands in the Philippines. . . . Can you help expidite [*sic*] this matter for me? Signed— Bill Baldwin KIWI Son #234.'"[25] Within 30 minutes, Baldwin was transferred to another ship and then transported away by a torpedo bomber, becoming "the first correspondent to return from the combat area."

Vincent Turner, whose father was Golden Dolphin 111, believes that
the opportunity to develop contacts across rank and military branches
made Chung's fictive kinship network particularly valuable for her
adopted sons.[26] Because rank defined one's status in the military, even
social functions separated enlisted men from officers. Consequently,
Chung's weekly dinners and her extended network allowed military
personnel across ranks and divisions greater opportunities for interaction. In other words, her kinship network countered the hierarchy of
the military family.

By creating an extra-institutional source of support for her soldier
sons, Chung demonstrated the mutuality of female domestic labor and
male military responsibilities. As a model mother, she nurtured good
citizens who could defend the nation. Prior to U.S. entry into the war,
Chung's "bastard" sons had no apparent father. After the United States
entered into political alliance with China, however, "Uncle Sam"
became the symbolic paternal figure for their family.[27] This interracial
political alliance encouraged Chung's participation in replenishing and
expanding the armed forces. While her alleged involvement in procur-
ing pilots for the Flying Tigers was not highly publicized, she was
described as a "one-woman flyers' recruiting force" for the American
military:

> From all over the country lads drop into San Francisco and phone Mom to
> help to get into some flying unit.
>
> She asks to see them. She's thorough about her investigation of the
> volunteer, but she's so casual and humorous that most time the lads don't
> know she's sizing them up.
>
> She's brisk when she thinks she's found a new flyer. She puts down
> whatever little rosewood or jade statue she's been fingering, writes out an
> address and says:
>
> "Here, take this to General so-and-so. Tell him Mom sent you. Tell him
> you're under age but that Mom says it won't matter."[28]

Chung's maternal identity helped to personalize the recruitment experience. She allayed fears about the bureaucratic nature of military processing by spending time with each potential flyer and providing a
personal referral for a high-ranking mentor. While her role as a mother
offered a sense of security, Chung's Chineseness, at least in the eyes of
the journalist who either noticed or imaged her fingering of oriental
trinkets, hinted at the possibility of exotic adventure. In entering the
military, young American soldiers joined a new family that necessitated

interaction and intimacy with people of diverse cultural and racial backgrounds.

THE LIMITS OF THE NATION

War, however, required not only the forging of new alliances but also the demonization of enemies. Chung advocated the inclusion of Chinese people into the Allied family in part by reinforcing racial hatred for those of Japanese ancestry. In exchange for her hospitality and support, she exacted a parting promise from her military sons: "Bring me back seven Jap scalps. Get seven for yourself. Good luck. Let me hear from you."[29] Chung, along with the mainstream American press, fueled these anti-Japanese sentiments to promote American support for the war in the Pacific. However, the use of racial rhetoric countered her attempts to promote more equitable treatment for Chinese people. Her sons continued to be influenced by racial attitudes that regarded all Asian people and all nonwhites as unwanted outsiders.

In their correspondence to Chung, her military sons expressed intense hatred for the Japanese, describing them as inhuman and deserving of extermination. As one wrote:

> Although I don't think I killed a Jap I saw many of them dead and bloating in the sun. They are hateful to see, and the worst smelling things one can imagine. They fight to the finish and do not surrender, so annihilation is the only solution to their folly. A few prisoners passed by our camp one day. They were very scrawny, monkey like creatures with extremely unintelligent faces.[30]

While Chinese food was rehabilitated for the American palate, the alleged eating habits of the Japanese served as evidence of their depravity and barbarism. As one of Chung's sons exclaimed, "For a long time I thought the Japs inhuman and now I know for sure. Had heard several tales as to their practicing canibalism [sic]. Will find that its true . . . I just hope there is soon a food shortage in Japan."[31]

These descriptions of the Japanese qualitatively differ from the sons' characterizations of European enemies.[32] While Chung's sons sought to exterminate the Japanese, they expressed admiration for Germans. As one expressed, "Those German pilots are really good and it is a shame that such talent should be expended on so unworthy a cause."[33] The Japanese, according to Chung's sons, were inherently evil and corrupt, whereas the Germans were misguided but worthwhile. Another son, stationed in the European theater, communicated his preference to fight against the Japanese: "I am in England. As you know my heart was set on something else but then I didn't have much to say in regard to where I would go. I figure its all the war anyway and finishing it up over here quickly will help to defeat Jap all the sooner."[34] While the author perceived the European and Asian war theaters as part of the same war, he clearly viewed Japan rather than Germany as the primary enemy.

The opinions of Chung's sons reflected popular wartime attitudes in the United States. The vilification of Japan stemmed not only from the perceived "sneak" attack on Pearl Harbor. Long before World War II, people of Japanese ancestry had been designated as unwanted aliens. Like the Chinese who arrived before them, they faced a series of legal restrictions that prevented immigration, land ownership, and citizenship. The Sino-Japanese conflicts and World War II allowed for the rehabilitation of the Chinese, but not the Japanese.

Chung endorsed, even promoted, these negative, racial attitudes toward the enemy of her ancestral nation. Her comments about the war, recorded in speeches, newspaper interviews, and correspondence, reveal her focus on the mortality rate of the Japanese. Instead of discussing the military's strategic position in the Pacific or the necessary but regrettable violence of war, she concentrated on head counts. Chung's request for Japanese scalps from her sons fighting in the Pacific evoked the savagery of racial conflicts between Native Americans and Anglos on the American frontier. She reinforced the belief that a barbarous technique was necessary to confront a barbarous enemy.

Her sons enthusiastically agreed with her call for extermination. One of her sons explained, "I decided I wouldn't report until I had something to report on and of course that only means one thing to you and I— Dead Japs."[35] The writer sought to affirm their mutual hatred for a nation and people that had attacked both the United States and China, her ancestral land by descent and his by adoption. Another reminded Chung, "Just wanted you to know that, as we go into action, I'm thinking of you and what you represent; and, when I've got one lined up in my sights, I'll be saying 'That's for Pearl Harbor; that's for Mom Chung; and that's for me, you son of a bitch!'"[36] One squadron, the Fighting Two, a.k.a. the Grim Reapers, even promised to shoot down two hundred Japanese planes for her as a Christmas present. The squadron exceeded their promise, meeting their goal by July, and eventually set new squadron and military records for downing enemy planes.[37] When interviewed about the exploits of the Fighting Two, Chung remarked, "It's Christmas in July, isn't it? . . . I wouldn't begin to guess how many planes I have had shot down, just for me, but I know Tokyo would be much happier if their pilots had never strayed into the path of my boys."[38] Her promotion of anti-Japanese sentiment personalized the conflict between nations. She demanded the killing of Japanese enemies as an act of personal loyalty to herself and political loyalty to the United States.

Chung's strategy reflected Chinese American tactics for promoting war morale. The Sino-Japanese War represented the most recent formulation of a long history of conflict between the two nations. Reports of atrocities committed during the 1930s invasion of China fueled anti-Japanese sentiment among Chinese American communities. In 1937, a *Chinese Digest* article that had originally appeared in the *New York Times Magazine* equated "Chinese Nationalism and Anti-Nipponism": "Strong racial hatred against the Japanese guarantees on the Chinese side a finest fighting morale any nation can hope for. Every Chinese coolie knows that Japan is China's enemy. . . . Whatever the Chinese lack, and however they may be abjected by force, they have racial pride."[39] The writer of the article advocated promoting "racial hatred against the Japanese" as a means of promoting "racial pride" among the Chinese.

This antagonism toward Japan extended to Japanese Americans as well. In the mid- to late 1930s, *Chinese Digest* articles reported the takeover of San Francisco's Chinatown businesses by people of Japanese ancestry. As one writer lamented,

> Since 1929 a dozen Chinese importers of antiques, curios, and objets d'art have liquidated their business and returned to other lines, while some have returned to their homeland. And as soon as one Chinese bazaar closed, a Japanese would move in, set up his goods, and seemingly prospered by selling the same kind of commodities in which the Chinese have failed. By this process the Japanese stores hace [sic] increased one by one, while the Chinese bazaars seem to vanish at the same rate.[40]

To position themselves as the rightful economic occupants of Chinatown, Chinese Americans depicted Japanese American merchants as representatives of Japan, not as independent agents residing in the United States. The writer noted: "The prospering Japanese bazaar trade in Chinatown is another evidence of Japan's world wide trade conquest in which no other country has been able to compete successfully."[41] The economic

conflict in Chinatown served as a domestic representation of the international conflict between Japan and China.

Even young children in the Chinatown community absorbed and
espoused this economic and national antagonism. For example, nine-
year-old Lorena How "became intensely anti-Japanese" during the
Sino-Japanese War.[42] When given a doll during a stay in the hospital,
the first thing she did was to check the label. She returned the doll
because it was made in Japan. She and her friends also boycotted
Japanese American stores in Chinatown. As she recalled, "My friends
and I would all run into the store and shout in our best English, 'Don't
buy here, ladies, this is a Japanese store.'"[43] Like her Chinese and white
American elders, she made little distinction between Japanese in the
United States and the Japanese engaged in fighting the war against
China and eventually the Allies. Chinatown residents had minimal to
no influence on the U.S. government's decision to intern Japanese
Americans, but the forced removal of Japanese Americans from
Chinatown to internment camps would eventually allow Chinese
American merchants to regain control in their designated ethnic
community.[44]

These attempts to exploit anti-Japanese sentiment to foster support
for the Chinese encountered setbacks due to the legacy of anti-Asian
sentiment that applied to both groups. Even wartime propaganda
attempting to educate the American public on the differences between
their Asian friends and their Asian enemies espoused this anti-Asian
undercurrent. An article in *Time* magazine published a few weeks after
the attack on Pearl Harbor was entitled "How to Tell Your Friends
from the Japs":

> Virtually all Japanese are short. Japanese are likely to be stockier and
> broader-hipped than short Chinese. Japanese are seldom fat; they often dry
> up and grow lean as they age. Although both have the typical epicanthic
> fold of the upper eyelid, Japanese eyes are usually set closer together. The
> Chinese expression is likely to be more placid, kindly, open; the Japanese
> more positive, dogmatic, arrogant. Japanese are hesitant, nervous in
> conversation, laugh loudly at the wrong time. Japanese walk stiffly erect,
> hard heeled. Chinese, more relaxed, have an easy gait, sometimes shuffle.[45]

According to the article, the distinguishing features between Japanese
and Chinese stem from biological factors—the stockier build of the
Japanese—as well as from personality differences—the placid and kindly
expression or the easy gait of the Chinese. The article's attempts to
identify differences between the two groups reveal two characteristics

of American racial thinking during World War II. First, the article does not seek to reject but merely to reinterpret racial distinctions. The writer seeks to ascribe essential characteristics, both biological and cultural, to particular national groups. Second, the contradictory descriptions of Chinese and Japanese demonstrate the difficulty of separating the two groups through a racialized lens. For example, the article begins by stating that "virtually all Japanese are short." However, the next sentence also describes Chinese as short.

Chung's sons, accustomed to prevailing racial attitudes, experienced difficulty distinguishing between allied and enemy Asians. One of her adopted children actually accosted Clifford Yip, the son of Chung's sister Anna, assuming he was Japanese.[46] Chung chastised her surrogate son for attacking her biological nephew. However, the encounter revealed the limitations of fostering race-based anti-Japanese sentiment to help Chinese Americans and China gain admission into the American and Allied family.

A WARTIME HOMEMAKER

Chung's status as a Chinese mother not only inspired her sons to fight on the battlefield. She also served as a role model for women, particularly those left on the home front. During the war, women as a group "remained more dovish than men."[47] For them, the departure of family members involved "not merely the fear of loss but also the daily problems of coping."[48] Women also faced increased demands, described as a "speed up," to perform both private and patriotic work.[49] Wartime propaganda promoted the figure of Rosie the Riveter to galvanize female entry into the blue-collar defense industry. However, women also were reminded to regard these positions as temporary, since homemaking still constituted their "natural" careers. As a professional woman who voluntarily chose to nurture a family, Chung demonstrated the mutuality of private and patriotic responsibilities and modeled the ability to balance the roles of homemaker and wage earner.

While most of Chung's activities focused on supporting male military personnel, she recognized the struggles of loved ones left behind. Separated from their husbands, these women often faced the difficult tasks of economically supporting their families, relocating, and even giving birth on their own. Chung provided support, advice, medical services, and sometimes food to her sons' wives and their children. One son thanked her for helping his wife adjust emotionally to their wartime separation: "Dotha seems to enjoy your most entertaining dinners, and writes long accounts of your times together. She needs a little cheering up, and any effort along that line is certainly appreciated."[50] Another made a simple request: "Watch after my Helen for me Mom."[51] Chung made a special effort to offer her support during holidays. Craig and Guy Clark, the children of Chung Golden Dolphin Lt. Commander Albert Hobbs Clark, recalled spending Thanksgiving and Christmas at her home during and even after the war.[52] With their father absent, initially fighting in the Pacific and then listed as missing in action, Chung encouraged the remaining members of the Clark family to regard her surrogate kinship network as theirs.

Chung also instructed women to fulfill their patriotic responsibilities. Unlike most Americans, who experienced war as a disruption to their home life, Chung's family was completely dedicated to the Allied cause. As one Navy publication explained, "'Mom' dearly loves her 'Sons' but above her love for them is her love for her country. 'I am an American, and deeply appreciative of that privilege. . . . I want to be of service to America. I want, in a measure, to repay my debt of gratitude to the America I love.'"[53] The lack of conflict between Chung's personal and political loves reminded other American women to place their country's needs ahead of their personal fears.

But how should women fulfill their patriotic duties? Chung's public persona as a maternal figure reminded women to contribute to the war by offering a comfortable home for their men. In preparing her weekly Sunday meals, Chung requested assistance from the wives and female family members of her sons. The division of labor resonated with idealized images of the "wartime homemaker."[54] In order to supply the armed forces and the struggling Allies, the American government instituted a rationing system to ensure "equitable" and adequate distribution of food. To promote compliance yet also allay fears of food shortage, wartime propaganda provided instruction on how to prepare nutritious meals with limited resources and also offered idealized depictions of home meals as a symbol of the nation's abundance. In the iconic family, inevitably white and middle class, the wife or mother's central role in preparing and serving food illustrated the woman's responsibility over the domestic realm. The ideal homemaker, sometimes assisted by a black maid, provided different types of physical nurturance for her family members, depending on their gender and age. Husbands and sons, perceived as central constituents of the fighting and workforce, received larger portions, especially of foods associated with physical strength, such as red meat.

To some degree, the figure of Mom Chung reinforced these assigned roles for women, especially women of color. As a nonwhite woman serving a white family, she resembled the figure of the black mammy, a common character that appeared in popular culture with increased frequency just as African American women were leaving domestic service to take advantage of higher paying and higher status jobs during the war.[55] The message that white families could count on the devotion of racialized women appeared in one of the most popular wartime movies, the 1944 production of *Since You Went Away,* directed by David O. Selznick. His 1939 epic *Gone With the Wind* had garnered Hattie McDaniel an Oscar for her portrayal of a black mammy who maintains her dedication to a Southern plantation family even after emancipation. The 1944 film, set during World War II, again features McDaniel as a maid. She demonstrates her patriotism and loyalty by working at a factory during the day and offering her cleaning services without pay for her former white employers in the evening.[56] As with the black maid, Chung's voluntary services as a war mother communicated her willingness to help share the burdens of white families during the war. Her role, which could be described as an "oriental" mammy, had a particular regional significance. In California, where African Americans did not constitute a sizable population until World War II, Asian American men as well as women more commonly filled the positions of cooks, gardeners, and servants.[57]

At the same time, Chung also challenged racial and gender hierarchies. Simply stated, the status of mother differed from that of maid. By serving as a model of patriotic motherhood, Chung demonstrated the superior ability of a nonwhite woman to serve her country. Both newspaper accounts and many of her friends remarked on her tireless energy and devotion to the war effort. Her accomplishments reminded other women that they should be able to make do. For example, one journalist commented that the lavishness and abundance associated with her weekly parties demonstrated to other women that "despite these days of shortages, substitutes, restrictions and rationing, it is still possible to throw a swell party."[58] Also, as the nonwhite female head of her extended family, she directed the labor of the more junior ranked but white women.[59]

Chung's much-publicized ability to maintain home and work did not take into account the fact that during the war, she reduced her medical clinic hours to two hours a day, and she devoted an increasing amount of her time and energies to supporting the Allied cause. The redecoration of her office in Chinatown reflects this shift in her professional identity. Chung created a "trophy room" in her medical clinic, filled with war-related souvenirs sent by her sons. The *National Geographic* described the room, where

> flags, pennants, insignia cover the walls. Here is a piece of shrapnel from a Jap plane which landed on the *U.S.S. Astoria* in the Coral Sea battle and was sent in by Rear Admiral W. W. Smith, Bastard No. 52, who watched it fall.
>
> When Lt. Comdr. "Red" Gill, No. 4, slid off the *Lexington* just before it went down in the Coral Sea, he automatically grabbed a couple of things that happened to be handy to stuff in his pockets. When he reached land, he sent them on to "Mom."
>
> "Mom" had already read about them. They were the now famous cans of Spam and Planters Peanuts. Dented and battered from concussion, they look very much at home among the tattered trophies of the Bastard Room.
>
> Most thrilling of all recent souvenirs, however, is a flimsy piece of red tin, which doesn't look like much until you read the tag that came with it:
>
> "The setting of the Rising Sun, emblem from the first Jap plane shot down at Pearl Harbor on the morning of December 7, 1941. Sent in by Capt. L. W. Ashwell, Bastard 509, U.S. Marine Corps, Unit #506. Officer of the day, December 7, 1941."[60]

The emphasis on displaying the physical evidence of war in Chung's office contrasts with her previous preference for "Orientalist" décor. In memorializing her family's contributions to the war, she highlighted her dual patriotism for China and the United States as well as her identity as a surrogate mother. The fact that Chung proclaimed their kinship relationship in her professional work place reveals a modification in her public identity from physician to political maternal figure.

It is unclear how Chung sustained herself economically during the war. As part of her efforts to promote humanitarian tourism in the late 1930s, she opened a Chinese art and curio business called the House of Chung. She also received payment for public appearances and talks. However, Chung frequently volunteered her services without remuneration and spent a considerable portion of her own savings. Some of her sons donated funds and perhaps even rationing coupons to help supply the large quantities of food at her parties. Acquaintances speculate that she received assistance from Chinatown restaurants, which like other businesses were exempt from rationing. Others suggest that the U.S. military helped sponsor her parties, since she occasionally served as a hostess for semi-official events. Most women did not have such resources to fulfill the multiplying and conflicting demands on their time during the war.

While Chung affirmed the naturalness of female and racialized labor in the home, she also used these traditional expectations to create new possibilities. Her sons' wives assisted Chung in cooking her weekly parties, but she also made sure that the men, especially those with the highest rank, cleaned up afterward. One newspaper article reported: "The rule is that the highest ranking are the helpers. So it is always admirals, commodores, captains and commanders who clear the table and wash the dishes while the lieutenants empty ash trays and run the vacuum."[61] Chung's sons agreed to her rules, which reversed gender and rank order. Even Admiral Nimitz, commander of the U.S. Pacific Fleet, participated in the cleanup process. In an interview about her involvement in the military, Commander Eleanor Rigby of the Navy Reserves recalled seeing Nimitz at one of Chung's parties: "That night I saw Admiral Nimitz there, naturally, being the highest ranking naval officer, he had to swab the kitchen floor, or deck. . . . He rolled up his trousers a bit, as I remember, and he knew how to handle the swab from his early midshipman days."[62] Women and low-ranked soldiers, frequently men of color in the military, traditionally performed the tasks of cooking and cleaning. By agreeing to share these responsibilities, Chung's white sons paid tribute to the contributions of women and nonwhites, not only to their night of entertainment but, more broadly speaking, to the war effort. The reversal of gender responsibilities and military rank suggested the possibility of transcending traditional social hierarchies. If white male officers could do "housework," then women and racialized individuals might venture outside of their assigned roles as well.

Chung's maternal identity and her surrogate kinship network mediated gender and racial tensions that resulted from the international conflicts of the 1930s and 1940s. Because moments of crisis engender new forms of alliances and antagonisms, Chung used the opportunity to expand the "imagined" national community.[63] Her focus on personal relationships to redefine political membership highlights the symbolic importance of the family for representing the polity. The language of kinship not only fosters a sense of belonging, it also assigns unequal forms of citizenship based on racial and gender differences. Like all propagandistic figures and like all individuals, Chung communicated complex and contradictory messages. Her persona as a war mother and her adopted family demonstrated how other Americans could reconcile conflicts between the demands for greater inclusion and the desires for maintaining existing social hierarchies.

CHAPTER 10

Creating WAVES

We, who are the beneficiaries of the American system, should
defend it with our heads as well as our hearts. We must not be
content with a passive patriotism. We must be active
Americans. . . . The seat of government may be in
Washington, but the heart of government is in your township.
And when that heart beats, Washington listens.

Margaret Chung, *Christian Science Monitor*, 1942

During the 1930s and early 1940s, Chung achieved recognition as a
symbol of the expanding American and Allied family. Her fame, however,
stemmed from her dedication to supporting the perceived central actors
in the U.S. polity. As a mother, she nurtured and inspired her children's
wartime achievements. As a person of Chinese ancestry, she encouraged
white Americans to develop interracial and international sympathies.
Not content with her derivative status, Chung aspired to offer direct
service to the American nation. In March 1942, a few months after the
attack on Pearl Harbor, she applied to join the U.S. Navy.

Chung decided to approach this particular branch of the military for
personal and political reasons. Most of her sons entered the navy as
pilots and submariners. In addition, sea power was absolutely essential
to the war in the Pacific. Chung's desire to become an official member
of the American fighting force stemmed from long-standing aspirations
to dedicate her life to a greater cause. Her previous efforts to become a
medical missionary in China, a reformer in Chinatown, and a humanitarian physician in war-torn Asia had met with obstacles. Even her bid
to enter the military during World War I did not succeed. However,
Chung's celebrity status during World War II provided her with the
social and cultural capital that she felt would grant her access into one
of the most honored arenas of citizenship.

Membership in the military for a woman, especially a nonwhite woman, was no easy matter. The armed forces historically constituted a male bastion where men—and only men—demonstrated their political allegiance through their fighting prowess.[1] Although women historically contributed to the military in a variety of ways, they did so primarily as civilians. During World War I, the army even recruited women but denied them official status, thereby rendering them ineligible for military rank, equal pay, health insurance, and a host of other benefits. Only the navy officially enlisted approximately thirteen thousand women, whites only, to ensure greater efficiency and control over this selectively expanded military labor force. This branch held the legal authority to do so, because the 1916 act that established the reserves allowed "any citizen of the United States" to join.[2] However, subsequent legislation, first revised in 1925 and then renewed in 1938, explicitly restricted the navy to men.[3] The military tended to either exclude nonwhites or assign them to the most menial and undesirable duties, though these practices were not legally mandated. The positions of women and people of color in relation to the armed forces correlated with their secondary status in American society. Consequently, the ability to perform valorous service for the nation symbolized the full attainment of citizenship for marginalized individuals.

In order to enter the U.S. Navy, Chung initiated and lobbied for congressional legislation to establish the WAVES (Women Accepted for Volunteer Emergency Services). Although wartime demands necessitated changes to the military, the prospect of altering the status quo incited fears of social disintegration. Faced with hostile resistance, Chung and other proponents of the WAVES attempted to minimize the perception that they were making waves in the figurative sense. In this context, Chung's public maternal persona and her adopted family served as crucial assets. Her network of surrogate children allowed her access into the inner circles of the national government. At the same time, these behind-the-scenes discussions remained largely hidden from the broader society. Chung provided reassurances that she intended to support, and not supplant, white male soldiers. Although she helped to create the Women's Naval Reserve, Chung ultimately received little public recognition for her role. Instead, she faced repeated rejections to her applications to serve in the organization that she had cofounded. Being a symbolic Chinese mother brought Chung close to the center of political power during World

War II but did not grant her authorized membership in the honored sanctums of the American polity.

MAKING WAVES

Chung's efforts to create the WAVES reflected a broader wartime movement to expand women's roles. Recognizing the disadvantaged status of female civilians during World War I, advocates for women sought official military status during World War II.[4] Even with the wartime need for labor, however, female entry into the traditionally male bastion required support among Washington politicians, military leaders, and the broader American public. Following a long tradition of maternalist reform, Chung used her influence as a mother to enact social change.

The politics surrounding the creation of the first female corps, the Women's Army Auxiliary Corps (WAAC), reveals the pervasive anxieties about women's entry into the military. The initial proposal, by Congresswoman Edith Nourse Rogers (R-Mass.), envisioned women as full members of the military. However, in May 1942, the Senate chose to approve the army plan, which limited the corps to auxiliary status.[5] After recognizing the administrative difficulties of coordinating a separate civilian corps with the military, the army requested legislation to integrate women as members of the military in 1943. However, Congress ensured that the newly formed Women's Army Corps (WAC) would not challenge the existing social hierarchy. Female soldiers held no military authority over men. Women also received fewer benefits, based on the assumption that they were helpmates rather than independent wage earners or primary breadwinners.[6] In addition, despite the active lobbying of African American leaders and organizations, the legislation declined to prohibit racial discrimination.[7] Instead, the military instituted a maximum 10 percent quota for African American women. Discriminatory recruitment procedures made it difficult to meet even this goal. Also, the female corps followed the army's policy of racial segregation.

In the midst of these debates and legislative initiatives, Chung decided to seek entry for herself in the U.S. Navy. During a trip to the nation's capital, in which she visited many of her adopted children, Chung approached her "Beloved Son #465," Captain McQuiston, "in the Navy Department and offered my services."[8] Upon learning that "in order to be able to accept your services and the services of other women it is necessary to have a Bill passed," Chung used her kinship network to lobby for the creation of the WAVES.[9] In recalling her efforts, she emphasized her inexperience but also her extensive contacts within the legislature. She explained that

> I knew nothing of laws, bills, and asked him [McQuiston] what was necessary to provide such a Bill. He said, "Well, Mom, you will have to get a Bill drafted, and have it brought before Congress for discussion and passage." I asked, "How are such things arranged?" Capt. McQuiston then said, "Do you know anyone in Congress who can introduce a Bill for you?" I answered, "Well, I have a son. . . . Congressman Melvin Maas, of Minnesota, who is a Colonel in the Marine Air Corps, and my 447th son. He is on the House Committee of Naval Affairs, and I am sure he would be happy to introduce a Bill for me."[10]

Chung immediately phoned and met with Maas (R.-Minn.), the chair of the House Naval Affairs Committee. During the war, Maas periodically requested leaves of absence from his congressional responsibilities in order to fulfill his Marine Corps duties in the Pacific. Chung likely met him during one of his visits to San Francisco. Maas responded enthusiastically to Chung's appeal. He had observed women's contributions to the military in Great Britain, while touring there. In response to Chung's request, Maas introduced House Bill 6807 for the creation of a Women's Naval Reserve. His committee approved the legislation "within less than half an hour's hearing" on 15 April 1942.[11] The next day, "it passed the House in about twenty minutes." Maas credited Chung with the idea of the Women's Naval Reserve, writing to her, "I am very proud to be the instrument in carrying out your brain-child as the legal sponsor of the Women's Naval Auxiliary."

Chung also initiated the process of introducing a bill in the Senate. She convinced Congressman Raymond Willis (R.-Indiana), Kiwi number 124, to introduce the Senate version of the Women's Reserve Bill. Chung attributed her success in lobbying Willis to his secretary, Ailene Loveland. It is unclear how Chung and Loveland met. However, as Kiwi number 120, Loveland had entered Chung's adopted family prior to Willis and most likely facilitated his introduction to their adopted mother. Chung also requested the support of Senator Albert "Happy" Chandler (D.-Kentucky), Golden Dolphin number 98. Chandler, the head of the Military Affairs Committee, shared political sympathies with Chung. He had long advocated focusing wartime resources on defeating Japan. He assured his adopted mother that "I shall remember your Navy bill and shall do everything I can for you."[12] Chandler eventually played an important role in negotiating the passage of the bill in the Senate, where the legislation met with more opposition than in the House.

Chung also enlisted the aid of influential contacts outside of Congress to build bipartisan support. She asked Alice Roosevelt Longworth (Kiwi number 49), the daughter of President Theodore Roosevelt and the widow of former speaker of the House Nicholas Longworth, to "contact the members of the Old Guard for me and ask them to help enact the Bill."[13] Chung also requested help from Mary Early Holmes (Kiwi number 130). As the sister of Steve Early, Franklin Roosevelt's executive secretary, she could lobby what Chung described as the "New Deal regime." Holmes created an effective forum for Chung by inviting prominent Democratic political leaders to a small dinner party:

> Mary Holmes had one end of the table, I was at the other end, and seated around us were the Democratic Whip of the House, Speaker Sam Ryburn [sic] a couple of Judge Advocates, some Senators from different states who could really swing the New Deal vote. As we finished the soup course, "Mom, tell these Gentlemen about your Bastards Club." Well, that settled them into listening, and I started to tell them the origin of the Bastards Club. Then Mary said, "Mom, tell these gentlemen what you are here in Washington for right now." Briefly, I told them that I was hoping to have a Bill introduced and passed with their help which would enable women to join the Armed Forces and serve their country. Mary said, "Don't you think that's a good idea?" They agreed that it was. Mary said, "When Mom's Bill comes up before you in the House and the Senate, would you all vote for it?" They said they would, so with the help of these gentlemen the Bill came into being.[14]

Chung's involvement in the passage of the WAVES bill demonstrates the transformation of her surrogate family from a political symbol into an active lobbying force. Her adopted children allowed her access to government officials who could author and implement national law. Chung gained the assistance of both men and women. The men occupied official positions of authority; the women held influence as assistants or family members of prominent men. The position of Chung's daughters mirrored her role as a maternal figure; both could inspire but not enact political change.

While Chung's maternalism represented an obvious political asset, her Chinese ancestry served as a more subtle resource. In lobbying individuals like Melvin Maas, she not only articulated the reasons for women's involvement in the military. She also cultivated these political ties by serving as a valued cultural guide. In his diary, Maas recalled visiting Chung in San Francisco, where she entertained him at restaurants and nightclubs in Chinatown.[15] In addition to the miniature buddhas that she bestowed on all of her sons, Chung also presented more expensive Chinese vases and bowls to the higher ranking and more prominent children. These maternal offerings of Oriental goods paved the way for political alliances.

NOT CREATING WAVES

While Chung portrayed and possibly perceived the WAVES as her idea, she was not alone in thinking about how to create opportunities for women in the military. In fact, her political effectiveness stemmed from her children's recognition that informal networks helped to circumvent institutional morass in Washington, D.C. Chung's identity as a Chinese mother proved especially valuable because she advocated for the expansion of the military while containing the threat to traditional gender and racial roles. In essence, her persona and surrogate family helped maintain social attitudes that ultimately limited structural transformation.

As the United States approached war, individuals in the navy began considering how to revise the existing gender-exclusive legislation, but met with repeated obstacles. The Bureau of Aeronautics led this campaign to incorporate women into the military. Joy Bright Hancock, who had previously served as a yeoman during World War I, worked within this department but was not an official member of the navy at the time. She recalled that their first appeal "met with singular disinterest[;] the Bureau of Navigation stat[ed] flatly that since no need for women was visualized, no legislation would be requested."[16] However, when Congresswoman Rogers initiated the effort to create the WAAC, the navy become subject to increased public and congressional pressures to establish a women's reserve. Concerned about the possibility of externally imposed legislation, the branch decided to survey its own divisions to determine the need for women's service. Again, all but two of the bureaus and offices expressed little interest in women's participation in the military.[17]

Despite this reluctance, the Bureau of Personnel eventually recommended the establishment of a women's reserve to the secretary of the navy. However, high-ranking officials in the navy and the president both criticized the proposal because it differed from the army bill. Whereas the WAACS represented civilians who would serve *with* the Army, the WAVES legislation defined women as members *of* the navy. Due to objections of women serving *in* rather than *with* the military, the navy declined to introduce the bill to Congress.

Chung played an important role in circumventing the bureaucratic stand-off. Her son, then Lt. Commander Irving McQuiston, was a member of the Bureau of Aeronautics, which had led the initiative to establish a women's reserve. Hancock recalled that when Chung approached McQuiston for an opportunity to serve in the military, he "described the foot-dragging process the Bureau of Aeronautics had to contend with" and requested that Chung use her contacts to introduce legislation in Congress. Unable to advance the cause of women's involvement in the military through proper navy channels, the Bureau of Aeronautics "decided to make an under-the-table effort," according to Hancock. The bills proposed by Maas and Willis, at the request of Chung, applied external pressure to the navy, essentially starting "the fires under the Navy Department's weak efforts."[18]

Once in Congress, the legislation for a women's reserve continued to meet with opposition, especially in the Senate, which debated the proposal for several months. Chung herself argued against traditional gender and racial beliefs to gain a sponsor for the bill. She recalled that Senator Willis "felt that a woman's place was in the home, and was not particularly enthusiastic about having a woman's auxiliary in the Navy."[19] In addition, the creation of a women's reserve raised concerns about disruption to the racial status quo. During Chung's lunch with Willis, his niece said, "I think you will have trouble getting this Bill passed, Dr. Chung, because the people of the South will object to having colored people in the Navy, and it is certain that as soon as the colored people hear about this, they will volunteer and want to join."[20] While these objections primarily focused on African Americans, the sentiments held implications for Asian American women as well.

The Senate debates revealed similar concerns about the perceived social threat of women in the military. In the hearings before the Committee on Naval Affairs, congressional representatives repeatedly questioned the need to create a women's reserve and criticized the proposal to provide equal pay and benefits for women.[21] They also raised the specter of women's presence in combat zones. As one senator expressed: "I do not believe your manpower is so low in this country that you cannot get that additional number of men into the navy when necessary."[22] Several committee members, including the chair, argued that men with physical disabilities that prevented them from meeting military requirements would be more appropriate than women in ful-filling the navy's needs.

In response to these criticisms, the legislation that eventually estab-lished the WAVES limited women's involvement in the navy in several ways. The original proposal, introduced by Maas, simply requested the formation of a women's reserve to "be administered under the same pro-vision in all respects . . . as those . . . with respect to the Volunteer Reserve."[23] Maas explained to Chung, "My bill places them [women] on the basis of absolute equality in the matter of rank, pay, and promo-tion, as well as in all other respects."[24] However, like the WACS bill, the final legislation ensured that women would not threaten men's preroga-tives or transgress traditional gender roles. The limited number of female officers commissioned for the WAVES would only hold authority over other women and could not achieve a rank above captain. Intended solely as replacements to "release male officers and enlisted men of the naval service for duty at sea," female reservists were restricted to shore duty within the continental United States.[25] The legislation also imposed admission requirements regarding age, education, marital, and mater-nity status. Some of these provisions assisted the navy in selecting quali-fied applicants. However, many of the limitations simply insured that the women's reserve would not "destroy . . . [women's] standings as 'good mothers.'"[26] According to the Bureau of Naval Personnel, "No woman is accepted as a WAVE who is the wife of a man in the armed forces, nor may she have children under the age of 18."[27]

Faced with this intense resistance, Chung resorted to defensive argu-ments. On the one hand, she emphasized the transformative impact of women's entry into the military. She pointed out that the women's aux-iliary "would give patriotic women an opportunity to serve their country in many vital capacities. . . . I envisioned the Waves as an organization of intelligent, refined, well-educated women, who would work with dignity and a full sense of responsibility, by the side of gallant men of the Navy."[28] At the same time, Chung also minimized the significance of the WAVES. She "envisioned a woman's auxiliary for the United States Navy composed of women who would free many a Navy man from humdrum or desk jobs for active duty at sea."[29] In essence, Chung described female reservists as serving in "vital capacities" by releasing men from "humdrum" desk jobs. While she applauded women's advancement in nontraditional realms, she also portrayed women as playing the secondary and supporting role to men, the primary actors in the war.

Chung's response to racial concerns reflected a similar use of utilitarian arguments. Instead of articulating an idealistic belief in equality, she emphasized the situational demands for wartime unity. In reaction to fears about racial integration in the military, Chung suggested that "the people from the South are going to have to make up their minds very soon as to whether they prefer to have colored people fighting for them or have the Japs and Germans in our hair."[30] In order to incorporate "colored people" into the U.S. military, Chung evoked not only American opposition to fascism but also American racism toward the Japanese.

THE LIMITS OF ORIENTALIZED MOTHERHOOD

The partial victories in the legislative realm translated into partial defeats in the administrative functioning of the WAVES. Chung, despite her many applications, never gained entry into the organization that she helped to create. The obstacles that she faced illuminate the ways in which institutions resist social change. In addition, her rejection reveals the limits of her authority as an Orientalized mother.

Chung expressed an early interest to help establish, administer, and serve in the WAVES. In April 1942, when the legislation was still under debate, she submitted an application to join the Women's Naval Reserve to Maas, the house sponsor for the bill:

> I am sending to you my application to join the Woman's Navy Auxiliary
> Corps of the United States, the moment the bill is passed and becomes effective. I am a native born American citizen, and am keenly aware of the privileges and opportunities which I have enjoyed here in this glorious country,
> which I would never have had elsewhere. This country has been exceedingly
> kind to me, and I am very anxious to show my gratitude and eager to get
> into the services of the United States of America.
>
> I have a pair of trained hands which I wish to place at the disposal of this
> beloved country. . . . I am a doctor of medicine and surgery. I am willing to
> work in this country or to do foreign duty, and I am willing to do whatever
> I can that will be of the most use of this country.[31]

Maas forwarded her letter to the Navy Department, assuring her that he had sent it "with a strong recommendation that you be the first to be considered for a commission as a woman in the Naval Reserve when the legislation is enacted."[32] Despite Maas's endorsement, Chung received a polite but routine response from the Navy's Bureau of Navigation. The letter asked her to wait for announcements in the press regarding application procedures after the reserve had been established.[33]

The deferral of Chung's application indicated the navy's reluctance to include her in the planning process of creating the WAVES. Even as the legislation was pending, the branch created an advisory council to develop an administrative plan for the Women's Naval Reserve. Council members consisted of prominent women from higher educational institutions, located predominantly in the East and Midwest. Mildred McAfee, the president of Wellesley, served as a member-at-large of the advisory council and eventually became the first director of the women's reserve. Other advisory council members included presidents and college deans of institutions such as Barnard, Radcliffe, the University of Pennsylvania, Sweet Briar College, Duke University, and the University of Michigan.[34] The navy's focus on recruiting the female leaders of institutions of higher learning reflected the elitist vision of the WAVES. While the Women's Army Corps had a more open recruitment policy, the WAVES from "the outset [became] defined as a specialist corps in which women with 'sound business and professional experience' were needed."[35] In contrast to WACS, who trained at army camps, the WAVES prepared at women's colleges and had access to "Elizabeth Arden beauty salons" and maid service. They also could purchase tailored uniforms in department stores rather than standard, government-issue attire. These touches helped to resolve the incongruity between being a "soldier" and a "lady."[36]

Aware of the ongoing planning process, Chung again attempted to participate in the development of the WAVES. In June 1942, Willis, the sponsor of the Senate legislation, spoke and wrote to the chief of the navy's Bureau of Navigation on her behalf:

> One of the most able exponents of the Womens' Navy Reserve, Dr. Margaret Chung . . . has been interested in this legislation from its inception. Her qualifications and experience make it natural for her interest in the measure. Dr. Chung is an outstanding surgeon with a special talent for plastic surgery. . . . She is noted for her lecturing ability, her leadership, her extensive philanthropic work and her large acquaintance and following.
>
>   In conclusion it is believed that it would be helpful in maintaining the support of the finest women in the country for naval service, if she would be invited to a conference either in Washington or at her home in San Francisco inasmuch as it is possible for her to offer much in valuable information as well as extensive leadership.[37]

Chung received another polite dismissal of her request. Again, she was asked to wait until after the reserve had been established and to learn about application procedures through the press.[38]

Following the signing of the WAVES bill on 30 July 1942, Chung made at least one more attempt to enter the Women's Naval Reserve. She approached Tova Petersen Wiley, an officer who worked in the Navy Procurement Department in San Francisco. Chung apparently made a deep impression on Wiley, who recalled her application during an oral history interview in 1969:

> Q: Didn't you often have to get in touch with Washington to say here's this situation, what do I do about it?
>
> *Wiley*: That's right.
>
> Q: Do you remember any of those?
>
> *Wiley*: . . . I remember we had a request from a very prominent woman Chinese doctor in San Francisco to become a WAVE. She felt that she had started the whole program by recommending it and she felt very close to it.
>
> Q: What do you mean—recommending it?
>
> *Wiley*: She said that she was very close to the Navy and knew a good many high ranking officers. She had suggested that women would be well able to handle many of these jobs. Whether or not she was the one who had sparked-plugged it or not, I don't know. She thought that she was.
>
> Q: Did she ever say who she had suggested it to?
>
> *Wiley*: No, not that I know of. She thought that she should go into the WAVES with a high rank right then and there without any indoctrination, as I had done. I didn't know quite what to do about that one. So, I wrote a letter back to Miss MacAfee and sent her the outline of her background and her career. I was so stirred up about it that I had neglected to notice her birthdate. Miss MacAfee wrote back and said, "She's not qualified. She's fifty-one years old."[39]

Born in 1889, Chung no doubt exceeded the age limit (fifty) for WAVES officers by more than a year. However, the repeated summary dismissals of her applications raise questions about the navy's motivations.

Chung's Chinese ancestry constituted an indirect factor in the rejection of her applications. Responding to fears of racial integration, the reserve initially denied black women's petitions and requests for entry into the service. The refusal of these applications rested on two premises. First, the Bureau of Naval Personnel cited the legislative mandate of the WAVES as replacements to release men for active sea duty. Second, the bureau decided that women of a particular racial background could only replace men of the same racial background. Following this line of reasoning, the navy, a traditionally more exclusive branch of the military than the army, had limited numbers of African American men to be released for active sea duty by African American women. In fact, black women only gained admission into the WAVES in January 1945, two and a half years after the creation of the Women's Naval Reserve. Filipino women faced the same combination of gender and racial arguments. As one denial explained, "Until recently the navy had accepted male Filipinos for duty in the messman branch only. However, male Filipinos are now being recruited for first enlistment ratings, and should it develop that the nature of their duties in the shore establishment is such that their release for sea duty is desirable, their replacement by women will be given due consideration."[40]

The navy's attitudes toward Chinese women differed somewhat from the attitudes toward black and Filipino women. In November 1943, Captain Darden of the Bureau of Naval Personnel suggested a general policy regarding the applications of Chinese American women:

> In connection with an application for appointment or enlistment in the Women's Reserve, the question has been brought up as to the general policy regarding American born Chinese women.
>
> It is recommended that Chinese women be accepted if they are citizens and meet all other requirements for appointment or enlistment in the Women's Reserve.
>
> It is not believed that this will have any effect upon the course being taken in the matter of accepting Negroes into the WAVES.[41]

In response to the recommendation to accept citizens of Chinese ancestry into the WAVES, Tova Peterson Wiley, who administered Chung's application, quickly endorsed the suggestion: "In Miss McAfee's absence I am replying for her in the affirmative because this office is certain that she agrees with this policy without reservation."[42]

The memorandum reflected the navy's ranking of the acceptability of racial and national groups. At the time that the recommendation was issued, the United States Congress also decided to repeal the Chinese Exclusion Act as a gesture of friendship to China. The Philippines as a U.S. Protectorate would not receive its independence until after the war. African Americans perceived as a racial minority rather than representatives of an African nation did not have the same international diplomatic leverage to promote greater racial equality in the United States.

Although Chinese American women appeared to be favored over other racial and ethnic groups, they were not necessarily embraced by the navy. The dates of the memos, over a year after the creation of the WAVES, indicate that some ambiguity regarding the eligibility of Chinese American women had existed previously. Furthermore, although Wiley enthusiastically supported the policy of admitting Chinese American women on McAfee's behalf, the attitudes of other members of the Naval Personnel Administration are unclear.[43] In general, fewer Chinese American men "served in the navy [compared to the army] because, until the end of May 1942, Chinese Americans were not allowed to enlist for naval positions other than mess stewards and cabin boys."[44] Some Chinese American women served in the WAVES. However, at least one individual enlisted in the WACS instead, because the "WAVES, known for being more discriminatory, turned her down."[45] The navy did not systematically exclude women of Chinese ancestry. However, as nonwhites, their acceptance depended on the racial attitudes of those processing their applications.

Chung's race clearly disadvantaged her initial request to help establish the reserve. All the appointed members of the advisory council were white. The navy's desire for female leaders from prominent educational institutions inevitably resulted in the exclusion of women of color. Even in schools that created positions of authority for women to oversee the intellectual development of female students, few nonwhite women could obtain presidencies and deanships. Although Chung had both "business and professional experience," she lacked the affiliation to demonstrate her capability of administrating complex institutions and could not harness the resources of elite establishments for the benefit of the military.

In addition to her race, Chung's sexuality also might explain her rejection from WAVES. The prospect of women entering a traditionally male institution incited fears of sexual abnormality.[46] Slander campaigns against female soldiers involved both charges of heterosexual promiscuity and allegations of lesbianism. In response, military commanders carefully screened female enlistees and closely monitored their on- and off-duty behavior. Publicly, Chung was perceived as a respectable professional woman. However, government investigations into her background and character, conducted as early as 1940, unearthed charges of lesbianism from Chinatown residents.[47] A report from the Naval Intelligence Service further indicated that due to these suspicions, Chung was "early in 1943, requested to resign from the Professional Women's Club of San Francisco."[48] The government memos include inaccurate information concerning basic biographical details about Chung. However, the recording of these rumors in official reports endowed the information with authority. Considering the political explosiveness of charges of sexual deviancy, the navy likely preferred not to recruit and involve someone rumored to be a lesbian.

Chung's exclusion and the lack of public recognition for her role in creating the Women's Naval Reserve resulted from a conscious decision rather than bureaucratic oversight. When Edith Stallings, Women's Reserve director of the Naval Air Operational Training Command in Florida, researched the history of the WAVES, she learned of Chung's efforts through informal communication. She cryptically wrote in one of her letters:

> It was at cocktails that very nite that Miss Loveland—if you recall—told me all about "Mom" and her initial interest and efforts for the Women's Reserve. . . . Admiral Mason asked Mel Maas to speak to us about the "Waves Bill". I had an opportunity to speak with him alone and know now why "Mom's" name was never mentioned in that connection and won't be thruout the present administration. Do I need to say I'll never rest content until—in some future time when I shall be a free agent—due recognition is given "Mom" for this *other* way she has served the Navy.[49]

Why the "present administration" decided to disassociate Chung from the WAVES is not clear. It is likely that the White House and the leaders of the navy did not appreciate Chung's role in introducing the Women's Naval Reserve legislation in Congress. Her contacts allowed her to develop an independent base of influence. However, once WAVES became an official navy unit, the bureaucrats perhaps did not look kindly upon someone who refused to follow institutional protocol.

The annoyance of the White House also may have stemmed from Chung's affiliation with the Republican Party. Her preference for the GOP most likely stemmed from local as well as historical reasons. The Republicans dominated San Francisco politics for most of the first half of the twentieth century.[50] In fact, the GOP historically had a better track record of attracting women and racial minorities. Only in the 1930s did African Americans begin to switch party identification, and not until the 1970s did the Democratic Party become more successful in advocating for women's needs. Although Chung adopted children affiliated with both parties, her Republican sons introduced the WAVES legislation, and a Democratic senator led the opposition to women's entry into the military.

While World War II is commonly viewed as a major impetus for the expansion of the American polity, the experiences of Margaret Chung demonstrate the persistence of racial, gender, and sexual constraints. She focused on developing informal networks among elite, white Americans, particularly men, to negotiate institutional constraints.

Chung achieved some success, but her strategy of creating political influence also resulted in a lack of historical and authorized recognition of her contributions. Within the military community, her adopted children and their acquaintances remember her fondly. However, their affection and support could not prevent her exclusion from the Women's Naval Reserve, which she helped to create. During World War II, the approximately 350,000 women in the military served in "nearly every activity short of combat." The largest group of women, 140,000, enlisted in the army, while the navy recruited the second most, with 100,000 women.[51] In Chung's public statements and in her autobiography, she proudly proclaimed her role in initiating the WAVES but declined to comment about her repeated rejections. However, she was well aware of the rebuff. When Stallings suggested that Chung adopt all members of the WAVES into her surrogate family, she responded: "You are very kind to wish that all the Waves were my adopted children; however, they might not share your enthusiasm."[52]

CHAPTER 11

"I'll Wait on You Forever"

The old woman who lived in a shoe may have had so many
children she didn't know what to do, but she had nothing on
Dr. Margaret Chung of San Francisco who claims close to
1,000 sons. . . .

Unmarried, this humane and generous woman believes
that every woman wants a home and children. "But some of
us get enmeshed in careers and others are not fortunate
enough to get these things," she observed.

Hilda Sidaras, *Miami Daily News,* 1946

Angel, it's wonderful having you to come home to! If you'll
stay—I'll always draw your bath and cook for you and wait
on you forever!

Margaret Chung, *Note to Sophie Tucker,* 1945

During Margaret Chung's reign as a celebrity surrogate mother, her lack
of romantic involvement appeared "natural" in the eyes of her friends
and family. As a middle-aged single professional woman dedicated to
the war cause, her asexuality seemed only fitting. Despite her status as
an unmarried woman, Chung publicly proclaimed her allegiance to
existing gender norms. She believed that "every woman wants a home
and children."[1] Since she described herself as not being "fortunate
enough" to attain these goals, Chung did the next best thing. She set out
to satisfy these presumably innate female desires through the creation of
an adopted family. Her perceived purity served as a crucial asset in this
endeavor, allowing her to foster close relationships with white men
without arousing suspicions of social transgression.

Although accepted as "natural," Chung's asexual persona resulted
from conscious effort. In a 1945 letter to singer and actress Sophie

Tucker about Tucker's autobiography, Chung expressed the belief that
certain experiences should not be discussed publicly:

> What a good girl you are! You *did* take my advice after all, you *did* delete
> the paragraph about 'doubling' up with [Frank] Westphal, and I appreciate
> the love and the friendship that prompted you to take that advice! As the
> book now stands, it is a terrific inspiration which any youth may read and
> emulate your life—you see, Boss—I love you deeply—I care very much what
> people say about you! I can't bear it if people criticize you—and that one
> little paragraph which is *not* essential to the interest of the book draws the
> censure of the blue noses and the ignorant.[2]

The opinions most likely reflected Chung's strategy for her own autobiography, which she began writing as the war drew to an end.

Chung's concern about self-image is understandable. She had experienced social censure due to perceptions about her sexuality. Similar
rumors, aired openly, could damage her ability to serve as a political
symbol for the national and Allied family. Consequently, as Chung
became a public figure, she increasingly adopted a more normative
gender presentation. Along with her new public persona as a mother,
she wore feminine and glamorous clothing. While her maternal identity
located her in the domestic sphere, her new and expensive attire facilitated entry into mainstream and upper-middle-class realms of recreation. Because Chung's new costumes and maternal persona fulfilled
conventional expectations, she gained the opportunity to explore new
emotional and erotic alternatives. Chung's perceived purity as an asexual
mother allowed her to articulate love and desire for another woman
while evading charges of lesbianism.

CELEBRITY PATRIOTISM

Given Chung's reserve about her romantic experiences, little evidence
remains in her papers regarding her desires and relationships. However,
her correspondence to Sophie Tucker, saved meticulously by the entertainer, offers a unique opportunity to explore Chung's private life.[3] They
first met in Los Angeles in 1913, when Chung was in medical school and
Tucker was on a vaudeville tour.[4] Born in Poland in 1884, five years
before Chung, Tucker arrived in the United States with her family as part
of the massive Jewish migration at the turn of the century.[5] Like many
other immigrant Jewish entertainers, she began her career by performing
in blackface makeup in New York City's theaters.[6] Struggling to make a
name for herself, Tucker, ever the self-publicist, kept lists of people she

met in various cities and sent postcards to remind them of her return performances. Chung likely attended Tucker's shows over the years, but their relationship did not appear to become more personal until World War II. Chung adopted many musicians and actors into her family. By January 1943, Tucker had become Kiwi number 107.

While Chung's fascination for entertainers is easy to understand, their willingness to participate in her surrogate network needs further exploration. Like her relationship with Tucker, some of Chung's friendships with actors and musicians stemmed from connections established before the war. Known for attending opening night performances of plays, musicals, and operas, Chung frequently invited the cast and crew for late-night suppers. Like her adopted sons in the military, touring performers welcomed her hospitality. Her acquaintances, many of whom eventually became her surrogate children, included such luminaries of the theatrical and musical worlds as opera singer Lily Pons and stage and film actresses Mary Martin, Helen Hayes, and Katherine Cornell.

These personal connections facilitated the formation of kinship ties as an expression of their common political support for the Allied cause. During World War II, the federal government enlisted the cooperation of the nation's most influential cultural producers, the entertainment industry, to mobilize the American public. Hollywood movie makers did not readily welcome state efforts to monitor their industry. However, they recognized the financial as well as political value of cooperation. Movies became even more popular during the war than during the depression. The significant presence of Jews in the film industry and their awareness of the atrocities in Europe also motivated their involvement in the war effort.[7]

During World War II, approximately one in three men in the movie industry entered the military, a ratio much higher than the national average of one in ten.[8] Chung's adopted sons included enlisted film stars, such as Ronald Reagan, Robert Young, Henry Fonda, and Robert Stack.[9] Actresses and female entertainers also did their part by selling war bonds, performing for troops, and even dancing with soldiers on leave at the Hollywood Canteen.[10] The call for patriotic service helped revive the careers of some entertainers, like Sophie Tucker, who recovered her popularity as a nightclub performer for both civilians and military personnel during the war.

The willingness of these famous individuals to become members of Chung's surrogate family represented an extension of their wartime responsibilities as celebrity patriots. Their appearances at her weekly Sunday dinners provided another venue to inspire American fighters on the war front as well as defense workers on the home front. In addition, the increasing fame of Chung and her surrogate family created publicity opportunities for entertainers associated with her kinship network. In turn, the presence of famous actors, singers, and personalities fueled media interest in Chung and her efforts to promote the war cause. Genuine friendship and political commitment provided the foundation for the relationship between Chung and her celebrity children. However, they also possessed a mutual awareness of the value of good publicity.

GLAMORIZING MOTHERHOOD

Chung not only befriended celebrities but also embraced the glamorous image of womanhood promoted by the movie industry. Along with her new maternal persona, she adopted an expensive, feminine fashion style. Her sister, Dorothy, recalled that Margaret's "clothing changed from almost mannish suits to more frivolous attire under the influence of 'stars.'"[11] Chung's favorite photograph during this time period, which appeared in a number of media publications, featured her in an evening gown and white ermine cape, with coifed hair and makeup. Apparently, the image accurately represented Chung's attire. By day, she sported a Red Cross military-like uniform, but for evening, Chinese American physician Bessie Jeong recalled, "Margaret used to drape herself in ermine and jewelry."[12]

Chung's new clothing both deflected criticisms regarding gender-appropriate attire and allowed her to maintain social freedoms previously associated with masculine dress.[13] The combination of femininity and independence reflected the emerging images of women from the entertainment world. Beginning in the 1930s, Hollywood increasingly focused on the lives of "strong, autonomous, competent, and career oriented" women.[14] Even the physical appearance of female movie stars changed. Instead of the waif-like look of Mary Pickford, the movie industry favored larger women, like Mae West, with "more flesh and physical strength."[15] The cinematic emphasis on women's autonomy reflected changing gender roles during the Great Depression. In response to the economic crisis, couples tended to delay marriage, and women engaged in a variety of paid and unpaid labor to support their families. Hollywood both addressed the realities that women faced and catered to their fantasies. Female entertainers donned glamorous and extravagant costumes to gratify audience desires for spectacle and escape from their economic woes.[16]

The new image of womanhood modeled the possibility of personal transformation for Chung. She remembered herself as a "homely little child" and became rather heavy in middle age. Nevertheless, she could acquire the clothes and accessories to emulate celebrity glamour. Also, her new costumes allowed Chung to socialize as a member of the white upper class. Serving as a hostess for her itinerant children, she welcomed them not only into her house but also to her adopted home city. She served as a tour guide, facilitating their visits to nightclubs, restaurants, and other popular destinations. Many of these locations specifically catered to military personnel seeking excitement and entertainment before and after their stints on the war front. Chung previously performed a similar role for Elsa Gidlow, introducing the writer to the "queer" speakeasy in "Dagoetown." Chung's maternal identity and glamorous attire cloaked such excursions as respectable yet still exciting acts of tourism.

Although Chung led an active social life, she took great care to protect her reputation. In contrast to the heterosexual image of celebrities, like Mae West, she projected a predominantly nonsexual quality due to her age, physical presence, and maternal identity. Letters from her sons, many of whom were half her age, demonstrate that they did not view her as a potential romantic partner. Although Chung entertained extensively in her home, her sons did not spend the night there except under emergency medical or similarly unusual circumstances. Normally, she only allowed female or married friends to sleep at her house. Chung also regulated the behavior of her houseguests. She monitored alcohol consumption within her home to ensure that the parties did not become uncontrollable. While she played matchmaker and arranged dates for her sons, she also guarded against inappropriate sexual behavior. She even intervened when a married man tried to seduce a younger, single woman.[17] The mixture of femininity and propriety perfectly suited Chung's lifestyle. She could enjoy the excitement of nightclubs and late nights with her sons with minimal damage to her reputation as a single woman.

MATERNAL HOMOEROTICISM

Even as Chung adopted glamorous new clothing and socialized in modern recreational settings, she projected a Victorian, maternal sensibility. Her acquaintances evoked traditional associations between womanhood, purity, and spirituality to describe her role as an "angelic" protectress, a "patron saint of flyers."[18] Such perceptions allowed her the freedom to explore possibilities for expressing romantic and erotic feelings for women.

Chung and Tucker became close companions when the singer returned to San Francisco for nightclub appearances in 1943. Chung regularly drove Tucker to her evening performances, usually attending the shows in company with large groups of her sons and then staying up late into the night playing cards with the performer.[19] During Tucker's stay in San Francisco, the two spent so much time together that one local gossip columnist referred to them as "me and my shadow."[20] Their intense relationship continued, even after Tucker left San Francisco. Chung occasionally traveled to watch her perform, and they regularly talked to each other on the phone and corresponded.

In one letter, written after the death of one of her adopted sons, Chung reflected on the unique closeness of her friendship with Tucker, who was known by her nickname "Boss":

> Hi Boss,
> Just got thru talking to you on the phone . . . and I just said "Thank you", to God for giving me a precious friend like you. . . . Your friendship . . . makes life very much richer and sweeter, gives me courage to take the hard socks on the chin with a smile, makes my daily tasks infinitely lighter, keeps me laughing with sheer happiness and a song in my heart.
>   You said last night on the phone, that you were not demonstrative. That is a masterpiece of understatement. And yet I understand you so well, Boss, and when you talked to me on the phone, suddenly light dawned and I realized that I wasnt just one of the many recipients of your gracious hospitality but that I was included in that enviable circle of your friends and that I have a little place in your heart that is all my own.[21]

Chung's correspondence and her actions reveal the depth of her feelings for Tucker. That Chung felt comfortable turning to Tucker for solace reveals the emotional intimacy between the two women. As one mutual friend explained, they "truly loved each other."[22]

While Chung expressed love for all her adopted children, her relationship with Tucker was laced with romantic undertones. When the performer returned to San Francisco in January 1945, she became a regular house guest of Chung's. Mutual friends recalled that the doctor reserved for Tucker a special bedroom with a large, pink, satin bed.[23] During her stay, Chung wrote affectionate good-night notes to Tucker, using romantic and comical endearments:

> Ah Boss- I surely do love you—and I'm so happy you are with me
>   (13 January 1945);
> Goodnight Sweet Heart (14 January 1945);
> Peek-a-boo—I love you (14 January 1945);

Hi, Angel! Love You (14 January 1945);
Hi-Stinky—Love You! (14 January 1945);
Love & Kisses Nightie Night (17 January 1945);
You are the most wonderful Pal in the whole world—and I adore you
   (19 January 1945).[24]

The content and frequency of these notes suggest an infatuation on Chung's part that blurred the boundary between platonic and romantic friendship.

Chung's desire for physical intimacy occasionally emerged in her correspondence. Unable to spend Christmas with Tucker in 1947, Chung sent her a series of presents, commenting on the meaning of the gifts: "The silver shell, I want you to keep with you always—on your desk to keep your little candle in—and to remind you of my shining love— Please wear the blue nightgown—Christmas night because it will be *close* to you—as I will be."[25] By describing her closeness to Tucker as comparable to the physical sensation of wearing a nightgown, Chung revealed the connection between emotional and sensual intimacy.

Chung's expressions of affection for Tucker frequently incorporated lyrics from popular music. In preparation for one of Tucker's departures from San Francisco, Chung wrote her a good-bye letter:

> My Beloved "Boss" -
> While you're getting dressed, and I'm waiting for you—I'm going to attempt to tell you how much the last two months with you has meant to me! There is a song which expresses my sentiments very aptly—"The hours I spent with thee! Dear Heart are as a string of pearls to me—I count them over every one apart!" They have been wonderful hours, Boss, whether we were laughing, kidding, joking, eating—or whether I was just napping or being in the same room with you—it was wonderful! Your companionship, your healthy, hearty laughter, your priceless humor, your ready wit, your loyalty, your friendship—these things, I love and cherish-
> I'm sad because you are leaving San Francisco—but you're really not leaving it—because you will always be deep in my heart. . . .
> Your adoring Mom[26]

The use of lyrics and song titles, such as "Deep in My Heart," reflected Chung's desire to communicate her feelings through a language common to both of them. Tucker as a performer and Chung as a patron both readily recognized the references to popular culture. Furthermore, by using songs that commonly express heterosexual romantic love, Chung borrowed recognizable and acceptable phrases to express her feelings for Tucker.[27]

Chung also articulated her feelings through maternal and religious language. In one goodnight note, she, as the mother, promised to care for all of Tucker's needs: "Angel, it's wonderful having you to come home to! If you'll stay—I'll always draw your bath and cook for you and wait on you forever!"[28] Chung, as the mother, offers to take care of Tucker, the adopted daughter. Chung sometimes reversed the relationship with herself as Tucker's "Baby." Chung also compared herself to the biblical figure of Ruth, the devoted daughter-in-law of Naomi:

> Boss, I don't want to be sent home with all the rest of your junk to be put away in storage!! *I want to go with you*—wherever you go—to be *your shadow*—Can't I ride with your music in the music case? "Cause I want to go where you go—do what you do—then I'll be happy"!—and you want your baby to be happy don't you?
> Remember what Ruth said to Naomi? "Whither thou goest, I will go—and thy people shall be my people—and thy god, my god."[29]

The expression of Chung's desires through maternal and religious language masked yet revealed the eroticism of her feelings. The Old Testament story of Ruth and Naomi demonstrates the love and loyalty between women of different national and religious backgrounds. Ruth, a Moabitess, marries into a Hebrew family but is subsequently widowed. Naomi, her mother-in-law, entreats Ruth to stay in Moab and find another husband. However, Ruth refuses to abandon Naomi, whose husband has also passed away. Instead, Ruth follows her into the land of Judah and cares for her. Chung used Ruth's words to express a lifelong commitment to Tucker. In the context of the biblical story, Chung's love could be interpreted as emotional, familial, or spiritual love. However, the same passage that Chung quotes also appears in marriage rites to profess the romantic union between two individuals. The multiple meanings embedded in the statement offered some protection for Chung. After all, the "transference of sexual tensions into the language of the family (and sexual love into the language of religion) . . . [helps] conceal the physical basis of so much . . . love."[30]

Chung's choice of language allowed her to express love for another woman and also avoid suspicions of lesbianism. Rather than accept modern theories that focus on sexual desire and behavior as indicators of normality and deviancy, Chung preferred Victorian beliefs that deemed females as naturally asexual and consequently permitted the development of intimate relationships between women. Her strategy resonated with the experiences of other middle-class women who came of age around the turn of the century. They were "raised with the sexual categories of an earlier culture" and then lived through "social changes that redefine[d] their behaviors" in a later era.[31] While one should caution against exaggerating the acceptability of romantic friendships during the Victorian era, Chung's choice of erotic expression suggests that the nineteenth-century notion of female "passionlessness" continued to provide some protection from social and perhaps even personal recognition of lesbian sexuality well into the twentieth century.[32]

ME AND MY SHADOW

Chung's selection of the Ruth and Naomi story reveals an additional dimension to her relationship with Tucker. As Chung negotiated shifting sexual norms, she also navigated cultural and racial barriers. Like Ruth, who abandoned her native land of Moab, Chung preferred white Americans as romantic partners and friends.[33] In fact, the two groups that she most adored, actresses and military heroes, epitomized mainstream cultural standards of femininity and masculinity. Her behavior and statements indicate her internalization of white definitions of beauty. She once told the child of an adopted son, "I wish I could wake up one morning and be blonde-haired and blue-eyed. All my troubles would go away."[34] The comment, which left a deep impression on her young listener, revealed a poignant sense of longing. Even as Chung altered her physical appearance, she could never achieve the white ideal because of her Chinese ancestry.

Tucker exhibited a similar struggle to embody mainstream conceptions of beauty. Like Chung, Tucker grew up recognizing that members of the opposite sex did not regard her as physically attractive. She recalled, "I wasn't the type of girl the boys like to play around with on tour. But they liked me as a pal, a good egg."[35] When the singer began performing in vaudeville at the turn of the century, the theater managers required her to appear in blackface makeup. One producer remarked, "This one's so big and ugly the crowd out front will razz her. Better get some cork and black her up."[36] The entertainment industry reinforced the connections between race and beauty. Only women who fit the existing standard of sexual attractiveness could appear as "white" on stage. Tucker acknowledged the regulation when she pleaded with the producer, "Let me work in whiteface. . . . Really, I'm not bad looking."[37]

Like other Jewish performers, adopting blackface makeup offered Tucker certain advantages. She initially achieved fame as a "world-renowned coon shouter."[38] When she eventually established a career as a white female performer, Tucker borrowed the style of African American blues to develop her stage personality as a "Red-Hot Mama."[39] She "learned her signature song 'Some of These Days' from her black maid" and took singing lessons from black performer Ethel Waters.[40] Temporarily relieved of the responsibility of maintaining white standards of femininity, Tucker could mine black culture to create a theatrical persona.

However, Tucker always insisted on "whiteness" as her real identity. At the end of her blackface performances as a "coon-shouter," Tucker would "peel off a glove and wave to the crowd to show I was a white girl."[41] In fact, considering the extent of anti-Semitism in the United States, even through much of World War II, the incorporation of Jews from a racial other to a white ethnic group was still incomplete.[42] However, by taking off her glove, basically by displaying herself as not black, Tucker attempted to include Jews as part of the American mainstream rather than being an in-between racial group. She explained to the audience during her first performance without blackface makeup: "You-all can see I'm a white girl. Well, I'll tell you something more: I'm not Southern. I grew up right here in Boston. . . . I'm a Jewish girl, and I just learned this Southern accent doing a blackface act for two years."[43]

Chung literally and figuratively attempted to emulate Tucker's ascension into whiteness. As a birthday surprise, Chung and a group of her sons flew to Las Vegas to visit Tucker. During the singer's performance at a nightclub, Chung adopted the costume of a black mammy figure as a prank and proceeded to serve cake to Tucker and audience members. By donning blackface makeup, Chung sought to remind Tucker and her fans of the origins of the entertainer's career and thereby highlight her success as a whiteface performer. In portraying Tucker's former self, Chung assumed the role of Tucker's "shadow." The part suited Chung, for she was a lesser-known celebrity than Tucker and a more readily racialized version of her. As a woman of Chinese ancestry, her incorporation into whiteness could never be as complete as Tucker's. Furthermore, the image of the black mammy captured Chung's own role as an Orientalized surrogate mother for her white children. By suggesting that she, like Tucker, was capable of removing blackface makeup, of becoming a "boss" in the social hierarchy, Chung also reminded audience members of her potential to move into the American mainstream.

Even as Chung and Tucker sought entry into a white mainstream, they nevertheless valued their cultural origins. Both women committed themselves to promoting causes that would benefit their ancestral people. In fact, Chung's reference to an Old Testament story to compare her relationship to Tucker indicates that she sought a common reference to recognize and bridge their religious and cultural differences. As an American-born Chinese Christian, she tried to identify similarities with Tucker's Jewish immigrant background. While they spent Christmas together, they also celebrated Jewish holidays. Separated during one Passover, Chung sent a telegram: "Happy Holidays to you and your family. Wish I were having matzofry with you in the kitchen. Am nostalgic with many beautiful and happy memories of seder and passover spent with you and yours. I cherish your friendship above all else and love you."[44]

Chung's attempts to assimilate yet also promote cultural pluralism reflect changing social attitudes during that era. World War II created opportunities for those traditionally marginalized, especially those of European ethnicity, to enter the mainstream. "What began in the 1910s and 1920s as a fascination with the exotic became by the 1940s and 1950s a desire to erase the exotic. . . . The 1950s were marked by a belief in America as potentially homogeneous, and . . . the desirability of the 'melting pot.'"[45] As some groups viewed themselves and became viewed as "white," they also struggled to retain a sense of ethnic identity. Chung's efforts to enter the white middle class and also embrace her Chinese ancestry paralleled this transformation. Her relationships with "white" individuals from immigrant and ethnic backgrounds reflected a mutual desire for, as well as sense of anxiety about, assimilation.

STRATEGIES OF DISCRETION

For the most part, Chung's efforts to protect herself from social censure appeared to have worked. Her adopted children knew that the two women were good friends and often asked about Tucker in their letters to Chung; some also wrote to Tucker about Chung. However, few expressed the opinion that Chung and Tucker were lesbians.[46] Because both women actively supported the war effort, it was fitting to view them as co-mothers. When Tucker sponsored and launched the military ship S.S. Grinnell Victory, Chung served as her "maid of honor."[47] One serviceman even jokingly requested that Tucker adopt her own group of sons, called the "S.O.B.s."[48]

The support for Chung's relationship with Tucker may have stemmed from the commingling of heterosexuals and non-heterosexuals within their social circle. Chung's adopted children included entertainers who became known as or who were rumored to be homosexual or bisexual, such as Tallulah Bankhead, Anna May Wong, Tyrone Power, and Liberace.[49] Although harder to identify, some of her military sons also likely considered themselves gay. Despite official policies that banned homosexuals, the same-sex environment necessitated by the war facilitated opportunities for experimentation.

In fact, San Francisco, a departure and demobilization location for the military, developed a reputation as a "mecca" for gays and lesbians seeking recreation and a sense of community.[50] The "queer" and bohemian bars and nightclubs in North Beach thrived during the 1930s and 1940s. One of Chung's sons, from a much less cosmopolitan community in Oklahoma, recalled his shock as well as his amusement in realizing that she had escorted him to see a floor show of female impersonators at Finocchio's.[51] Bars in Chinatown, like Li-Po's and the Rickshaw, also developed a "swish crowd."[52] Gay servicemen seeking a less exhibitionist environment might socialize more discreetly at the bar of the Mark Hopkins, one of the city's most luxurious hotels, located on Nob Hill.[53]

Lesbians of middle- and upper-class background, rather than frequent bars that catered predominantly to a working-class clientele, continued to socialize privately in homes with their own networks of homosexual as well as heterosexual friends. Paralleling Chung's decisions regarding gender attire, the middle-class lesbian subculture rejected the adoption of butch or masculine roles that was practiced in working-class bar culture. Instead, they sought integration into the existing heterosexual culture and emphasized dressing "appropriately" and behaving with "sufficient, though never excessive, femininity."[54] This pattern of coexistence, which continued through the war and into the 1950s, provided middle-class women who pursued same-sex relationships with a degree of protection from social persecution.

The commingling of straight and gay communities during the war permeated much of military and popular culture, the two arenas closely affiliated with Chung's adopted family. One of Ronald Reagan's movies, for example, served as a template for GI drag. Reagan, who eventually established his political career on a platform of promoting normative "family values," acted in the most successful movie of the 1940s, the musical *This Is the Army* (1943). The film featured a standard heterosexual love story: "the plot revolves around the efforts of the central character's sweetheart to persuade her reluctant soldier to marry her."[55] Her success by the end of the film, "just before the hero leaves to fight on foreign shores," projects the nuclear family as "the vision for what the men are fighting for."[56] However, this musical "became the prototypical World War II soldier show and established the . . . basic wartime styles of GI drag."[57] Because of the immense popularity of *This Is the Army,* the musical was performed in all the arenas of the war—the United States, North Africa, Europe, and the Pacific. The multiple stagings allowed men in the military of varying sexual identifications and practices to perform and enjoy performances of female impersonation.

Tucker herself might have benefited from the coexistence of heterosexual and homosexual cultures in the entertainment industry. The availability of Chung's letters allow for the possibility of reconstructing her feelings for Tucker. However, the entertainer's perspective remains difficult to decipher. Tucker's autobiography ends during World War II and omits any mention of Chung. The singer did express negative view regarding male homosexuals in the book; while visiting Europe in 1922, Tucker criticized "the cheap morale of Berlin," commenting on "the number of 'fag joints,'" male cross-dressers, and prostitutes.[58] Married and divorced three times before she met Chung, Tucker had a bawdy, heterosexual stage persona. Ironically, because of her glamorous and sexually charged image, she was widely impersonated by male performers at establishments like Finocchio's. Her imitators no doubt recognized that Tucker's gender persona constituted an act of masquerade. Like other women, she had to use extensive makeup and costuming to achieve an ideal image of female beauty. Notwithstanding Tucker's negative comments regarding homosexuality, there were quite a few lesbian or bisexual blues and jazz singers, such as Bessie Smith, Josephine Baker, Gladys Bentley, and Tucker's former teacher Ethel Waters, who adopted "a heterosexual public persona, most favoring a 'red hot mama' style . . . [to keep] their love affairs with women a secret."[59]

Tucker's actions demonstrate that she greatly cared for and respected Chung. They spent a considerable amount of time together both in San Francisco and in other parts of the country. At the end of the war, Chung was on the verge of losing her house due to her inability to pay the mortgage. Her sons had provided the down payment for this home on Masonic Avenue as a token of their love and appreciation. To save Chung's home, Tucker contacted the sons again to raise money for the mortgage as a Christmas present. Chung's thank you letter expressed her deep appreciation:

> Well, I'm a flabbergasted wide-eyed, speechless Chinaman! You've got me embarrassed, bewildered and topped for a fare-thee well! I knew you were up to something—wanting a roster of my sons, but I never dreamt in all the whole wide world that you were going to pay off the mortgage on my [crossed out] our house! . . . Wish I could run and jump on your lap and put my arms around you and kiss your dear cheeks—or pinch them hard for you—wish you could look into my eyes and see the mute gratitude there. . . . I'm the luckiest person in the world, to have your friendship! I love you, for sure & for keeps.[60]

Perhaps due to Tucker's schedule as a performer or to her lack of desire to do so, the two women did not live together on a permanent basis. However, Chung wanted to share her home with Tucker, and their friendship lasted for the rest of Chung's life.

"There Will Never Be Another Mom Chung"

On 14 August 1945, at 4 P.M. Pacific time, Chung heard of Japan's surrender over the radio. In the midst of composing a letter to son number 600, Admiral William Halsey Jr., the commander of naval forces in the South Pacific, she interrupted her train of thought to write, "I have just dropped to my knees in thanksgiving to God and to you."[1] Having dedicated fourteen years of her life to the war cause, Chung must have found it fitting that one of her adopted sons, William Sterling Parsons, had served as bomb commander on the Enola Gay; involved in the testing and development of atomic weaponry at Los Alamos Scientific Laboratory, he personally assembled the trigger of "Little Boy," the bomb dropped on Hiroshima on 6 August 1945.[2] There is no indication of what Chung thought of the destruction, which must have surpassed even her desires for "Jap" scalps. Instead, she expressed gratitude for the end of the war that had ravaged her ancestral homeland and transformed the land of her birth.

As the war drew to a close, Chung received official commendations for her patriotic service. The Chinese government had previously rejected her offer to provide medical aid in war-torn Asia. However, in June of 1945, she became the first American woman to receive the "People's Award" of China. Her adopted son Paul Yu-pin, the country's first Catholic bishop, presented Chung with the honor during a ceremony at her home on Masonic Avenue.[3] She also received a citation from the American Red Cross for "meritorious personal service performed in behalf of the nation, her Armed Services, and suffering humanity in the Second World War."[4] Chung helped establish the San Francisco Downtown Disaster Station in 1939 and volunteered on its medical staff.[5] The certificate of acknowledgment, signed by President Truman, perhaps soothed some of the pains of rejection she had suffered at the hands of the armed forces. The tributes served the dual purposes of celebrating symbolic advancements and masking persistent institutional obstacles. Chung accepted these partial recognitions with pride.

After World War II, Chung continued some of her professional and political activities. Whereas during the war she had limited her medical practice to focus on supporting the Allied cause, afterward she clung to her professional identity.[6] By 1951, she had moved her practice out of 752 Sacramento, the site of her Chinatown medical practice for nearly twenty years, and opened a new office in the nearby tourist and financial districts.[7] The location of Chung's clinic geographically symbolized the in-between status that she had long occupied between Chinese and mainstream America. Although recurring health problems in the late 1940s and 1950s curtailed her postwar professional activities, Chung leased office space for a medical practice until her death.

Despite her removal from the immediate vicinity of the Chinatown community, Chung continued to express interest in political developments in China. She corresponded with Madame Chiang Kai-shek in the early 1950s. The two women most likely met in March 1943, when Chung served on the city's welcome committee for the first lady of China.[8] Chung sent gift packages to Chiang and inquired about the political status of the Republic of China after the takeover of the mainland by Mao's supporters. Considering Chung's elite social status and her idealization of American values, it is not surprising that she allied herself with the Nationalist, rather than Communist, forces. In fact, her political statements during World War II foreshadowed the anti-Communist rhetoric of the Cold War. In a 1942 address, she warned that "the greatest danger which imperils the American way of life is ... the miserable, fifth column termites within our own structure, destroying our very foundations."[9] Although Chung was referring to the need for "active Americanism," for internal vigilance against those who did not support the war, the same language would soon be used to refer to suspected Communist saboteurs in the United States. Chung expressed interest in visiting Taiwan and publicized the plight of "Free China" by speaking on anti-Communist propaganda broadcasts in the United States.[10]

Despite her concern about the situation in China, Chung's correspondence revealed her sense of removal from the immediate political turmoil there. While the exiled Republic of China engaged in a struggle to legitimize its existence, Chung enjoyed the material luxuries of a sophisticated lifestyle in the United States. In addition to sending boxes of candies and gifts, she also shared her interest in expensive clothing with Madame Chiang. The latter expressed her annoyance politely, thanking Chung for "the clippings about the sapphire mink coat. It looks very lovely, but I am afraid I am in no position to buy any furs. As you know, we are making every effort to get back to the mainland and whatever resources we have will all be directed towards that one object."[11]

Chung also continued monitoring American military developments and international policies, relying on her surrogate network to inform her of important changes. She followed the Korean conflict, receiving updates from Rear Admiral Arleigh Burke, a veteran of the World War II, a future chief of naval operations, and one of her adopted sons stationed in Asia as part of the United Nations Command.[12] She tracked the progress of the WAVES as well. In a 1946 newspaper interview, she explained proposed legislation that would transform the women's reserve into a permanent, rather than just an emergency, branch of the navy.[13] The new plan also allowed female officers to achieve ranks above captain. Republican representative Margaret Chase Smith of Maine successfully maneuvered these proposals through Congress in 1948 and became known as "Mother of the Waves."[14] Chung, the Chinese American mother, remained unrecognized.

Though Chung followed political developments after the war, she mainly focused her energies on maintaining her network of surrogate kin by providing support for their postwar transition. She expressed an interest in creating a rest and rehabilitation center for her returning sons. The proposed home would provide free lodgings until they "can find themselves a niche in the business world." Recalling the economic hardships that Americans experienced following World War I and prior to World War II, Chung explained, "None of my boys will be forced to sell apples on street corners."[15] Concerned about job prospects for discharged military personnel, she personally sought and "received promises of 20 postwar jobs for her boys."[16] Chung's plan to purchase an estate for the home never materialized, probably due to the cost. Because of her generosity during the war, she faced economic difficulties and maintained ownership of her house only with the financial support of her adopted children.

Unable to realize her goal of a rest center, Chung continued to provide hospitality and maternal comfort for her sons at her home. She sustained her schedule of weekly parties. These events, at first well attended but increasingly less so, served as reunions for military personnel, some of whom had retired and returned to civilian life after the war. As Chung's sons turned their attention to their own conjugal and biological families, their surrogate mother became less central in their lives. However, just as Chung insisted on maintaining her professional career, even in a limited capacity, she persisted in her maternal responsibilities. She left instructions to her sisters to always welcome any of her adopted children to her home on Masonic Avenue, even after her death.

Chung maintained an active social life during the post-World War II era. She continued corresponding, and as late as December 1954, she still sent out thousands of Christmas presents.[17] In addition to hosting friends and family members in San Francisco, she traveled frequently throughout the country. She also continued attending concerts and plays, enjoying the talents and company of her celebrity adoptees. As she became increasingly ill, her children, including conductor Andre Kostelanetz and opera singer Girgio Tozzi, visited and even performed by her bedside.[18] She maintained her close friendship with Sophie Tucker. When the singer came to San Francisco to perform, Chung moved into Tucker's hotel suite, explaining, "My doctors insist I work only two hours a day and keep regular hours. . . . But they's [sic] be crazy if they think I can keep regular hours with Sophie Tucker in town."[19] Following Chung's death, Tucker planted trees in Israel in honor of her friend.[20]

In her rounds of socializing following the war, Chung frequently was accompanied by two of her favorite companions, Mickey Hamilton and a pet parakeet named Sweetheart. Sweetheart, reportedly housebroken, attended social functions with Chung, frequently perched on her glasses or transported in a cage with its own ermine cape covering.[21] Mickey, daughter of an adopted son and a Kiwi in her own right since her first birthday in 1941, stayed with Chung frequently throughout her childhood.[22]

Chung's statements and activities during this period of her life reveal her enthusiasm for memorializing the accomplishments of the war generation. She began writing her autobiography with the encouragement of her adopted children. She jokingly complained that actress Ruth Chatterton, scholar Carl Van Doren, and his wife Jean "practically nagged and brow beat me into writing this book."[23]

In her memoirs, Chung used her life and accomplishments as a tribute to America. In recounting the hardships of her childhood and education, she did not discuss structural discrimination against women and racial minorities. Instead, she emphasized the rewards of hard work and diligence. Her patriotism and idealism explain her decision to focus most of the manuscript on her adopted sons and her war activities. She wrote one and a half chapters on her early childhood, education, and early medical career. The remaining five and a half chapters traced the development of her surrogate family, her role in recruiting the Flying Tigers, and her support for the WAVES. In describing the manuscript, Chung sometimes even eclipsed herself as a subject, referring to the work as "a book about my beloved sons, as a tribute to each one of you who fought so valiantly in this last war."[24] This characterization, along with the contents of the manuscript, indicates that she viewed her maternal identity as the most important or at least the most marketable aspect of herself. As a surrogate Chinese American mother, she touched the lives of others and engaged in the most significant political events of her time.

Reports of book and movie contracts for Chung's autobiography circulated in the newspapers and among her circle of friends and family members. Both MGM and Twentieth-Century-Fox reportedly approached her about the memoir. One newspaper even indicated that Barbara Stanwyck had expressed interest in portraying Chung.[25] In the end, neither a book nor a biographical movie resulted from all the discussions and speculations.

Chung's inability to find a forum to publicize her life story seems puzzling considering her extensive entertainment industry contacts and her wartime fame. The reticence of book publishers and movie producers probably stemmed from the altered political culture of the Cold War, which valued different types of role models from those of the Sino-Japanese conflict and World War II.

During the 1930s and the first half of the 1940s, Chung achieved prominence as a symbol for U.S.-China unity. She even inspired a fictional movie based on her life as well as a comic book biography. In 1939, Paramount released *King of Chinatown*, starring Chung's friend Anna May Wong as an idealistic Chinese American surgeon committed to helping war-torn China. Although made and released before the United States officially entered the war, the film reflected the growing support among mainstream Americans for China. Prior to the Sino-Japanese War, depictions of Chinese in U.S. popular culture tended to emphasize their servility, depravity, and foreignness. Anna May Wong's early movie career, in which she played evil, exotic, enslaved, and sensual women, reflected and reinforced the mainstream perception of Asians as threatening foreigners incapable of assimilation. However, Japan's invasion of Manchuria and the publication of Pearl S. Buck's *The Good Earth* aroused American concern for the plight of China.[26] Sympathetic portrayals of the Chinese increasingly appeared in movies. Although these roles tended to be played by white actors in "yellowface" makeup, Asian American actors and actresses like Wong also had opportunities to portray noble leading characters.

The fictional character based on Margaret Chung, Dr. Mary Ling, is a respected surgeon who seeks to give up her successful career in the United States to offer her services to China. However, she becomes ensnared in an attempted murder investigation and a romantic triangle involving a Chinese American lawyer and a European ethnic crime boss. Ironically, the plot device illustrates the dilemmas that Chung herself faced. In the movie, Ling, despite her professional status, spends much of her time caring for her patient and potential lover in a manner reminiscent of a domestic servant.[27] Similarly, Chung achieved her greatest accolades not as the first known American-born Chinese female physician but as a hostess and surrogate mother. She, like Ling, developed feelings for an individual of European ethnic background, but for a female rather than a male.[28] The film's ending, with Ling marrying her Chinese American fiancé and traveling to China, closes off the transgressive possibilities in the plotline. The conclusion affirms the desirability of marriage between people of the same ethnicity and class status. The movie also emphasizes that Chinese Americans, no matter how American, belong in their ancestral homelands. The fictional character Mary Ling accomplished what Margaret Chung was unwilling and unable to do. Chung never fulfilled her dream of going to China. She also refused to accede to the social demands for a respectable marriage.

In addition to the film inspired by Chung's life, *Real Heroes,* a comic book series, featured a story on her in 1943.[29] During the late 1930s and first half of the 1940s, described as a "Golden Age" for comics, the genre achieved widespread popularity.[30] Sales averaged 200,000 to 400,000 copies per issue, not only for "superhero" comics but also for publications that featured "true adventure" stories. From 1941 to 1946, Parent's Magazine Press cashed in on this multi-million-dollar industry by publishing a series entitled *Real Heroes,* which promised stories "not about impossible supermen, but about real-life heroes and heroines."[31]

Seeking to promote role models for young boys and girls, the comic book featured the lives of famous politicians, military leaders, reformers, musicians, and scientists. Although most of the featured heroes tended to be white men, the accomplishments and experiences of women and people of color also appeared in the segments. The racial and gender inclusivity of *Real Heroes* reflected the wartime context. By 1943, the publication date of Chung's comic book biography, not only had the United States entered into an alliance with China, but Madame Chiang Kai-Shek was making public appearances throughout the country, calling for increased attention to and resources for the war in the Pacific.[32] Her unprecedented address before both houses of Congress on 18 February 1943 aroused strong support for China and eventually led to the repeal of the Chinese Exclusion Act of 1882. Just as government propaganda emphasized the need to involve all Americans—men and women, whites and nonwhites, in the war effort—so *Real Heroes* attempted to inculcate those values in its young readers by featuring individuals like Margaret Chung. Because comic books tended to be popular among military personnel as well, the biography of Chung found a receptive audience.

The comic book version of Chung's life surprisingly captured some of the complexities of her identity but also exaggerated certain facets of her persona to fulfill wartime propagandistic needs. For example, while *Real Heroes* depicted Chung's efforts to enter the American professional class through her educational achievements, it also tended to highlight her difference from the mainstream. In the very first frame, her name appears in bold, Chinese calligraphy-like brush strokes next to a picture of a jade Buddha. Although Chung adopted self-Orientalizing strategies to enhance her value to white America, the comic book version exceeded her actual practices. Whereas Chung wore Western clothing, her character appears in Chinese costume in almost every panel. Furthermore, the biography identified where Chung resided as a child but did not specify the location of her birth. Published before the repeal of the Chinese Exclusion Act, the comic book chose not to include information that would clearly mark Chung as an American citizen. Instead, the publication created a version of Chung that evoked stereotypical tropes associated with the Orient for its intended mainstream audience.

The comic book also tended to reinforce conventional gender roles. On the one hand, the biography gave some attention to Chung's medical career. It also depicted her adopted sons engaged in domestic duties under her supervision, such as washing and mending their clothes,

activities that no doubt resonated with the military audience of the publication. On the other hand, the biography underscored the message
that Chung's most important accomplishments stemmed from her
maternal identity. As in her eventual autobiography, much of the comic
book segment featured Chung performing traditionally female responsibilities, such as serving food and nursing her sons. In addition, the
comic book sought to encourage its young readers to admire Chung for
her presumed physical beauty. The real Chung did alter her appearance
to emulate feminine standards of attractiveness. However, she did not
achieve what the comic book depicted. During the 1930s and 1940s,
Chung was a large person and in her forties and fifties. The illustrator
drew her as a relatively young and very slender woman.

The comic book version of Chung, like the Hollywood rendition, tit-
illated the intended audience of predominantly male adolescents and
military personnel with the possibility of interracial romance. In the
drawings, she appears as an attractive Chinese woman surrounded by
similarly aged, good-looking white men. However, just as Chung chose
to cultivate an asexual image to deter social criticism, the comic
affirmed the platonic nature of her relationship with her sons. Instead of
using the phrase "Fair-Haired Bastards," the publisher adopted the
more respectable term "Foster Sons."

The portrayals that Chung inspired during the 1930s and World War II
explain why she increasingly received less attention during the late
1940s and 1950s. Cold War hostilities complicated American attitudes
toward China and people of Chinese ancestry. While the public recognized a distinction between Nationalist and Communist China, there
also was a tendency to suspect all Chinese, including those with
American citizenship, as agents of the Red Menace. With Chinese soldiers fighting American troops in Korea and threatening to invade other
Asian nations, anti-Chinese sentiment, fostered by the "red" hysteria of
the 1950s, was comparable to anti-Japanese attitudes of World War II.

Government documents reveal that Cold War politics influenced
perceptions of Chung. A 1953 report to the Department of Justice inti-
mates that she supported a front organization for the Communist Party
because of her sponsorship of a 1947 fund-raising event for Spanish
refugees who had fought against fascism.[33] The State Department also
denied her 1947 request for a passport to travel to Europe. No clear
explanation was given for the refusal, although the paperwork indicates
that Chung was "now under investigation" and instructed that future
inquiries should be referred to the "Fraud Section."[34] The surveillance

and portrayal of her activities resonate with the increased suspicion of Chinese people during the postwar era. In this context, the movie industry and book publishers chose not to promote Chung as a symbol of American patriotism or a friendly China.

Furthermore, Chung's maternal persona, so useful for her efforts to negotiate social expectations in the earlier era, diverged from Cold War depictions of Asia. Following World War II, popular plays and films like *South Pacific,* one of Chung's personal favorites, explicitly portrayed Asian women as love interests of American GIs and Asian children as adoptees for white mother figures. These cultural representations both promoted and encouraged acceptance of the postwar trends of interracial marriage and transnational adoption. These new configurations of family also reinforced a self-serving image of the United States. As a liberal, democratic, and prosperous nation, America could nurture the victims and outcasts of Asia and incorporate them into the U.S. national family.[35] In the interracial and international family of the Cold War, there was little room for someone like Chung. In reality, she chose not to be a love interest to a white man. She also claimed the authority of motherhood for herself. Her public persona, which had provided comfort during World War II, seemed like an indirect challenge to white paternalism and maternalism during the Cold War. And if Chung's homoerotic relationships with white women had been more widely known, her life might have gained notoriety but not respectability in the midst of the homosexual witchhunts of the 1950s.

While Chung received little popular attention due to the reconfiguration of social hierarchies during the Cold War, her neglect in academic circles stems from different political reasons. Chung died just as the mass movements of the postwar period began to transform American social attitudes and practices about race, gender, and sexuality. Inspired by the politics of the Civil Rights and 1960s eras, the scholarly fields that emerged in the following decades called for more innovative and inclusive studies that would recognize the diversity of American society. Chung, however, did not interest academics in the fields of women's, Asian American, and what would become known as sexuality studies. Instead of focusing on exceptional individuals, the early works in these subjects sought to recover the lives of everyday, and especially working-class, people. Seeking to promote group solidarity among oppressed groups, scholars called attention to the structural forces that fostered systems of inequality in American society. They were less concerned with elite individuals, including extraordinary minorities or women, who appeared to have "sold out" or who identified with the dominant culture. Furthermore, racial bias in women's and sexuality studies as well as gender and heteronormative bias in ethnic studies combined to result in few studies regarding women of color who sought alternatives to heterosexuality.

While Chung's life could be interpreted as a model of assimilation and integration, her achievements derived from an ability to reconcile symbolically contradictory social roles. As she attempted to transcend certain gender boundaries and sexual norms, she also embraced a traditional female identity of asexual motherhood. Chung devoted her life to China and Chinese American communities. At the same time, she felt more comfortable in the company of European Americans and catered to their fantasies about the Orient. Her adoption of multiple identities allowed her to develop alliances and create opportunities across social divides. However, her personal strategies ultimately could not transform her liminal status into complete acceptance.

Throughout her life, Margaret Chung displayed a keen awareness of the need to create certain types of identities to fulfill the desires of her audience. Even her funeral demonstrated this sense of performance. Chung died on 5 January 1959, at the age of sixty-nine. She had been aware of her impending death. In August of 1958, she underwent an operation at Franklin Hospital in San Francisco to treat ovarian cancer, an illness that tends to afflict childless women. A month later, her adopted son Vice Admiral Charles Lockwood recorded a visit to her in his diary: "Shoved off and called on Mom Chung at 0930. Found her in good spirits but looking very badly . . . She says that she has 5 months to live but she's not perturbed by it."[36] Preparing for her death, Chung made the arrangements for her funeral. One of her friends described and reflected upon the experience in a diary: Margaret "had planned it just as she wanted it. The music was light opera followed by hymn tunes. The minister sincere and a good speaker."[37] Chung's selection of music reflected her early religious training as well as her love of classical music. Her maternal authority and influence were displayed by the presence of her pallbearers; all white men, they included an ensign and two privates as well as two admirals and the mayor of San Francisco.[38] The diversity of rank among the pallbearers, along with their sameness in race and gender, communicated Chung's ability to inspire individuals from different backgrounds as well as her success in gaining the respect of the central members of the American polity.

As she planned her final performance, Margaret Chung most likely anticipated the impact of her death on the people who would come to pay their respects. She would have been pleased by the observations that she inspired. On her medical certificate, the attending physician, a friend as well as a male doctor who was most likely white, indicated her "color or race" as "white."[39] Never completely successful in her efforts to "pass" during her life, Chung finally attained whiteness in death. At the same time, others viewed her as a symbol of the diversity of the American people. The wife of Admiral Nimitz recorded in her diary that "all creeds, all colors, all types of people, rich and poor came to pay homage."[40] Two days after the funeral, Lockwood reflected on Chung's uniqueness as an individual. In his journal, he represented her death as the close of "a very delightful and inspiring chapter in our lives. God bless and rest her very beautiful soul. There will never be another Mom Chung."[41]

Acknowledgments

Reflecting on my motivations for writing a biography of Dr. Margaret Chung (1889–1959), I immediately think of a cartoon displayed in the halls of my graduate history department. The maître d' of a fine dining establishment, accepting a reservation over the phone, asks for clarification of the caller's title: "Is that a *real* doctor, or just a PhD?" The social respect accorded to physicians is one of the reasons that my parents, like many other Americans of Asian ancestry, encouraged their children to pursue medicine as a career. Formerly health professionals in Taiwan, my parents experienced the common immigrant phenomenon of occupational downgrading. In the United States, they worked long hours in restaurants and convenience stores to finance their children's education. Because of these hardships, they valued the prestige and economic security associated with the medical profession. While my brother became a dentist, I, always the more rebellious one, chose to pursue my interest in the humanities. In college, I enrolled in the minimum number of science courses to fulfill graduation requirements. I thought of myself as marching to the beat of a different drummer and looked with disdain upon students who were preparing for medical school. To me, they represented the conventional, the status-hungry, the obedient ones.

I first discovered Margaret Chung through the recommendation of Wei-chi Poon, librarian of the Asian American Studies Collection in the Ethnic Studies Library at the University of California, Berkeley. Because of my interest in U.S. gender and race relations, Poon suggested that I examine the Margaret Chung Collection and write her life story. The collection, which includes an unpublished autobiography, reveals that Chung could not easily be categorized as conventional. Her life experiences challenged me to rethink my understanding of the past.

Biography is in many ways a foreign genre to me. Before I decided to write about Margaret Chung, I seldom read biographies for professional or personal interest. As my project progressed, I encountered two central challenges. First, because of my training in social history, I wanted my study of Chung to illuminate broader trends in U.S. history. At first glance, this seemed rather difficult. The existing studies on Asian American women tend to emphasize class exploitation, racial segregation, and gender oppression, especially during the years before World War II. Chung's ability to transcend social boundaries made her seem like a historical anomaly. She appeared to be an exceptional, elite individual, not at all "representative" of other Asian American women. However, a closer examination of Chung's life and a more nuanced understanding of historical changes allowed me to use her experiences as a window onto the shifting margins and changing mainstreams of American society.

Second, I needed to bring my subject to life. A more experienced biographer once asked if I was trying to write a history or a biography. When I replied, "both," she explained that I might have to choose between the two. This book is my attempt to weave together history and biography. I tried to balance academic analysis with a more empathetic approach that would allow me to understand and portray Chung as a person. My training as a historian helped me to gather and scrutinize the variety of sources about Chung's life. While her own autobiography was an invaluable source, I frequently discovered that materials found outside of her collection were equally if not more illuminating. In addition to the textual sources, visual portraits of Chung offered fascinating insights into her consciously crafted public personas. To convey the complexities of Chung's identity in an accessible manner, I relinquished some conventional ways of writing scholarly monographs. The end result, I hope, is a book that engages readers in the life and times of Margaret Chung.

It has been a much longer journey than I anticipated, and I owe thanks to many who helped me along the way. I am grateful to Margaret Chung for having lived such a rich and unusual life. I particularly want to thank her family and friends, who shared their intimate memories of her and encouraged my interest with their fond and friendly curiosity.

Clifford and Dorothy Yip initially put me in contact with the rest of the Chung family. Rodney Low, who grew up with "Auntie Doc," generously shared his stories and family mementos. Gilbert and Kay Siu kindly gave me permission to examine the private papers of Dorothy Siu, Margaret's youngest sister, who died shortly before I began my research. Elmo Gambarano, a longtime friend of Dorothy's, not only helped me sort through her collection but also restored my flagging energies by serving tea and cookies. I was fortunate to have the opportunity to interview Lucile Chung, Margaret's sister-in-law, before her death. Roger Chung, William Chung, and Patricia and Harry Mixer also freely offered their time and memories. Terry Cimino, the granddaughter of Dorothy Siu, greatly assisted my efforts to complete the book manuscript by locating photographs and encouraging me with her enthusiasm.

Members of Margaret Chung's adopted family, including Dick Bingham, Betsy Bingham Davis, Craig Clark, Guy Clark, Norman Clerk, Eleanor and Kenneth Eymann, Bob Flowers, John Garling, Elizabeth Peck Hutchins, Dick Rossi, Dick and Barbara Sewall, Karen Garling Sickel, Vincent Turner, and Bill Wildey, shared their affectionate stories of "Mom Chung." It is a testament to her that many of these individuals, the children of her adopted children, have such glowing and warm memories of her. In fact, several sought me out to learn more about their adopted "grandmother." I particularly want to thank Gail Dormer Smith, who vividly brought Margaret Chung to life for me.

I benefited tremendously from the perceptive insights of numerous scholars. My dissertation advisors, Gordon Chang and Estelle Freedman, continue to offer not only intellectual and professional guidance but also personal support. Mary Louise Roberts kindly served on my committee and made valuable suggestions to develop my ideas about history and biography. The Stanford Women's History Workshop and the Biographers' Group also provided helpful forums for my research. I am grateful for the support of my former graduate student colleagues, many of whom continue to serve as mentors and fellow commiserators as we advance along our respective careers. I especially want to thank Jennifer Gee, who offered insightful comments for my manuscript, brought important documents to my attention, and, most importantly, reminded me to keep a sense of humor and perspective about this endeavor.

Peggy Pascoe and Judy Yung encouraged my interest in Margaret Chung and also directed me to valuable primary sources. Carson Anderson, Randy Carol Balano, Linda Bentz, Nan Alamilla Boyd, Roberta S. Greenwood, Bert Hansen, Chad Heap, Gregory Kimm, and

Him Mark Lai generously shared their research as well. I thank Rachel
Buff, Susan K. Cahn, Nancy Cott, Evelyn Nakano Glenn, Eric Goldstein,
Gayatri Gopinath, Shirley Hune, Victor Jew, Moon-Ho Jung, Tom
Klubock, Shawn Lahr, Bob Lee, Karen Leong, Shirley Jennifer Lim, Mary
Lui, Valerie Matsumoto, Mae Ngai, Gail Nomura, Gary Okihiro, Liz
Pleck, Leslie J. Reagan, David Roediger, Vicki Ruiz, Nayan Shah, Susan
L. Smith, Marc Stein, Jack Tchen, K. Scott Wong, Alice Yang-Murray,
and Henry Yu for their insightful comments on my work.

Since I arrived at Ohio State University, my intellectual and social life
has been greatly enriched by my faculty and student colleagues. In particular, I thank Steve Conn, Mark Grimsley, and David Hoffmann for
helping me negotiate the sometimes challenging transition to life as a
faculty member. Victoria Getis and Kevin Boyle, two of the most recent
additions to the OSU history community, have been most generous with
their time and suggestions. I also have benefited tremendously from the
community of women's historians, particularly Susan Freeman, Stephanie
Gilmore, Donna Guy, Susan Hartmann, Heather Miller, Carla Pestana,
Leila Rupp, Birgitte Soland, and other members of the OSU Women's
History Workshop. My research assistants, Kevin Fujitani, Choon Kun
Lee, Takashi Nishiyama, and Christianna Thomas, patiently tracked down
sources, made countless copies, and offered valuable suggestions for my
manuscript. I particularly want to recognize the members of the history
department's "first book club," Leslie Alexander, Nick Breyfogle, Robin
Judd, and Lucy Murphy. The stimulating conversations over fabulous
meals have improved the quality of my work as well as my life at OSU.

Many colleagues and friends outside of the history department also
offered their support and intellectual firepower. I thank Sam Choi,
Mary Margaret Fonow, Ken Goings, Logan Hill, Jill Lane, Pamela
Paxton, Kira Sanbonmatsu, and Barry Shank for helping me think
through difficult issues. Members of the Asian American Studies Reading Group—Oona Besman, Roland Sintos Coloma, Kristina de los
Santos, Jeong-Eun Rhee, Binaya Subedi, and especially Steve Yao—
fostered a politically as well as intellectually supportive community at
OSU. Roland also patiently and carefully proofread and helped to index
this manuscript.

I would not have been able to devote my time and energies to writing
this biography without receiving generous financial and emotional support. I thank the Andrew W. Mellon Foundation for providing a
summer research/travel grant as well as a dissertation award, Stanford
University for the Graduate Research Opportunity Fund, the American

Historical Association for the Albert J. Beveridge Grant, the Stanford Institute for Research on Women and Gender for the Graduate Dissertation Fellowship Award, the Margaret Chase Smith Library's Ada Leeke Fellowship, and the Ohio State University for the Humanities Fellowship, the Seed Grant Program, the Grant-in-Aid fellowship, and the Elizabeth D. Gee Fund for Research on Women. I also benefited tremendously from unofficial subsidies by friends and relatives who provided free food, transportation, and lodgings! Pat Anderson, the captain of my tennis team, offered enthusiastic support for my intellectual as well as athletic endeavors.

I also want to thank the wonderful editors at the University of California Press, Monica McCormick, Randy Heyman, and Mary Severance, who have guided and supported me in the publication process. I've particularly enjoyed conversing with Monica at various conferences during the past few years. Her enthusiasm and probing questions encouraged me to rethink and rewrite my manuscript. I also want to express my appreciation to the reviewers for their critical and helpful comments. I was very fortunate to have Sue Carter as my copy-editor. She not only sharpened my analysis and writing but also contributed her keen insights about Mom Chung.

Finally, I want to acknowledge those who are closest to my heart. I owe almost all of my accomplishments to my parents, Betty Chao-Hua Huang Wu and John Yu-Pu Wu. Although I disregarded their advice in my career choice and in many other matters, they continue to express their unwavering love and support. As we all grow older, I gain greater appreciation for their ability to make difficult life transitions with energy and patience. Christel and Manfred Walter are ideal parents-in-law who have welcomed me warmly into their family. They also offered their physical and creative energies to help us create and maintain our home. From Christel, I have learned valuable skills that helped me to survive the writing process, namely the ability to quilt and knit. My life partner, Mark, has put up with my foul moods as well as my giddy exuberance ever since we met at faculty orientation. He first attracted me with his smooth tennis strokes, homemade cookies, and shy but sharp sense of humor. His own professional dedication also reminds me of the fulfillment that one can achieve through discipline and hard work. I look forward to sharing the next stage of our lives together, namely the adventures of parenthood.

Notes

INTRODUCTION

1. The following works include discussions of Margaret Chung as part of broader studies. See Judy Yung, *Unbound Feet: A Social History of Chinese Women in San Francisco* (Berkeley and London: University of California Press, 1995); Yung, *Unbound Voices: A Documentary History of Chinese Women in San Francisco* (Berkeley and London: University of California Press, 1999); and Leila J. Rupp, *A Desired Past: A Short History of Same-Sex Love in America* (Chicago: University of Chicago Press, 1999).

2. For overviews of Asian American history, see Ronald Takaki, *Strangers from a Different Shore: A History of Asian Americans* (Boston: Little, Brown, 1989); and Sucheng Chan, *Asian Americans: An Interpretive History* (Boston: Twayne Publishers, 1991).

3. In her study of Chinese women in San Francisco, Judy Yung notes that 1.7 percent of the foreign-born women and 0.6 percent of the native-born worked as teachers, nurses/midwives, or in another professional occupation in 1900. By 1920, the numbers had risen to 3.9 and 4.4 percent, respectively. See Yung, *Unbound Feet,* p. 299.

4. For a sample of the extensive scholarship on the concept of separate spheres, see the following: Barbara Welter, "The Cult of True Womanhood, 1820–1860," *American Quarterly* 18, no. 2 (Summer 1966): 151–74; Nancy Cott, *The Bonds of Womanhood: "Woman's Sphere" in New England, 1780–1835* (New Haven, Conn.: Yale University Press, 1977); and Linda Kerber, "Separate Spheres, Female Worlds, Woman's Place: The Rhetoric of Women's History," *Journal of American History* 75, no. 1 (June 1988): 9–39.

5. This work is inspired by the methodologies of the "new biography." Traditional biographies, closely associated with a triumphant narrative of history, focused on the public accomplishments of prominent individuals, most

of whom were elite men. The new biographies incorporate the approaches developed by new social history, ethnic studies, women's studies, and gay/lesbian studies. These works are more likely to focus on lesser known individuals, especially those who experienced marginalization. The new biographies also highlight the importance of gender, sexuality, race, and class as significant categories that shape the identities and experiences of their subjects. Furthermore, some authors incorporate postmodernist theories regarding the conception of self by emphasizing the constructed and fragmented nature of identity. See the following: Sara Alpern, Joyce Antler, Elisabeth Israels Perry, and Ingrid Winther Scobie, eds., *The Challenge of Feminist Biography: Writing the Lives of Modern American Women* (Urbana: University of Illinois Press, 1992); Teresa Iles, ed., *All Sides of the Subject: Women and Biography* (New York: Teachers College Press, 1992); Linda Wagner-Martin, *Telling Women's Lives: The New Biography* (New Brunswick, N.J.: Rutgers University Press, 1994); Gwendolyn Etter-Lewis and Michéle Foster, *Unrelated Kin: Race and Gender in Women's Personal Narratives* (New York: Routledge, 1996); Jo Burr Margadant, ed., *The New Biography: Performing Femininity in Nineteenth-Century France* (Berkeley and London: University of California Press, 2000); and Jill Lepore, "Historians Who Love Too Much: Reflections on Microhistory and Biography," *Journal of American History* 88, no. 1 (June 2001): 129–44.

6. For a sample of the extensive literature on maternalism, see Seth Koven and Sonya Michel, *Mothers of a New World: Maternalist Politics and the Origins of Welfare States* (New York: Routledge, 1993).

7. The Margaret Chung Collection, which includes an unpublished autobiography, is housed in the Asian American Studies Collection, Ethnic Studies Library, University of California, Berkeley.

CHAPTER 1: "THE MEDICAL LADY MISSIONARY"

1. The total number of missionaries who served abroad grew from 934 in 1890 to over 9,000 in 1915. American women constituted the majority, in some countries nearly two thirds, of the missionaries stationed abroad. Their endeavors were supported by female missionary societies in the United States that by 1915 had grown to 3 million members. See Patricia R. Hill, *The World Their Household: The American Woman's Foreign Mission Movement and Cultural Transformation, 1870–1920* (Ann Arbor: University of Michigan Press, 1985), p. 3.

2. Mrs. P.D. Browne, "The President's Address: Are Foreign Missions a Success," *Tenth Annual Report of the Occidental Board of the Woman's Foreign Missionary Society of the Presbyterian Church of the Pacific Coast* (San Francisco: A.J. Leary, 1883), p. 15.

3. I thank Peggy Pascoe for generously sharing the findings of her research on the Chinese Presbyterian Mission Home in San Francisco. She identified Chung's mother as Ah Yane. Chung's mother used several different names with various spellings. During her stay at the Chinese Presbyterian Mission Home, she was referred to as Ah Yane or A Yane. On official documents after her marriage, she identified herself as Minnie and her maiden name as Chin or Chan.

4. Judy Yung, *Unbound Feet: A Social History of Chinese Women in San Francisco* (Berkeley and London: University of California Press, 1995), pp. 29 and 32.

5. Sucheng Chan, "The Exclusion of Chinese Women, 1870–1943," in *Entry Denied: Exclusion and the Chinese Community in America, 1882–1943,* edited by Sucheng Chan (Philadelphia: Temple University Press, 1991), pp. 94–146.

6. Margaret Chung, who filled out her mother's death certificate in 1914, had no knowledge—not even the names—of her mother's parents (Los Angeles County, "Certificate of Death for Minnie Chung," Local Register No. 3466). Margaret's youngest sister, Dorothy, claimed that their mother's mother resided in the United States. This is not verified by other sources. Ah Yane passed away when Dorothy was just six years old. (Dorothy Siu, Oral History, interviewed by Jean Wong, 12 January 1979 and 6 November 1980, in *Southern California Chinese American Oral History Project,* Department of Special Collections, University Research Library, University of California, Los Angeles.)

7. There is some uncertainty about when Ah Yane arrived at the Mission Home. An account published in 1884 dates her arrival in October 1880. However, she first makes an appearance in the *Occidental Board Annual Report* in 1882, suggesting that she may have entered the Mission Home in 1881. See "Report of the Mission Home," *Ninth Annual Occidental Board Report* (1882), p. 14; "Mission Home," *Eleventh Annual Occidental Board Report* (1884), p. 24; and Chun Fah to Mr. Hunter, *Twelfth Annual Occidental Board Report* (1885), p. 58.

8. "Mission Home," *Eleventh Annual Occidental Board Report* (1884), p. 24.

9. Lucie Cheng Hirata, "Free, Indentured, Enslaved: Chinese Prostitutes in Nineteenth-Century America," *Signs* (Autumn 1979): 4.

10. Yung, *Unbound Feet,* p. 37. Yung argues that the numbers of *mui tsai* were probably undercounted by the 1870 census, which lists only "2 percent of Chinese women . . . as 'young servants.'"

11. Ibid., p. 39.

12. "Report of the Mission Home," *Ninth Annual Occidental Board Report* (1882), p. 14.

13. Dorothy recalled that she spoke the Sze Yup dialect with her family. Chinese immigrants from the Sze Yup region constituted a group with fewer resources than those from the Sam Yup region. Whereas the former became laborers, domestic servants, and small shop owners, the latter became important merchants within the Chinese American community. See Sucheng Chan, *This Bitter-Sweet Soil: The Chinese in California Agriculture, 1860–1910* (Berkeley and London: University of California Press, 1986), p. 18.

14. On Chung Wong's death certificate, his oldest son, Andrew, indicated that he did know the names of his father's parents. Los Angeles County, "Certificate of Death for Chung Wong," Local Register No. 5665. Dorothy Siu recalled that the family did not know of any relatives in China until the late 1920s: "Someone went to my sister the doctor in San Francisco and told her they had found our grandmother. I think on my father's side in China, and that

she was very poor. So my sister gave him some money to give her. Then later we found out our grandmother was dead and this guy was just pocketing the money." Dorothy Siu, Oral History.

15. Ira M. Condit to F. F. Ellinwood, 7 February 1887, Board of Foreign Missions (PCUSA) Secretaries' Files, 1829–1895, Record Group 31, box 45, folder 16, Presbyterian Historical Society, Philadelphia. These files will be hereafter cited as BFMSF. The Presbyterian Historical Society will be referred to as PHS.

16. Margaret Culbertson came west from New York State in 1878 and became the first superintendent of the Presbyterian Chinese Mission Home in 1881. Margaret Culbertson Biographical File, PHS.

17. Peggy Pascoe, *Relations of Rescue: The Search for Female Moral Authority in the American West, 1874–1939* (New York: Oxford University Press, 1990), p. 104.

18. "Report of the Mission Home," *Ninth Annual Occidental Board Report* (1882), p. 14.

19. For a discussion of the multiple meanings of motherhood, see Pascoe, *Relations of Rescue*, pp. 103–4.

20. Chun Fah to Mr. Hunter, *Twelfth Annual Occidental Board Report* (1885), p. 58.

21. "Mission Home," *Eleventh Annual Occidental Board Report* (1884), p. 24.

22. Ah Yane to Mr. Hunter, 3 March 1885, published in *Twelfth Occidental Board Report* (1885), p. 59.

23. Pascoe, *Relations of Rescue*, p. 108.

24. Margaret Culbertson, "Mission Home," *Fourteenth Occidental Board Report* (1887), p. 42.

25. Pascoe, *Relations of Rescue*, p. 113.

26. Ah Yane, "Report of 'The Tong Oke' or Light House Band," *Thirteenth Occidental Board Report* (1886), p. 55.

27. For accounts of Ah Yane's services as an interpreter, see Culbertson, "Report of Mission Home," *Thirteenth Occidental Board Report* (1886), pp. 47–49; Culbertson, "Report of Mission Home," *Fifteenth Occidental Board Report* (1888), pp. 54–56; and Culbertson, "Report of Chinese Mission Home," *Sixteenth Occidental Board Report* (1889), pp. 48–49.

28. Culbertson, "Report of Mission Home," *Fifteenth Occidental Board Report* (1888), p. 56.

29. Culbertson, "Report of Mission Home," *Thirteenth Annual Occidental Board Report* (1886), p. 41.

30. "Chinese in America Annual Report," 1 December 1915 to 30 November 1916, The United Presbyterian Church in the United States of America Commission on Ecumenical Mission and Relations, Secretaries Files, RG 81, box 1, folder 2, PHS.

31. Missionary activity in China peaked in the 1920s with an estimated 6,500 individuals stationed there. Of that total, approximately 70 percent were American and 60 percent were women. An estimated total of 50,000

missionaries served in China from 1809 to 1949. Kathleen L. Lodwick, *Educating the Women of Hainan: The Career of Margaret Moninger in China, 1915–1942* (Lexington: University Press of Kentucky, 1995), p. 2 and footnote 3.

32. Ira M. Condit and Alexander J. Kerr, "To the General Assembly of the Presbyterian Church in Saratoga Convened" [May 1884], BFMSF, RG 31, box 45, folder 12, PHS.

33. Culbertson, "Our City of Refuge," *Occidental Leaves* (San Francisco, 1893), p. 18.

34. Culbertson, "Mission Home," *Eleventh Annual Occidental Board Report* (1884), p. 25.

35. Peggy Pascoe, "Gender Systems in Conflict: The Marriages of Mission-Educated Chinese American Women, 1874–1939," in *Unequal Sisters: A Multicultural Reader in U.S. Women's History*, edited by Ellen Carol DuBois and Vicki L. Ruiz (New York: Routledge, 1990): 123–40.

36. Ah Yane to President et al., *The Occident*, 12 December 1888, p. 11.

37. Culbertson, "Report of Chinese Mission Home," *Sixteenth Annual Occidental Board Report* (1889), p. 50.

38. "Monthly Meeting of the Occidental Board," *The Occident*, 14 May 1890, p. 11.

39. "Items from Santa Barbara," *Occidental Leaves* (1893), p. 48.

40. Margaret Chung, "Autobiography," Margaret Chung Collection, box 1, folder 1, Asian American Studies Collection, Ethnic Studies Library, University of California, Berkeley. The collection contains a typed manuscript and some handwritten notes to the autobiography. The unpublished work is not paginated. The collection will hereafter be cited as the Chung Collection, and her autobiography as Chung, "Autobiography."

41. Yong Chen, *Chinese San Francisco, 1850–1943: A Trans-Pacific Community* (Stanford, Calif.: Stanford University Press, 2000), p. 25.

42. Lucy S. Bainbridge, *Woman's Medical Work in Foreign Missions* (New York: Women's Board of Foreign Missions of the Presbyterian Church, 1886), pp. 9, 14.

43. Mrs. J.B. Stewart, "Medical Missions," *Occidental Leaves* (San Francisco, 1893), p. 38.

44. Ibid.

45. Single women, married women, and married men were serving as missionaries in nearly equal numbers in China by 1919. Jane Hunter, *The Gospel of Gentility: American Women Missionaries in Turn-of-the-Century China* (New Haven, Conn.: Yale University Press, 1984), p. 52.

46. Weili Ye, "Crossing the Cultures: The Experience of Chinese Students in the U.S.A., 1900–1925," PhD diss., Yale University, 1989, pp. 263–82. The first Chinese woman to receive a medical degree in the United States, King Ya-Mei (Jin Yunmei), had been adopted as a small child by American missionaries after the death of her Christian parents. She graduated from the Woman's Medical College in New York in 1885 and returned to China under the sponsorship of the Woman's Board of the Dutch Reformed Church in 1888. Other early

Chinese female physicians include Hu King-Eng and Li Bi Cu, who graduated from the Philadelphia Woman's Medical College in 1894 and 1905, respectively, and Mary Stone (Shi Meiyu) and Ida Kahn (Kang Cheng), who graduated from the University of Michigan in 1896. All were members of Chinese Christian families and gained opportunities to study medicine in the United States through their connections with western missionaries. Ida Kahn was also adopted by a missionary. For more information, see Elizabeth Lee Abbott, "Dr. Hu King Eng, Pioneer," in *The Life, Influence and the Role of the Chinese in the United States, 1776–1960* (San Francisco: Chinese Historical Society of America, 1976), pp. 243–49; Margaret E. Burton, *Women Workers of the Orient* (New York: The Woman's Press, 1919).

47. Ellen S. More, *Restoring the Balance: Women Physicians and the Profession of Medicine, 1850–1995* (Cambridge, Mass.: Harvard University Press, 1999), p. 99. After peaking at 6 percent in 1910, the percentage of female physicians in the United States fluctuated between 4 and 5 percent until World War II.

48. For information about La Flesche, see Pascoe, *Relations of Rescue;* and Benson Tong, *Susan La Flesche Picotte, M.D.: Omaha Indian Leader and Reformer* (Norman: University of Oklahoma Press, 1999).

49. Annie M. Houseworth, "Report of Home School," *Fifteenth Annual Occidental Board Report* (1888), p. 61.

50. Minnie Robertson Browne, "Report of Assistant Matron," *Twenty-Second Annual Occidental Board Report* (1895), pp. 55–56.

51. Culbertson, "Annual Report for 1890," *Eighteenth Annual Accidental Board Report* (1891), pp. 48–49.

52. Culbertson, "Report of Missionary," *Twenty-Third Annual Occidental Board Report* (1896), p. 65.

53. Quoted in Isabel Stewart, "Young People's Presbyterial Society of S.F.," *Fourteenth Annual Occidental Board Report* (1887), pp. 33–34.

CHAPTER 2: LIVING THEIR RELIGION

1. Albert Camarillo, *Chicanos in a Changing Society: From Mexican Pueblos to American Barrios in Santa Barbara and Southern California, 1848–1930* (Cambridge, Mass.: Harvard University Press, 1979).

2. New Directory of the City of Santa Barbara (Independent Publishing Co., 1888), p. 144.

3. The Chinese population in Santa Barbara is difficult to determine. The U.S. census lists 227 Chinese in Santa Barbara in 1880, 581 in 1890, and 224 in 1900. Other sources estimate approximately 300 residents in Santa Barbara Chinatown in the 1880s and 700 in the entire city in the late 1800s. See Camarillo, *Chicanos in a Changing Society,* p. 117; Maryann Hellrigel, "A Social History of Presidio Area Occupants 1900 to the Present," in *Santa Barbara Presidio Area 1840 to the Present,* edited by Carl V. Harris, Jarrell C. Jackman, and Catherine Rudolph (Santa Barbara: Presidio Research Center, 1993), p. 28; and Richard Piedmonte, "The Chinese Presidio Community," in *Santa Barbara Presidio Area 1840 to the Present,* pp. 119–20; and Ella Yee Quan,

"Santa Barbara Chinatown: The Early Years," *Gum Saan Journal* 5, no. 2 (November 1982), p. 1.

4. Some of Chung Wong's products, such as the "ladies' underwear," might have catered to the vice economy. Lisa See describes similar stores in the Los Angeles area during the early twentieth century that sold garments to prostitutes. Lisa See, *On Gold Mountain: The One-Hundred-Year Odyssey of My Chinese-American Family* (New York: Vintage Books, 1995).

5. City Directory of Santa Barbara (Press Publishing Co., 1893), p. 82. The next available city directory, published in 1897, lists a Chung Tong residing in Carpenteria and working as a farmer. This could refer to Margaret's father, whose full name is Chung Wong Tong. City Directory of Santa Barbara (W.H. Arne, 1897), p. 113.

6. Office of Collector of Customs, Port of San Francisco, "Chinese Merchants Santa Barbara," 22 August 1894, Santa Barbara Historical Society.

7. Chung, "Autobiography." The words in brackets were crossed out in the handwritten version of the autobiography.

8. "Chinese Woman of Santa Barbara in Fight for Country," Newspaper clipping found in the Margaret Chung file, Santa Barbara Historical Society.

9. Sucheng Chan, *This Bitter-Sweet Soil: The Chinese in California Agriculture, 1860–1910* (Berkeley and London: University of California Press, 1986), pp. 117, 119.

10. Paul Chung was one of the four Chung children who died during infancy.

11. "Chinese Merchants Santa Barbara," p. 32.

12. Ibid., pp. 5, 17. The survey of Chinese merchants refers to an individual named Wong Chong, which most likely referred to Chung Wong.

13. William A. Edwards, "In the Days of Pon Sue," *Noticias* 13, no. 4 (Autumn, 1967).

14. The Mexican American community in Santa Barbara grew from 932 in 1880 to approximately 1,500 in 1900. A controversy over bilingual education in the mid-nineteenth century eventually resulted in the removal of Spanish-speaking students to a parochial day school. See Camarillo, *Chicanos in a Changing Society*, pp. 16–17, 116–17, 200–201.

15. Chung, "Autobiography."

16. Margaret, the eldest, was born in 1889. Dorothy, the youngest, was born in 1908. Other siblings included Bertha Grace (1895), Paul (1897), Andrew (1898), Anna [1899], Virgil [1901], Mildred Venus (1902), and Florence (1903). The dates in brackets indicate an estimated year of birth based on census records. Two other children were born and died with no surviving records of their names.

17. Culbertson left the Presbyterian Chinese Mission Home and San Francisco in 1897 after developing a serious illness. She was replaced by her assistant, Donaldina Cameron, who served as the home's superintendent from 1900 to 1934.

18. "75 years ago," 28 December 1973, clipping found in the archives of the Santa Barbara News Press.

19. Chin Mooie came from an impoverished family in China who decided to send her to the United States to live with her uncle. Because of her uncle's unwillingness to take care of her, Chin Mooie was raised at the Presbyterian Chinese Mission Home. Gregory Kimm, "This Remarkable Couple: The Story of Ng Hon Gim and Chin Mooie," unpublished paper, 1995.

20. Chun Fah to Chin Mooie, 2 October 1893, Ng Family Papers.

21. Kimm, "This Remarkable Couple." The Congregational and Presbyterian churches appeared to cooperate in their mission activities, especially in regions that were sparsely populated by Protestant Christians. During the Chung family's stay in Ventura County, they most likely attended the Chinese Congregational Mission, located in San Buenaventura Chinatown. The mission, established in 1889, was the largest in the county. Although San Buenaventura was relatively far from where the family resided, Margaret Chung recalled that one of her earliest jobs was moving chairs for the Congregational Church.

22. Judy Yung, *Unbound Feet: A Social History of Chinese Women in San Francisco* (Berkeley and London: University of California Press, 1995), pp. 94–95.

23. Peggy Pascoe, *Relations of Rescue: The Search for Female Moral Authority in the American West, 1874–1939* (New York: Oxford University Press, 1990), p. 158.

24. Yung, *Unbound Feet*, pp. 42–43.

25. See, *On Gold Mountain*, discusses women's roles in family businesses. Although she is describing the activities of her white great-grandmother, who married a Chinese merchant, it is likely that Chinese American women assumed similar responsibilities. Lisa See, *On Gold Mountain: The One-Hundred-Year Odyssey of My Chinese-American Family* (New York: Vintage Books, 1995).

26. Tomás Almaguer, *Racial Fault Lines: The Historical Origins of White Supremacy in California* (Berkeley and London: University of California Press, 1994), pp. 75–104; Linda Bentz, "The Overseas Chinese of Ventura," Honors thesis, University of California, Los Angeles, 1994; Roberta S. Greenwood and James J. Schmidt, "Data Recovery at the Soo Hoo Property, Ventura" (Pacific Palisades, Calif.: Greenwood and Associates, 1993); Margaret Jennings, "The Chinese in Ventura County," *Ventura County Historical Society Quarterly* 29, no. 3 (spring 1984): 3–31.

27. The Broome family, who hired Chung Wong, bought the ranch in 1880. William Richard Broome, a native of England, came to Santa Barbara as a health tourist, seeking to recover from tuberculosis. He died in 1891, leaving his ranch to his wife, Frances, and their three children. They apparently had enough respect for Chung Wong's abilities to employ him as a ranch manager rather than as a ranch hand. However, his stay in Ventura County lasted only a couple of years. See Almaguer, *Racial Fault Lines*, p. 76; Mark T. Swanson, "From Spanish Land Grants to World War II: An Overview of Historic Resources at the Naval Air Weapons Station, Point Mugu, California," report prepared for Naval Air Weapons Station, Point Mugu (Tucson: Statistical Research, 1994), p. 15.

28. Chung, "Autobiography."

29. Ibid.

30. Ibid.

31. Ibid.

32. Ibid.

33. Ventura County, Superintendent of Schools Office, San Buena Ventura District Promotion Record 1898–99.

34. From 1873 to 1894, Mexican Americans constituted between 14 and 16 percent of the voting population in Ventura County. Almaguer, *Racial Fault Lines*, p. 87.

35. Ventura County, Superintendent of Schools Office, Ocean View District Promotion Record 1901.

36. Camarillo, *Chicanos in a Changing Society*, p. 200.

37. From 1900 to 1930, the number of Japanese in Los Angeles increased from 150 to 11,000, the number of African Americans grew from 2,000 to nearly 16,000, and the number of Mexican Americans multiplied tenfold, from 3,000–5,000 to 30,000–50,000.

38. George J. Sánchez, *Becoming Mexican American: Ethnicity, Culture and Identity in Chicano Los Angeles, 1900–1945* (New York: Oxford University Press, 1993), p. 87.

39. Chung, "Autobiography."

40. Alan Trachtenberg, *The Incorporation of America: Culture and Society in the Gilded Age* (New York: Hill and Wang, 1982).

41. Sánchez, *Becoming Mexican American*, p. 105.

42. During the late nineteenth century, almost half of the Chinese population in Los Angeles lived in the East Adams area. See Chan, *This Bitter-Sweet Soil*, pp. 117, 119.

43. Small numbers of Chinese began appearing in Los Angeles in the 1850s, mostly in the undesirable vice district known as Negro Alley. The neighborhood was the site of an anti-Chinese riot and massacre in 1871, but the Chinese population continued to reside there. *Linking Our Lives: Chinese American Women of Los Angeles* (Los Angeles: Chinese Historical Society of Southern California, 1984); Raymond Lou, "The Chinese American Community of Los Angeles, 1870–1900: A Case of Resistance, Organization, and Participation," PhD diss., University of California, Irvine, 1982; See, *On Gold Mountain*, pp. 61–65; Kim Fong Tom, "The Participation of the Chinese in the Community Life of Los Angeles" (master's thesis, University of Southern California, 1944; reprint, San Francisco: R and E Research Associates, 1974).

44. Sánchez, *Becoming Mexican American*, pp. 71–75.

45. Eventually, the plans to build a union station near the Plaza area forced the relocation of many Chinese residents and businesses, creating both New Chinatown and China City in the 1930s. Dorothy Siu, Oral History, interviewed by Jean Wong, 12 January 1979 and 6 November 1980, *Southern California Chinese American Oral History Project*, Department of Special Collections, University Research Library, University of California, Los Angeles; Suellen Cheng and Munson Kwok, "The Golden Years of Los Angeles Chinatown: The Beginning," In *Chinatown Los Angeles: The Golden Years, 1938–1988* (Los Angeles: Chinese Chamber of Commerce, 1988), pp. 39–40.

46. Siu, Oral History.

47. Chung, "Autobiography."

48. Ibid.

49. This small percentage is actually more than double the national average of 7 percent. Victoria Bissell Brown, "The Fear of Feminization: Los Angeles High Schools in the Progressive Era," in *Gender and American Law: The Impact of the Law on the Lives of Women,* edited by Karen J. Maschke (New York: Garland Publishing, Inc., 1997), p. 495.

50. "Chinese Girl Enters," newspaper clipping, Ng Family Papers.

51. To prepare those with middle-class ambitions for business and white-collar professions, private business schools were established and commercial courses were introduced into public high schools around the turn of the century. Ironically, the "frontier" West, traditionally a site of opportunity for men, boasted more women in professional and white-collar positions than any other part of the country due to the region's rapid economic growth. See Brown, "The Fear of Feminization," pp. 111–36; John Leslie Rury, "Women, Cities and Schools: Education and the Development of an Urban Female Labor Force, 1890–1930," PhD diss., University of Wisconsin, Madison, 1982.

52. Regina Markell Morantz-Sanchez, *Sympathy and Science: Women Physicians in American Medicine* (New York: Oxford University Press, 1985), p. 107.

53. Dr. Ida V. Stambach began her practice in Santa Barbara the same year that Margaret Chung was born. Stambach is listed on the birth certificates of Bertha Grace Chung, born 14 September 1895, and Paul Chung, born 18 February 1997, both of whom died before adulthood.

54. Helen Satterlee, "The Story of a Persevering Chinese Girl Who Reached the Heights of Surgical Fame," *Los Angeles Times Sunday Magazine,* 25 June 1939.

CHAPTER 3: WHERE WOMANHOOD AND CHILDHOOD MEET

1. It is not clear whether Chung attempted to receive a tuition reduction on the basis of her religious aspirations. During her first year, the cost of her education was $67 for two semesters of tuition plus approximately $20 worth of fees. By her senior year, the tuition had been raised to $80 for two semesters plus the additional fees. Students interested in working for the ministry needed to receive a recommendation from a quarterly conference. For young women, an additional approval from the Conference Board Deaconesses was required. By Chung's senior year, however, only children of ministers received tuition reductions. *University of Southern California Bulletin, College of Liberal Arts Year Book, 1907–1908* (Los Angeles: University of Southern California, 1908), pp. 89 and 188. Hereafter cited as *USC Bulletin.* Also see *USC Bulletin, 1910–1911,* p. 248.

2. The USC School of Medicine was established in 1885 at 445 Aliso Street, on the site of a former vineyard, in downtown Los Angeles just south of the Plaza. In 1896, the school relocated to 737 Buena Vista Street, now North Broadway, just a block or two north of the Plaza. In 1909, the School of

Medicine severed its relationship to the University of Southern California and affiliated instead with the University of California. That same year, USC developed ties with the College of Physicians and Surgeons of Los Angeles. Started in 1903 by Charles W. Bryson, the college was located at 516 East Washington, close to the San Pedro City Market area. *USC Medicine, Centennial Historical Issue* 33, no. 2 (1985): 2–11.

3. Lynn D. Gordon, *Gender and Higher Education in the Progressive Era* (New Haven, Conn.: Yale University Press, 1990), p. 1.

4. I used university bulletins and school annuals to determine the gender and racial composition of Chung's classes.

5. Victoria Bissell Brown, "Golden Girls: Female Socialization in Los Angeles, 1880 to 1910," PhD diss., University of California, San Diego, 1985.

6. It is possible that Chung played in a lower division or recreationally.

7. Victoria Bissell Brown, "The Fear of Feminization: Los Angeles High Schools in the Progressive Era," in *Gender and American Law: The Impact of the Law on the Lives of Women,* edited by Karen J. Maschke (New York: Garland Publishing, Inc., 1997), pp. 111–36.

8. *El Rodeo 1909, Class Annual of the University of Southern California,* 1908, p. 300. Hereafter cited as *El Rodeo.*

9. Chung claimed that the *Los Angeles Times* scholarship helped pay for the first two years of preparatory, and that oratorical scholarships financed the last two years. I was not able to find external confirmation of Chung winning the scholarship from the *Los Angeles Times.* In other sources, Chung stated that the *L.A. Times* scholarship only provided one year of tuition. During her sophomore year, the *USC Bulletin* reported that the Declamation Prize of $10 was awarded to Katherine Chang. Chung had a classmate by the name of Katherine Chan, but it is also possible that the *Bulletin* misreported the name of the winner (*USC Bulletin, 1909–1910,* p. 204). For representing USC at the Interscholastic Oratorical Contest during her junior year, Chung received a one-semester tuition scholarship (*USC Bulletin, 1910–1911,* p. 247). There is no record of Chung participating in similar contests during her senior year.

10. Chung's name appears as a freshman in 1911 and 1912. After 1910, the USC College of Physicians and Surgeons required an extra year of preparation in the sciences and foreign language in addition to a high school diploma.

11. Thomas Neville Bonner, *To the Ends of the Earth: Women's Search for Education in Medicine* (Cambridge, Mass.: Harvard University Press, 1992), p. 142.

12. Susan La Flesche graduated from the Woman's Medical College of Pennsylvania in 1889. Rebecca Lee, the first black woman physician, graduated from the New England Female Medical College in Boston in 1864. She was followed by Rebecca J. Cole, who graduated from the Woman's Medical College of Pennsylvania in 1867, and Susan Smith McKinney Stewart, who completed her studies at New York Medical College for Women in 1870. See Darlene Clark Hine, *HineSight: Black Women and the Re-construction of American History* (Brooklyn: Carlson Publishing, 1994), p. 148. For information about Chinese female doctors, see chapter 1, footnote 47.

13. Paul Starr, *The Social Transformation of American Medicine: The Rise of a Sovereign Profession and the Making of a Vast Industry* (New York: Basic Books, 1982), p. 117.

14. Bonner, *To the Ends of the Earth*, p. 155. The Woman's Medical College of Pennsylvania did not become coeducational until 1971.

15. Ellen S. More, *Restoring the Balance: Women Physicians and the Profession of Medicine, 1850–1995* (Cambridge, Mass.: Harvard University Press, 1999).

16. Bonner, *To the Ends of the Earth;* Regina Markell Morantz-Sanchez, *Sympathy and Science: Women Physicians in American Medicine* (New York: Oxford University Press, 1985); More, *Restoring the Balance;* William G. Rothstein, *American Medical Schools and the Practice of Medicine: A History* (New York: Oxford University Press, 1987); Starr, *The Social Transformation of American Medicine.*

17. Although the process occurred over the course of the late nineteenth and early twentieth centuries, the comprehensive evaluation of medical schools by Abraham Flexner, published in 1910, is commonly perceived as the catalyst for institutional reform. Similar to the AMA review, conducted four years earlier, Flexner identified "A" schools that still needed to be strengthened, "B" schools that could be raised to the higher standard, and "C" schools that should be extinguished. The 1906 AMA report reviewed 160 schools, rated 82 as Class A, 46 as Class B, and 32 as Class C. By 1915, the number of schools had fallen from 131 to 95. Starr, *The Social Transformation of American Medicine,* p. 118.

18. The Flexner report rated the USC College of Physicians and Surgeons as Class B. The rating reflected, among other factors, the low admission standards, which had facilitated Chung's entry into the school. By 1914, the medical school required at least one year of college work as a prerequisite for medical study. By 1916, two years of college were required for enrollment into medical school.

19. The total number declined from 5,574 to 3,536, while female graduates decreased from 198 to 92. More, *Restoring the Balance,* p. 98. The gender contrast is particularly striking among African Americans. While the total number of black physicians increased from 909 in 1890 to 3,885 in 1920, the number of African American female physicians decreased from 115 to 12. Hine, *Hine-Sight,* p. 148.

20. Morantz-Sanchez, *Sympathy and Science,* p. 249.

21. *El Rodeo,* 1915 (Los Angeles: University of Southern California). Vern and Bonnie Bullough define cross-dressing as a "symbolic incursion into territory that crosses gender boundaries." Because dress represents a visible marker of gender differences, cross-dressing challenges the naturalness of "social conceptions of masculinity and femininity." Vern L. Bullough and Bonnie Bullough, *Cross Dressing, Sex, and Gender* (Philadelphia: University of Pennsylvania Press, 1993), p. viii. Chung's masculine gender presentation will be analyzed in more detail in chapter 7.

22. Lillian Faderman, *Odd Girls and Twilight Lovers: A History of Lesbian Life in Twentieth-Century America* (New York: Columbia University Press, 1991), p. 21.

23. P. M. Suski, *My Fifty Years in America*, English Summary (1960; reprint, Hollywood: Hawley Publications, 1990), p. 21. I thank Susan L. Smith for bringing this source to my attention.

24. *El Rodeo, 1915*, pp. 212, 220, and 232–33. Seven women founded the USC chapter of Nu Sigma Phi.

25. "Friendship Theme of Y.W. Address," *The Daily Southern Californian*, 30 October 1913, pp. 3–4.

26. The picture for Chung's senior class suggests that at least three people of Asian descent graduated from the academy that year. Katherine Chan, who attended the preparatory school with Chung during the previous three years, did not enroll for her senior year. *El Rodeo, 1912*.

27. George F. West, "Battlefields of China Call Dr. Margaret Chung," Clipping found in the private collection of Dorothy Siu.

28. Bertha Van Hoosen, *Petticoat Surgeon* (Chicago: Pellegrini & Cudahy, 1947), p. 219.

29. Chung, "Autobiography."

30. Ibid.

31. Mariko Tse, "Made in America," Research Project for East West Players on Chinese in Southern California, unpublished paper, June 1979, private collection of Judy Yung, p. 10.

32. Gerald J. O'Gara, "Interesting Westerners: A Chinese Woman Surgeon," *Sunset* 53, no. 6, December 1924, p. 28.

33. *The Daily Southern Californian*, 23 November 1914, p. 4.

34. *El Rodeo, 1917*, p. 18.

35. "Poon Chew on New Democracy," *The Daily Southern Californian*, 25 October 1912; and "Ng Poon Chew Addresses of W.," *The Daily Southern Californian*, 28 October 1912.

36. See the following articles: "Y.W.C.A. to Study Chinese Revolution" and "China Making Rapid Growth: Western Civilization Being Rapidly Assimilated," *The Daily Southern Californian*, 18 October 1912; "Mrs. Stuart Talks to Y.W.C.A. on 'China,'" *The Daily Southern Californian*, 20 February 1913; "Miss Baugh Talks to Girls," *The Daily Southern Californian*, 20 March 1913.

37. *El Rodeo, 1910*, p. 368.

38. *El Rodeo, 1911*.

39. Manuel P. Servin and Iris Higbie Wilson, *Southern California and Its University: A History of USC, 1880–1964* (Los Angeles: Ward Ritchie Press, 1969), p. 60.

40. Roberta S. Greenwood examined the burial records of the Evergreen Cemetery. I thank her for sharing her research with me. She published part of her results in *Cultural Resources Impact Mitigation Program: Los Angeles Metro Rail Red Line Segment 1* (Los Angeles: Los Angeles County Metropolitan Transportation Authority, 1993), p. 69.

41. *USC Bulletin, 1907–1908*, p. 100.

42. *USC Bulletin, 1914–1915*, pp. 28–29.

43. *USC Medicine, Centennial Historical Issue* 33, no. 2 (1985): 2–11.

44. Chung, "Autobiography."

45. Helen Satterlee, "The Story of a Persevering Chinese Girl Who Reached the Heights of Surgical Fame," *Los Angeles Times Sunday Magazine,* 25 June 1939, p. 20.

46. *Forty-Seventh Occidental Board Report* (1920), pp. 48–54. The Occidental Board sponsored a total of 137 missionaries from 1875 to 1920. Cecilia Tsu has identified second-generation Chinese Americans who served as missionaries in China. However, their names do not appear in the listings of the Presbyterian Missionary Board. Cecilia M. Tsu, "'Winning These Americans for Christ': Protestant Women and the Vision of Chinese American Assimilability in California, 1870–1920," unpublished paper, Berkshire Conference on the History of Women, 6–9 June 2002.

47. Jane Hunter, *The Gospel of Gentility: American Women Missionaries in Turn-of-the-Century China* (New Haven, Conn.: Yale University Press, 1984).

48. Tse, "Made in America," p. 10.

49. *El Rodeo, 1917,* p. 432. I thank Samuel Choi for identifying the poem and sharing his interpretation of it.

50. Henry Wadsworth Longfellow, "Maidenhood," in *Ballads and Other Poems* (Cambridge, Mass.: John Owen, 1842), p. 125.

51. Ibid., p. 128.

CHAPTER 4: "A NOBLE PROFESSION"

1. *USC Bulletin,* 1911–1912, p. 26.

2. *USC Bulletin,* 1916–1917, pp. 83, 85, 86.

3. According to the AMA, only 50 percent of medical students obtained hospital training after graduation in 1904. However, by 1914, 75 to 80 percent of physicians took internships. Paul Starr, *The Social Transformation of American Medicine: The Rise of a Sovereign Profession and the Making of a Vast Industry* (New York: Basic Books, 1982), pp. 123–24.

4. For three of the more influential works on Progressivism, see Richard Hofstadter, *Age of Reform* (New York: Knopf, 1955); James Weinstein, *The Corporate Ideal in the Liberal State* (Boston: Beacon Press, 1968); and Robert Wiebe, *The Search for Order, 1877–1920* (New York: Hill and Wang, 1967).

5. David J. Rothman, *Conscience and Convenience: The Asylum and Its Alternatives in Progressive America* (Boston: Little, Brown and Company, 1980), pp. 293–323.

6. Mary Roth Walsh, *"Doctors Wanted: No Women Need Apply": Sexual Barriers in the Medical Profession, 1835–1975* (New Haven, Conn.: Yale University Press, 1977), pp. 219–21; Darlene Clark Hine, *HineSight: Black Women and the Re-construction of American History* (Brooklyn: Carlson Publishing, 1994).

7. One source refers to Agnes Scholl as the first female intern at the hospital; Barbara Bronson Gray, *120 Years of Medicine: Los Angeles County 1871–1991* (Houston: Pioneer Publications, Inc.), pp. 43–44. Another source identifies Lulu Peters as the first female intern. She held an appointment in pathology in 1910 at the Los Angeles County Hospital, but the same source suggests that the position may not have been a regular internship. Helen

Eastman Martin, *The History of the Los Angeles County Hospital (1878–1968) and the Los Angeles County-University of Southern California Medical Center (1968–1978)* (Los Angeles: University of Southern California Press, 1979), p. 73.

8. Chung, "Autobiography."

9. Regina Markell Morantz-Sanchez, *Sympathy and Science: Women Physicians in American Medicine* (New York: Oxford University Press, 1985), p. 168.

10. Woman's Medical College of Pennsylvania, *62nd Annual Announcement, 1911–1912* (Philadelphia: The Woman's Medical College of Pennsylvania), p. 43.

11. Bertha Van Hoosen, *Petticoat Surgeon* (Chicago: Pellegrini & Cudahy, 1947), p. 218.

12. The 1916 Chicago Medical Directory lists Lin Hie Ding, who graduated from the University of Illinois in 1915, as an affiliate of the Mary Thompson Hospital.

13. Van Hoosen, *Petticoat Surgeon,* p. 297.

14. Chung, "Autobiography."

15. From 1870 to 1920, the population of Chicago grew from 300,000 to 2.7 million.

16. The number of wage-earning women living apart from family and relatives in Chicago grew from approximately 31,500 in 1910 to an estimate of 49,100 in 1930. Joanne J. Meyerowitz, *Women Adrift: Independent Wage Earners in Chicago, 1880–1930* (Chicago: University of Chicago Press, 1988), p. 5.

17. From 1880 to 1930, the female labor force in Chicago grew from 35,600 to 407,600. Nationally, the number increased from 2.6 to 10.8 million during the same period. Meyerowitz, *Women Adrift,* pp. 5 and xvii.

18. Chung, "Autobiography."

19. Victoria Bissell Brown, "The Fear of Feminization: Los Angeles High Schools in the Progressive Era," in *Gender and American Law: The Impact of the Law on the Lives of Women,* edited by Karen J. Maschke (New York: Garland Publishing, Inc., 1997), p. 112; Meyerowitz, *Women Adrift,* p. 7.

20. Tin-Chiu Fan, "Chinese Residents in Chicago," PhD diss., University of Chicago, 1926; Susan Lee Moy, "The Chinese in Chicago: The First One Hundred Years, 1870–1970," M.A. thesis, University of Wisconsin, Madison, 1978; Paul C.P. Siu, *The Chinese Laundryman: A Study of Social Isolation,* edited by John Kuo Wei Tchen (New York: New York University Press, 1987).

21. Fan, "Chinese Residents in Chicago," pp. 37, 40.

22. Approximately 30 percent of the Chinese in Chicago operated businesses in non-Chinese neighborhoods. Siu, *The Chinese Laundryman.*

23. Council of the Chicago Medical Society, *History of Medicine and Surgery and Physicians and Surgeons of Chicago* (Chicago: Biographical Publishing Corporation, 1922), p. 256.

24. Mary Harris Thompson, "The Chicago Hospital for Women and Children," in *In Memoriam, Mary Harris Thompson,* edited by Maria S. Iberne (Chicago: Board of Managers, 1896), p. 59.

25. Rose V. Mendian, "Bertha Van Hoosen: A Surgical Daughter's Impressions," *Journal of American Medical Women's Association* (April 1965): 349.

26. Lori D. Ginzberg, *Women and the Work of Benevolence: Morality, Politics, and Class in the Nineteenth-Century United States* (New Haven, Conn.: Yale University Press, 1990).

27. Constance M. McGovern, "Bertha Van Hoosen," in "Bertha Van Hoosen Biography File," Chicago Historical Society; Mabel E. Gardner, "Bertha Van Hoosen, M.D.: First President of the American Medical Women's Association," *Journal of the American Medical Women's Association* 5, no. 10 (October 1950): 413–14.

28. Judith Walzer Leavitt, "Birthing and Anesthesia: The Debate over Twilight Sleep," in *Mothers and Motherhood: Readings in American History,* edited by Rima D. Apple and Janet Golden (Columbus: Ohio State University Press, 1997), pp. 242–58.

29. Starr, *The Social Transformation of American Medicine;* and Charles E. Rosenberg, *The Care of Strangers: The Rise of America's Hospital System* (New York: Basic Books, Inc., 1987).

30. Chung, "Autobiography."

31. Van Hoosen, *Petticoat Surgeon,* p. 219.

32. "Manuscript," Bertha Van Hoosen Papers, Bentley Historical Library, University of Michigan, Ann Arbor, box 2, file 1, p. 440.

33. "Margaret Jessie Chung," Application for a Certificate from the Illinois State Board of Health, Illinois State Archives, Department of Registration and Education, Register of Licensed Physicians and Surgeons, 208.28. Hyman L. Meites, ed., *History of the Jews of Chicago* (Chicago: Chicago Jewish Historical Society and Wellington Publishing, Inc., 1990; facsimile of the original 1924 edition), p. 409.

34. Marilyn Elizabeth Perry, "Rachelle Yarros," Jane Addams Memorial Collection, University of Illinois at Chicago.

35. James R. Barrett and David Roediger, "Inbetween Peoples: Race, Nationality and the 'New Immigrant' Working Class," *Journal of American Ethnic History* 16, no. 3 (spring 1997): 3–44; Karen Brodkin, *How Jews Became White Folks and What That Says about Race in America* (New Brunswick, N.J.: Rutgers University Press, 1998); and Matthew Frye Jacobson, *Whiteness of a Different Color: European Immigrants and the Alchemy of Race* (Cambridge, Mass.: Harvard University Press, 1998); and David R. Roediger, *The Wages of Whiteness: Race and the Making of the American Working Class* (New York: Verso Press, 1991).

36. Michael Rogin argues that activism on behalf of racial equality and exploitation of racial stereotypes might be two sides of the same coin. Jewish participation in NAACP and the Civil Rights Movement, as well as Jewish adoption of blackface in entertainment, both use racial masquerade to achieve their acceptance in mainstream American society. Michael Rogin, *Blackface, White Noise: Jewish Immigrants in the Hollywood Melting Pot* (Berkeley and London: University of California Press, 1996).

37. Quoted in Martha Douglas Bost, "History of Mary Thompson Hospital, 1865–1973," paper, December 1973, Chicago Historical Society, p. 2.

38. Chung, "Autobiography." This quote incorporates the handwritten as well as the typed versions of Chung's autobiography.

39. Ibid.

40. Ibid.

41. Ibid.

42. "Manuscript of Autobiography," 403, Bertha Van Hoosen Papers, box 3, folder 1.

43. Carroll Smith-Rosenberg, *Disorderly Conduct: Visions of Gender in Victorian America* (New York: Oxford University Press, 1985); Bert Hansen, "American Physicians' 'Discovery' of Homosexuals, 1880–1900: A New Diagnosis in a Changing Society," in *Framing Disease: Studies in Cultural History*, edited by Charles E. Rosenberg and Janet Golden (New Brunswick, N.J.: Rutgers University Press, 1992): 105–33.

44. Dorothy Siu, Oral History, Interviewed by Jean Wong, 12 January 1979 and 6 November 1980, in *Southern California Chinese American Oral History Project*, Department of Special Collections, University Research Library, University of California, Los Angeles.

45. Gilbert Siu, conversation with author, 24 June 2001, Los Angeles.

46. Mariko Tse, "Made in America," Research Project for East West Players on Chinese in Southern California, unpublished paper, June 1979, p. 10.

47. Stuart K. Jaffary, *The Mentally Ill and Public Provision for Their Care in Illinois* (Chicago: University of Chicago Press, 1942), pp. 20–21.

48. Morantz-Sanchez, *Sympathy and Science*, p. 153.

49. Anthony M. Platt, *The Child Savers: The Invention of Delinquency* (1969; rev. ed. Chicago: University of Chicago Press, 1977), pp. 75–100.

50. Victoria Getis, *The Juvenile Court and the Progressives* (Urbana: University of Illinois Press, 2000); Robert M. Mennel, *Thorns and Thistles: Juvenile Delinquents in the United States, 1825–1940* (Hanover, N.H.: University Press of New England, 1973).

51. Louise de Koven Bowen, *Growing Up with a City* (New York: Macmillan, 1926), p. 103.

52. State of Illinois, Department of Mental Health, "Employment Record for Dr. Margaret J. Chung," number 84350. Chung was appointed assistant physician at Kankakee on 1 November 1917. She was transferred to the Division of Criminology on 16 December 1917 and appointed as a resident at Cook County Psychopathic Hospital, which housed the Juvenile Psychopathic Institute. (State of Illinois, Department of Public Welfare, RG 206, "Minutes of Meetings," 5 December 1917; Herman M. Adler, "The Juvenile Psychopathic Institute and the Work of the Division of the Criminologist," *The Institution Quarterly* 9, no. 1 (31 March 1918): 6–10.

53. Singer, born in 1875, received his medical training at the University of London and worked in Nebraska and Illinois in the field of psychiatry.

54. Adler received his medical degree from Columbia and served as chief of staff of the Boston Psychopathic Hospital as well as assistant professor of psychiatry at Harvard Medical School. Invited to review the institutions for criminals and delinquents in Illinois, Adler was appointed to succeed William Healy, the first director of the JPI, in 1917.

55. David A. Hollinger, *Science, Jews, and Secular Culture: Studies in Mid-Twentieth-Century American Intellectual History* (Princeton, N.J.: Princeton University Press, 1996), p. 25.

56. Tse, "Made in America," pp. 10–11. Adler, born in 1876, was thirteen years older than Chung. He married Frances Porter in March 1917.

57. Chung, "Autobiography."

58. From 1915 to 1919, approximately one in five juvenile delinquency cases involved girls. Helen Rankin Jeter, *The Chicago Juvenile Court*, U.S. Department of Labor, Children's Bureau, Publication no. 104 (Washington: Government Printing Office, 1922), p. 18.

59. From 17 December 1917 to 30 September 1918, the JPI processed 939 cases. *The Institution Quarterly* 9, no. 3 (30 September 1918): 59. For a discussion of Adler's accomplishments at the JPI, see Getis, *The Juvenile Court and the Progressives*, pp. 92–97.

60. All of Chung's quotes in this paragraph come from her autobiography.

61. Elizabeth Lunbeck, *The Psychiatric Persuasion: Knowledge, Gender, and Power in Modern America* (Princeton, N.J.: Princeton University Press, 1994), pp. 118–19.

62. Getis, *The Juvenile Court and the Progressives*, pp. 122–27; and Lunbeck, *The Psychiatric Persuasion*, pp. 121–26.

63. Reflecting the demographics of Chicago as well as the community surrounding Cook County Hospital, the overwhelming majority of Chung's patients at the JPI were southern and eastern European immigrants, along with sizable populations of Irish, native-born whites, and African Americans. During Chung's residency there, no Chinese and only one individual of Mexican descent were processed. Cook County Hospital, Annual Reports (Chicago, 1918), p. 230.

64. *Twelfth, Thirteenth, and Fourteenth Annual Reports of the Municipal Court of Chicago* (2 December 1917–6 December 1920), Chicago Historical Society.

65. Lunbeck, *The Psychiatric Persuasion*, p. 34.

66. Margaret Chung resided in Chicago before the era that Henry Yu analyzes in his work on Asian American intellectuals during the immigration exclusion, from 1924 to 1965. Most of these individuals were either trained or influenced by the University of Chicago's School of Sociology, which was shaped by the research agenda of the Juvenile Psychopathic Institute. There are interesting connections as well as dissonances in the experiences of the exclusion era intellectuals and Margaret Chung's earlier career in Chicago. The fields of social science and social work evolved from the religious and Progressive movements of the late nineteenth and early twentieth centuries. Both Chung and the later generation of Asian American professionals gained entry into scientific and reform communities due to political and research interest in migration and cultural contact. Both encountered obstacles and limitations because of the persistent structures of racial and gender hierarchy. Yu emphasizes the dominance of white, native-born Protestant men in academia; Chung's professional training,

though, was assisted by the presence of female and Jewish reformers in Progressive medicine. Furthermore, while Chung primarily provided services for or studied non-Chinese patients, scholars of Asian descent during the exclusion era became valuable researchers as well as subjects because of the interest in researching communities of Asian ancestry. Asian Americans, as both an immigrant and a racialized group, became ideal populations for testing and developing Robert E. Park's theories on assimilation and discrimination. Individuals of Asian ancestry gained entry into academia because of their perceived status as ethnic/racial "insiders" who possessed valuable knowledge about their subjects. During Chung's tenure in Chicago, the research agenda on studying "Orientals" had not yet developed. However, the perception of her unique access to "Oriental" culture and communities would become an integral aspect of her professional, political, and personal identities. Henry Yu, *Thinking Orientals: Migration, Contact, and Exoticism in Modern America* (New York: Oxford University Press, 2001).

67. Emma Wheat Gillmore, "An Unprecedented Opportunity for Women," *Southern California Practitioner,* October 1918, p. 133.

68. Chung was granted an indefinite military leave from her position as an assistant physician with the Department of Public Welfare's Division of Criminology. In one interview, Chung claimed to be a member of the Canadian Reserves, but there is no additional evidence to support her statement. As late as June of 1919, she was listed as a member of the Chicago Medical Society, an organization that she joined in October 1918. However, it is likely that she left Chicago soon after receiving her military leave.

CHAPTER 5: "THE BEGINNING OF A NEW ERA"

1. Samuel N. Clark, "Letter," 19 June 1919, "Margaret J. Chung" file, Department of Consumer Affairs, State Board of Medical Examiners, Deceased Physicians Files, California State Archives, Sacramento.

2. Mae N. Ngai, "The Architecture of Race in American Immigration Law: A Reexamination of the Immigration Act of 1924," *Journal of American History* 86 (June 1999): 67–92. The 1924 immigration act did not target Filipinos for complete exclusion because they originated from an American territory.

3. Chung had fond memories of her earlier work at the Santa Fe Railroad Hospital, recalling that even though she was officially a nurse, she "was generally first assistant, and also did all the dressings in the surgical wards"; the skills she developed there, she wrote, were to "stand me in good stead when I reached Chicago." Chung, "Autobiography."

4. Glenn Danford Bradley, *The Story of the Santa Fe* (Boston: Gorham Press, 1920); Keith L. Bryant Jr., *History of the Atchison, Topeka and Santa Fe Railway* (New York: Macmillan, 1974); James H. Ducker, *Men of the Steel Rails: Workers on the Atchison, Topeka and Santa Fe Railroad, 1869–1900* (Lincoln: University of Nebraska Press, 1983); Donald Duke and Stan Kistler,

Santa Fe: Steel Rails through California (San Marino, Calif.: A Golden West Book, 1963); James Marshall, *Santa Fe: The Railroad That Built an Empire* (New York: Random House, 1945); Ward McAfee, *California's Railroad Era, 1850–1911* (San Marino, Calif.: Golden West Books, 1973); *The Santa Fe Trail: A Chapter in the Opening of the West* (New York: Random House, 1946).

5. Stuart D. Brandes, *American Welfare Capitalism, 1880–1940* (Chicago: University of Chicago Press, 1970); C.D. Selby, *Studies of the Medical and Surgical Care of Industrial Workers*, Treasury Department, United States Public Health Service, Public Health Bulletin no. 99 (Washington, D.C.: Government Printing Office, 1919); *Medical Care of Industrial Workers* (New York: National Industrial Conference Board, Inc., 1926); T. Lyle Hazlett and William W. Hummel, *Industrial Medicine in Western Pennsylvania, 1850–1950* (Pittsburgh: University of Pittsburgh Press, 1957); Henry B. Selleck and Alfred H. Whittaker, *Occupational Health in America* (Detroit: Wayne State University Press, 1962); Pierce Williams, *The Purchase of Medical Care through Fixed Periodic Payment* (New York: National Bureau of Economic Research, Inc., 1932).

6. Chung, "Autobiography."

7. Ibid.

8. George H. Kress, *A History of the Medical Profession of Southern California* (Los Angeles: Times-Mirror Printing and Binding House Press, 1910), p. 196; *The Bulletin of the Los Angeles County Medical Association* 48, no. 15 (December 1918), p. 4.

9. Chung, "Autobiography."

10. Helen Satterlee, "Two Remarkable Women," *Los Angeles Times Magazine*, 25 June 1939, p. 5.

11. Chung, "Autobiography."

12. Satterlee, "Two Remarkable Women," p. 5.

13. Ibid.

14. Dorothy Siu, Oral History, interviewed by Jean Wong, 12 January 1979 and 6 November 1980, *Southern California Chinese American Oral History Project*, Department of Special Collections, University Research Library, University of California, Los Angeles.

15. George J. Sánchez, *Becoming Mexican American: Ethnicity, Culture and Identity in Chicano Los Angeles, 1900–1945* (New York: Oxford University Press, 1993), p. 75.

16. Carl Yetzler, "San Bernardino Proud to Be a Railroad City," *San Bernardino Sun-Telegram*, clipping found in San Bernardino Public Library.

17. Albert Camarillo, *Chicanos in a Changing Society: From Mexican Pueblos to American Barrios in Santa Barbara and Southern California, 1848–1930* (Cambridge, Mass.: Harvard University Press, 1979), pp. 206–8.

18. Satterlee, "Two Remarkable Women," p. 5.

19. Howard J. Nelson, *The Los Angeles Metropolis* (Dubuque, Ia.: Kendall/Hunt Publishing Company, 1983), p. 254.

20. *U.S. Census, 1920*, California, vol. 62, E.D. 216, sheet 16, line 94.

21. Robert M. Fogelson, *The Fragmented Metropolis: Los Angeles, 1850–1930* (Cambridge, Mass.: Harvard University Press, 1967), p. 147.

22. Jules Tygiel, "Introduction," *Metropolis in the Making: Los Angeles in the 1920s,* edited by Tim Sitton and William Deverell (Berkeley and London: University of California Press, 2001), p. 2.

23. Fogelson, *The Fragmented Metropolis,* p. 147.

24. I thank Carson Anderson for sharing the findings of his research. According to his analysis of the 1920 census, only fourteen Chinese families resided in Pasadena.

25. Gerald J. O'Gara, "Interesting Westerners: The Ministering Angel of Chinatown," *Sunset Magazine,* December 1924, pp. 28–29.

26. Joe Shoong owned the China Toggery. One of the wealthiest Chinese American entrepreneurs, Shoong gained fame and notoriety for creating the chain of National Dollar Stores. For an account of the 1938 strike by Chinese American women against the store, the longest labor protest in the history of San Francisco Chinatown, see Yung, *Unbound Feet,* pp. 210–22.

27. Clark Davis, "The View from Spring Street: White-Collar Men in the City of Angels," *Metropolis in the Making,* p. 184.

28. Bertha Van Hoosen, *Petticoat Surgeon* (Chicago: Pellegrini & Cudahy, 1947), p. 219.

29. Pearl P. Puckett, "She's Mom to Two Thousand American Flyers," *Independent Woman,* January 1946, p. 32.

30. Chung, "Autobiography."

31. Siu, Oral History.

32. Steven J. Ross, "How Hollywood Became Hollywood: Money, Politics, and Movies," in *Metropolis in the Making,* p. 255.

33. Michael Rogin, *Blackface, White Noise: Jewish Immigrants in the Hollywood Melting Pot* (Berkeley and London: University of California Press, 1996); Max Vorspan and Lloyd P. Gartner, *History of the Jews of Los Angeles* (Philadelphia: Jewish Publication Society of America, 1970), pp. 129–34.

34. Chinese Historical Society of Southern California, *Linking Our Lives: Chinese American Women of Los Angeles* (Los Angeles: California Historical Society of Southern California, 1984), pp. 4–5.

35. Siu, Oral History.

36. Icy Smith, *The Lonely Queue: The Forgotten History of the Courageous Chinese Americans in Los Angeles* (Gardena, Calif.: East West Discovery Press, 2000), p. 55.

37. George P. West, "Battlefields of China Call Dr. Margaret Chung," Dorothy Siu Collection. I am indebted to the scholarship of Karen Leong and Shirley Jennifer Lim, both of whom conducted extensive research on Anna May Wong. See Karen Janis Leong, "The China Mystique: Mayling Soong Chiang, Pearl S. Buck and Anna May Wong in the American Imagination," PhD diss., University of California, Berkeley, 1999; and Shirley Jennifer Lim, "Girls Just Wanna Have Fun: The Politics of Asian American Women's Public Culture, 1930–1960," PhD diss., University of California, Los Angeles, 1998.

38. Neil Okrent, "Right Place, Wong Time: Why Hollywood's First Asian Star, Anna May Wong, Died a Thousand Movie Deaths," *Los Angeles Magazine*, May 1990, pp. 84+.

39. "Born in Los Angeles—Reared in Oriental Fashion," in *Orientals and Their Cultural Adjustment: Interviews, Life Histories, and Social Adjustment Experiences of Chinese and Japanese of Varying Backgrounds and Length of Residence in the United States* (Nashville, Tenn.: Social Science Institute, Fisk University, 1946), p. 25. The interview subject claims to be a relative of Chung's but does not appear to be one of her siblings. It is possible that the subject is descended from one of the Presbyterian Chinese Mission Home sisters of Ah Yane.

40. Roberta S. Greenwood, communication to author, 29 October 1997. Only the records after 1914 include attending physicians.

41. Siu, Oral History.

42. Gina Marchetti, *Romance and the "Yellow Peril": Race, Sex, and Discursive Strategies in Hollywood Fiction* (Berkeley and London: University of California Press, 1993); Robert G. Lee, *Orientals: Asian Americans in Popular Culture* (Philadelphia: Temple University Press, 1999), p. 119.

43. Edward Said, *Orientalism* (New York: Random House, 1978). For discussions of American Orientalism, see Anthony W. Lee, *Picturing Chinatown: Art and Orientalism in San Francisco* (Berkeley and London: University of California Press, 2001); John Kuo Wei Tchen, *New York before Chinatown: Orientalism and the Shaping of American Culture, 1776–1882* (Baltimore: John Hopkins University Press, 1999); Mary Yoshihara, "Women's Asia: American Women and the Gendering of American Orientalism, 1870s–WWII," PhD diss., Brown University, 1997; and Henry Yu, *Thinking Orientals: Migration, Contact, and Exoticism in Modern America* (New York: Oxford University Press, 2001).

44. Marchetti, *Romance and the "Yellow Peril,"* pp. 81–84.

45. The titles of D. W. Griffith's one-reel films before 1915 reveal his fascination with the themes of race and sex: *The Red Man and the Child, The Hindoo Dagger, The Mexican Sweethearts, A Child of the Ghetto, The Greaser,* and *The Chinaman and the Sunday School Teacher.* Griffith also produced one of the earliest features on Asian-white relations, entitled *Broken Blossoms* (1919, United Artists). Lee, *Orientals,* pp. 119–20.

46. Kevin J. Mumford, *Interzones: Black/White Sex Districts in Chicago and New York in the Early Twentieth Century* (New York: Columbia University Press, 1997).

47. Lisa See, *On Gold Mountain: The One-Hundred Year Odyssey of My Chinese-American Family* (New York: Vintage Books, Inc., 1995). See describes herself as a hybrid anthropologist/storyteller. For a discussion of her methodology, see the forward and acknowledgements to this fascinating and engrossing family history.

48. Ibid., p. 136.

49. In 1922, the neighborhood spanned two streets and thirteen thoroughfares with 184 shops, most of them with living quarters in the back. Chinese Historical Society of Southern California, *Linking Our Lives,* p. 14.

50. See, *On Gold Mountain*, pp. 197–98.

51. Smith, *The Lonely Queue*, pp. 63–66.

52. Ivan Light, "From Vice District to Tourist Attraction: The Moral Career of American Chinatowns, 1880–1940," *Pacific Historical Review* 43, no. 3 (1974): 367–94.

CHAPTER 6: "THE MINISTERING ANGEL OF CHINATOWN"

1. Chung, "Autobiography."

2. The Chinese constituted the largest nonwhite group in San Francisco and would continue to do so until the influx of African Americans during World War II. The numbers for people of Mexican ancestry are difficult to identify, because it was not until the 1960 census that individuals with Spanish surnames were counted separately. It is likely that Mexican Americans constituted a sizable presence in San Francisco. In 1920, the next largest racial minorities after Chinese Americans were Japanese Americans (slightly over five thousand) and African Americans (approximately twenty-five hundred). World War II internment removed people of Japanese ancestry from San Francisco; the number of African Americans dramatically increased from approximately five thousand in 1940 to nearly forty-four thousand in 1950. Brian J. Godfrey, *Neighborhoods in Transition: The Making of San Francisco's Ethnic and Nonconformist Communities* (Berkeley and London: University of California Press, 1988), pp. 68, 97.

3. Out of 7,744 Chinese, 6,020 were male and 1,724 were female. Judy Yung, *Unbound Feet: A Social History of Chinese Women in San Francisco* (Berkeley and London: University of California Press, 1995), p. 296.

4. The physical boundaries of Chinatown shifted over time, and people of various racial backgrounds resided in the neighborhood. However, the designation of a racially segregated community emerged. During the predepression era, Chinatown was understood as the area bound by Powell, Broadway, Kearny, and Bush streets. Nayan Shah, *Contagious Divides: Epidemics and Race in San Francisco's Chinatown* (Berkeley and London: University of California, 2001), p. 236. Also see Mary Ting Yi Lui, "'The Real Yellow Peril': Mapping Racial and Gender Boundaries in New York City's Chinatown, 1870–1910," *Hitting Critical Mass: A Journal of Asian American Cultural Criticism* 5, no. 1 (spring 1998).

5. Chung, "Autobiography."

6. Shah, *Contagious Divides*.

7. Elsa Gidlow, "Original Manuscript" of Gidlow's autobiography, p. 100, Elsa Gidlow Papers, box 7, Gay and Lesbian Historical Society of Northern California, San Francisco.

8. Joseph Lee, trained in homeopathy at the University of California, established the first Western medical practice in San Francisco Chinatown in 1918. There are conflicting accounts about when Chung arrived. One source dates her practice as starting in 1920, but her name does not appear in the San Francisco city directory until 1924. Chung herself dates her history in the city to 1922. *The Dawning* (San Francisco: Chinese Hospital Medical Staff Archives, 1978), p. 3.

9. Chung, "Autobiography."

10. Male immigrants could join family and district associations, societies based on common lineage and region of emigration. These groups provided basic welfare services, such as shelter and employment contacts. They also formed the foundation of the most important community organization, the Six Companies, which served as the primary political voice for Chinatown. Men, but not women, born in the United States could become a member of the Chinese American Citizens Alliance, a group formed in 1895 to advance the concerns of the second generation.

11. Yung, *Unbound Feet,* p. 293.

12. Yung, *Unbound Feet.*

13. Chung, "Autobiography."

14. Pearl P. Puckett, "She's Mom to Two Thousand American Flyers," *Independent Woman,* January 1946, p. 32.

15. Chung, "Autobiography." Other Chinese doctors supported Chung's interpretation. James Hall, a Chinese immigrant who began medical practice in Chinatown a year after Chung, recalled that a "Chinatown practice did not look promising . . . since 50 to 70% of the Chinese still use[d] Chinese herbs. Also there were already many Americans practicing in Chinatown." Hall uses the term "Americans" to refer to "white" physicians, a linguistic practice common among both Chinese and non-Chinese that equated nationality with race. I thank Him Mark Lai for generously sharing this source with me. Philip Choy and Him Mark Lai, "Summary of Interview with Dr. James Hall," 23 August 1970, Belmont, California.

16. Cathy Luchetti, *Medicine Women: The Story of Early-American Women Doctors* (New York: Crown Publishers, Inc., 1998), p. 132. Luchetti led me to the useful Helen MacKnight Doyle autobiography, *A Child Went Forth* (New York: Gotham House, 1934).

17. I thank Lucy Murphy for suggesting this insight. In Helen Doyle's memoirs about practicing in Chinatown, she indicated that white female physicians developed knowledge about Chinese cultural beliefs regarding health and death. When she and a colleague assisted the birth of a deformed Chinese child, they expected the husband, who was a merchant, to blame them for the physical defect. She writes, "The Chinese considered a deformed child a curse upon the house, and that the doctor was held responsible for any deviation from the normal." However, the Chinese merchant found fault with a Chinese midwife, rather than the two white physicians. Race and professional status protected Doyle and her colleague. Doyle, *A Child Went Forth,* pp. 278–79.

18. Pardee Lowe, "Business Establishments," information quoted from "The Chinese Community of S.F." (Lee & Lee, 1929), Pardee Lowe Papers, Hoover Institution of War, Revolution and Peace, Stanford University. Hereafter cited as PLP.

19. Haiming Liu, "The Resilience of Ethnic Culture: Chinese Herbalists in the American Medical Profession," *Journal of Asian American Studies* 1, no. 2 (1988): 177. Also see Christopher Muench, "Chinese Medicine in America: A Study in Adaptation," *Caduceus* 4 (1988): 5–35; and Henry G. Schwarz, ed.,

Chinese Medicine on the Golden Mountain: An Interpretive Guide (Seattle: Wing Luke Memorial Museum), 1984.

20. George Kao, "Tung Wah Hospital," in *Cathay by the Bay: San Francisco Chinatown in 1950* (Hong Kong: Chinese University Press, 1988), p. 92.

21. Lowe, "Death a Commonplace in Chinatown," box 326, folder "Death," pp. 8–9, PLP.

22. Shah, *Contagious Divides.*

23. Joan B. Trauner, "The Chinese as Medical Scapegoats in San Francisco, 1870–1905," *California History* 57, no. 1 (spring 1978): 70–87.

24. Charles E. Rosenberg, *The Care of Strangers: The Rise of America's Hospital System* (New York: Basic Books, Inc., 1987), pp. 109–13.

25. Board of Medical Examiners Reports, California State Archives, Sacramento.

26. Nayan Shah, "San Francisco's 'Chinatown': Race and the Cultural Politics of Public Health, 1854–1952," PhD diss., University of Chicago, 1995, p. 52.

27. Chung, "Autobiography." In one interview, it was reported that Chung saved a "critically ill Chinese man whom she had brought in from the street." See Puckett, "She's Mom to Two Thousand American Flyers," p. 32. In another version, "the friends of Jennie Fung" brought her to Chung's office. See Gerald J. O'Gara, "Interesting Westerners: The Ministering Angel of Chinatown," *Sunset Magazine*, December 1924, p. 28. An additional version has Chung eating in the restaurant, when a Chinese American woman became sick. These differences may result from journalistic error as well as from Chung's variations in narration. Despite the differences, these accounts all emphasize the emergency circumstances surrounding the case and its beneficial impact on her medical practice.

28. Chung, "Autobiography."

29. Members of the Square and Circle Club, conversation with author, 17 July 1999, San Francisco; Members of the Berkeley Chinese Community Church Senior Center, conversation with author, 6 July 1999, Berkeley; and Dr. Edmund Jung, interview with author, 21 July 1999, San Francisco.

30. Shah, *Contagious Divides,* p. 207. As a result of the high reproduction rate as well as efforts to use immigration loopholes, the Chinese population in San Francisco more than doubled between 1920 and 1930, reaching over sixteen thousand. The gender gap also steadily decreased and had almost reached parity by the time Chung died in the late 1950s.

31. Siu, Oral History," Interviewed by Jean Wong, 12 January 1979 and 6 November 1980, in *Southern California Chinese American Oral History Project,* Department of Special Collections, University Research Library, University of California, Los Angeles.

32. "Local News," *Chung Sai Yat Po,* 4 August 1922.

33. The founding of the Chinese Hospital reflected the cooperation between established immigrant organizations and emerging second-generation civic groups. In 1918, the Chinese Six Companies sought the cooperation of fourteen

community organizations, representing various social, civic, religious, and political interests, to remodel and update the medical facility, resulting in the founding of the Chinese Hospital in 1925. The sponsors included family and district associations and political organizations focused on Chinese national reform, as well as the Chinese Chamber of Commerce, Chinese American Citizens Alliance, Chinese Christian Union, and Chinese Y.M.C.A. *The Dawning;* T.J. Gintjee and Howard H. Johnson, "San Francisco's First Chinese Hospital," *The Modern Hospital,* October 1925, pp. 283–85; Kao, "Tung Wah Hospital," pp. 91–94; Shah, "San Francisco's 'Chinatown'"; Trauner, "The Chinese as Medical Scapegoats in San Francisco, 1870–1905."

34. Lowe, "Chinese Hospital—Herb Treatments Forbidden, 1925," passage quoted from "Chinese Hospital Records, Dec. 1925," PLP.

35. "The Opening of the Chinese Hospital," Chinese Historical Society, San Francisco Collection, box 3, folder 11, Asian American Studies Collection, Ethnic Studies Library, University of California, Berkeley.

36. Lowe, "Personal History of a Chinese Doctor," box 192, folder "Medicine-Western," p. 15, PLP.

37. Ibid.

38. Shah, *Contagious Divides,* p. 226.

39. Lowe, "Medicine and Health—Doctors in Chinatown, 1934," box 125, folder "Medicine-Health," PLP.

40. Ibid.

41. "Margaret J. Chung," Deceased Physicians Files, 1902–1977, Department of Consumer Affairs, State Board of Medical Examiners, California State Archives. Chung's files also contain some complaints and inquiries from non-Chinese patients and their relatives about her qualifications to practice medicine. The state board responded succinctly to all queries by confirming her credentials.

42. Community historian Him Mark Lai confirmed that this organization did not exist.

43. It is unlikely that a non-Chinese individual wrote the letter; assuming a Chinese identity would not have enhanced the credibility of the charges.

44. Darlene Clark Hine, *HineSight: Black Women and the Re-construction of American History* (Brooklyn, N.Y.: Carlson Publishing, 1994), p. 153.

45. Dr. Bessie Jeong, Oral History, interviewed by Suellen Cheng and Munson Kwok, 17 December 1981 and 17 October 1982, in *Southern California Chinese American Oral History Project,* Department of Special Collections, University Research Library, University of California, Los Angeles.

46. Lai and Choy, "Hall" interview.

47. Justice B. Detwiler, ed., *Who's Who in California: A Biographical Directory, 1928–1929* (San Francisco: Who's Who Publishing Company, 1929).

48. Shah, *Contagious Divides,* p. 217.

49. *The Dawning,* pp. 7–8.

50. Ibid., p. 8.

51. Both oral histories and a photograph of Wong reveal her presentation to be masculine or androgynous. The picture, which appears in Shah's book, features Wong with two nurses, a Chinese female client, and two children. Wong,

unlike the other women in the picture, is distinctly not feminine. All the medical professionals wear white uniforms that distinguish them from the client and her children. However, the two nurses pull back their hair to accommodate their caps. In contrast, Wong's hair, like Chung's, is slicked back in a masculine style. Shah, *Contagious Divides*, p. 217. Descriptions of Wong's appearance were communicated to the author during a community presentation of her research in San Francisco Chinatown, Chinese Historical Society of San Francisco, 26 June 1999.

52. D.M. Ladd, "Memo to A.H. Belmont," 12 October 1953, "Dr. Margaret Chung," file 65–35400, U.S. Department of Justice, Federal Bureau of Investigation.

53. Jeong, Oral History.

54. L.B. Nichols to Tolson, memorandum, 9 October 1940, Federal Bureau of Investigation file on "Dr. Margaret Jesse Chung," Department of Justice.

55. See oral histories in *Following the Dawn* (San Francisco: Chinese Hospital Medical Staff Archives, 1979). According to the research of Pardee Lowe, non-Chinese patients represented a majority or at least a significant minority of the clients for Chinatown physicians. In handwritten notes, Lowe indicates that one physician reported 65 percent of his patients as "American." PLP. Also see Shah, *Contagious Divides*, p. 212.

56. Shirley Radke, "We Must Be Active Americans," *Christian Science Monitor*, 3 October 1942.

57. Lowe, "Chinafication Desired by S.F. People, 1934," box 126, "Chinafication" Section, PLP.

58. Bertha Van Hoosen, *Petticoat Surgeon* (Chicago: Pellegrini & Cudahy, 1947), p. 219.

59. Lowe, "Chinafication Desired by S.F. People, 1934," PLP.

60. Gloria Heyung Chun, *Of Orphans and Warriors: Inventing Chinese American Culture and Identity* (New Brunswick, N.J.: Rutgers University Press, 2000); and Henry Yu, *Thinking Orientals: Migration, Contact, and Exoticism in Modern America* (New York: Oxford University Press, 2001).

61. Yung, *Unbound Feet*, p. 136.

62. Liu, "The Resilience of Ethnic Culture," pp. 181–82.

63. Lowe, "Chinafication Desired by S.F. People, 1934," PLP.

64. I thank Leslie J. Reagan for suggesting this argument and referring me to the autobiography of Charles Eastman. Charles A. Eastman, *From the Deep Woods to Civilization: Chapters in the Autobiography of an Indian* (Boston: Little, Brown, and Co., 1920), p. 137.

65. Elsa Gidlow, *Elsa: I Come with My Songs* (San Francisco: Booklegger Press, 1986), p. 207.

66. Gidlow, *Elsa*, p. 255. Chung's method of referral was representative of physicians who engaged in this practice. See Leslie J. Reagan, *When Abortion Was a Crime: Women, Medicine, and Law in the United States, 1867–1973* (Berkeley and London: University of California Press, 1997).

67. Percival Dolman, "Letter to Frederick N. Scatena," 29 July 1950, Margaret J. Chung File, Deceased Physicians File. It is striking that this concern

about Chung's involvement in facilitating abortions did not surface in state medical records until 1950, an era of renewed cultural emphasis on family formation in American society.

68. Yung, *Unbound Feet*, p. 174.

69. Lowe lists a "Birth Control Clinic" on 754 Oak St., operated by Dr. Pennington on Tuesdays. Pardee Lowe, "Chinatown Study: Persons & Organizations Contacted," PLP.

70. Ibid.

71. Shah, *Contagious Divides*, p. 207.

72. Initially underground antigovernment organizations in China, tongs in the United States offered mutual aid and protection for immigrants. Some tongs became involved with a variety of illegal activities, such as gambling and prostitution. Occasionally, conflicts between tongs escalated to violence and attracted the attention of the mainstream public. See Ronald Takaki, *Strangers from a Different Shore: A History of Asian Americans* (Boston: Little, Brown, 1989), p. 118.

73. Yong Chen, *Chinese San Francisco, 1850–1943: A Trans-Pacific Community* (Stanford, Calif.: Stanford University Press, 2000).

74. Basil Woon, *San Francisco and the Golden Empire* (New York: Harrison Smith and Robert Haas, 1935), p. 52.

75. O'Gara, "Interesting Westerners," p. 28.

76. Ibid.

CHAPTER 7: A SISTER LESBIAN?

1. Justice B. Detwiler, ed., *Who's Who in California: A Biographical Directory 1928–1929* (San Francisco: Who's Who Publishing Company, 1929), p. 55.

2. Chung's autobiography and papers contain scant evidence about her romantic desires, behavior, or attitudes. There is no reference to Gidlow in her writings or collection. I accidentally discovered their relationship by browsing through Susan Stryker and Jim Van Buskirk, *Gay by the Bay: A History of Queer Culture in the San Francisco Bay Area* (San Francisco: Chronicle Books, 1996), pp. 21–23. The book featured a photograph of Chung and identified her as Gidlow's friend.

3. Kevin J. Mumford, *Interzones: Black/White Sex Districts in Chicago and New York in the Early Twentieth Century* (New York: Columbia University Press, 1997), p. 20. Alternatively, these communities could be characterized as "port cultures," a concept developed by John Tchen to describe the "mixing and shifting amalgam of individuals and groups from many places" that characterized lower Manhattan throughout the nineteenth century. John Kuo Wei Tchen, *New York before Chinatown: Orientalism and the Shaping of American Culture, 1776–1882* (Baltimore: John Hopkins University Press, 1999), p. 71. Also see Mary Ting Yi Lui, "'The Real Yellow Peril': Mapping Racial and Gender Boundaries in New York City's Chinatown, 1870–1910," *Hitting Critical Mass: A Journal of Asian American Cultural Criticism* 5, no. 1

(spring 1998); and Nayan Shah, *Contagious Divides: Epidemics and Race in San Francisco's Chinatown* (Berkeley and London: University of California, 2001).

4. Given the difficulties of uncovering past sexual lives, scholars have focused on the figure of the "mannish" woman as a signifier of the sexually assertive lesbian. For discussions of the methodological approaches of lesbian/ sexuality studies, see Lisa Duggan, "The Trials of Alice Mitchell: Sensationalism, Sexology, and the Lesbian Subject in Turn-of-the-Century America," *Signs* 18, no. 4 (1993): 791–814; Martha Vicinus, ed., *Lesbian Subjects: A Feminist Studies Reader* (Bloomington: Indiana University Press, 1996); and Elizabeth Lapovsky Kennedy, "'But we would never talk about it': The Structures of Lesbian Discretion in South Dakota, 1928–1933," in *Inventing Lesbian Cultures in America,* edited by Ellen Lewin (Boston: Beacon Press, 1996), 15–39.

5. Bertha Van Hoosen, *Petticoat Surgeon* (Chicago: Pellegrini & Cudahy, 1947), p. 219.

6. Chung, "Autobiography."

7. Ibid.

8. Ibid.

9. Even after Ford introduced the affordable Model T in 1908, only one in five people in the country owned an automobile. Virginia Scharff, *Taking the Wheel: Women and the Coming of the Motor Age* (New York: The Free Press, 1991), pp. 113 and 117.

10. Xiaojian Zhao, *Remaking Chinese America: Immigration, Family, and Community, 1940–1965* (New Brunswick, N.J.: Rutgers University Press, 2002), p. 50.

11. Bertha Van Hoosen, "Travel Letters through the Orient: Personal Observations and Experiences of Dr. Bertha Van Hoosen," *The Medical Woman's Journal* 30, no. 3 (March 1923): 77.

12. Edmund Jung, interview with author, 2 July 1999, San Francisco. Chung's nephew, Rodney Low, also recalled his aunt's pride in her cars. On one road trip together, Chung explained to the male gas attendant that there was no need to wash the windshield because her car was equipped with automatic wipers. Rodney Low, interview with author, 20 December 1997 and 2 January 1998, San Francisco.

13. Van Hoosen, *Petticoat Surgeon,* p. 219.

14. Bessie Jeong, interview by Suellen Cheng and Munson Kwok, 17 December 1981, and 17 October 1982, Southern California Chinese American Oral History Project, Special Collections, University of California, Los Angeles. For biographical information about Jeong, see Yung, *Unbound Feet: A Social History of Chinese Women in San Francisco* (Berkeley and London: University of California Press, 1995), pp. 131–33.

15. Jeong, interview.

16. Even sexologists attempted to make some refinements in their distinctions between women who wanted male privileges and those who exhibited masculine desires for women. Richard von Krafft-Ebing, in his late-nineteenth-century

publication *Psychopathia Sexualis,* first discussed the gradations of homosexuality, which he defined in terms of gender roles, not necessarily sexuality. The "Mannish Lesbian," whom he viewed as "the extreme grade of degenerative homosexuality," demonstrated her "sexual perversion" by desiring male power and adopting male dress. Havelock Ellis extended Krafft-Ebing's work by arguing that "a woman's love for other women was both sexual and degenerate." He argued that the true "invert" was biologically predisposed and unchangeable. However, other women merely "possessed a genetic predisposition, a weakness, for the advances of other women" and were in fact "potential heterosexuals." These summaries and quotes about sexology are based on my reading of Carroll Smith-Rosenberg, "Discourses of Sexuality and Subjectivity: The New Woman, 1870–1936," in *Hidden from History: Reclaiming the Gay and Lesbian Past,* edited by Martin Bauml Duberman, Martha Vicinus, and George Chauncey Jr. (New York: New American Library, 1989), pp. 269–71.

17. Jeong, interview.

18. Elsa Gidlow, "Journal," 13 and 25 January, 30 August 1928, Elsa Gidlow Papers, box 1, Gay and Lesbian Historical Society of Northern California, San Francisco. Hereafter cited as EGP. The poems that Gidlow wrote about Chung include "Chinese Lotus," "For a Gifted Lady, Often Masked," "Miracle," and "Surgeon's Hands," box 11.

19. Gidlow, *Elsa: I Come with My Songs* (San Francisco: Booklegger Press and Druid Heights Books, 1986), p. 208.

20. Gidlow, "Journal," 28 August 1928.

21. Ibid., 30 August 1928.

22. Ibid., 12 May 1931.

23. Ibid., 28 May 1931.

24. Ibid.

25. Ibid., 4 July 1931.

26. Ibid., 13 August 1931.

27. Mary Lui argues that race, gender, and class influenced an individual's ability to travel within urban spaces. See "'The Real Yellow Peril'."

28. Gidlow, "Original Manuscript," box 7, p. 158, EGP.

29. Gidlow, "Journal," 28 August 1928.

30. James R. Barrett and David Roediger, "Inbetween Peoples: Race, Nationality and the 'New Immigrant' Working Class," *Journal of American Ethnic History* 16, no. 3 (spring 1997): 3–44.

31. Gidlow, "Journal," 30 August 1928.

32. David F. Myrick, *San Francisco's Telegraph Hill* (Berkeley, Calif.: Howell-North Books, 1972), pp. 105–15.

33. Nan Alamilla Boyd, "Homos Invade S.F.! San Francisco's History as a Wide-Open Town," in *Creating a Place for Ourselves: Lesbian, Gay, and Bisexual Community Histories,* edited by Brett Beemyn (New York: Routledge, 1997), p. 80.

34. Stryker and Buskirk, *Gay by the Bay,* p. 26.

35. Ibid., p. 23.

36. Gidlow, "Original Manuscript," p. 200.

37. Russell Leong, "Home Bodies and the Body Politic," *Asian American Sexualities: Dimensions of the Gay and Lesbian Experience* (New York: Routledge, 1996), p. 11.

38. Gidlow wrote and published various versions of this poem. The earliest typed version was entitled "An Exercise in Free Verse, Dashed off for Doctor Margaret Chung," 22 September 1927, box 11, EGP.

39. Edward W. Said, *Orientalism* (New York: Vintage Books, 1979), pp. 1–3.

40. Gidlow, "Journal," 4 and 13 July 1931.

41. Ibid., 10 November 1928.

42. Ibid.

43. Yung, *Unbound Feet,* p. 165. See John D'Emilio and Estelle B. Freedman, *Intimate Matters: A History of Sexuality in America* (New York: Harper and Row, 1988).

44. Lucile Chung, interview with author, Vista, California, 28 January 1996.

45. Pardee Lowe, "Americanization: Intermarriage: Limited Families: Write up on M. Ch—family," PLP. Virgil married a woman of German ancestry. Venus's second husband was white as well. Neither couple had children.

46. See Karen Isaksen Leonard, *Making Ethnic Choices: California's Punjabi Mexican Americans* (Philadelphia: Temple University Press, 1992).

47. Second-generation Chinese Americans successfully lobbied for the repeal of this provision in 1931. See Yung, *Unbound Feet,* pp. 168–69.

48. Lucile Chung, interview with author.

49. Peggy Pascoe, "Gender Systems in Conflict: The Marriages of Mission-Educated Chinese American Women, 1874–1939," in *Unequal Sisters: A Multicultural Reader in U.S. Women's History,* edited by Ellen Carol DuBois and Vicki L. Ruiz (New York: Routledge, 1990), p. 125.

50. Regina Markell Morantz-Sanchez argues that the marriage rates were disproportionately higher for female physicians than for other female professionals. However, approximately two thirds of female physicians did not marry during the first three decades of the twentieth century. Morantz-Sanchez, *Sympathy and Science: Women Physicians in American Medicine* (New York: Oxford University Press, 1985), pp. 135–37.

When Van Hoosen was asked by her college classmates at their fiftieth anniversary reunion why she had never married, she replied: "Well if the boys when I was of a marriageable age had been like the boys of today, I would have set up a male harem." Christopher Matthew, "Doctor in Petticoats: 84 Year Old Chicago Surgeon Tells the Story of Her Life in a Frank and Refreshing Book," clipping, 24 August 1947, Bertha Van Hoosen Collection, 80–133, box 1, folder 3, University of Illinois at Chicago, Department of Special Collections.

51. Robert G. Lee, conversation with author, summer 1999, Palo Alto.

52. Lowe, "Sex—Homosexuality in C.T.," PLP.

53. A.H. Belmont to D.M. Ladd, Memorandum, 12 October 1953, Federal Bureau of Investigation File on "Dr. Margaret Jesse Chung," Department of Justice.

54. I situate Margaret Chung's sexuality historically by differentiating between the concept of lesbianism that developed during the turn of the century and other forms of homoeroticism. See Leila J. Rupp, "'Imagine My Surprise': Women's Relationships in Mid-Twentieth Century America," in *Hidden from History: Reclaiming the Gay and Lesbian Past,* edited by Martin Bauml Duberman, Martha Vicinus, and George Chauncey Jr. (New York: New American Library, 1989), pp. 395–410; and Estelle B. Freedman, "'The Burning of Letters Continues': Elusive Identities and the Historical Construction of Sexuality," *Journal of Women's History* 9, no. 4 (1998): 181–200.

55. See Judy Tzu-Chun Wu, "Was Mom Chung a 'Sister Lesbian'? Asian American Gender Experimentation and Interracial Homoeroticism," *Journal of Women's History* 13, no. 1 (spring 2001): 58–82; *Amerasia Journal: Dimensions of Desire* 20, no. 1 (1994); David L. Eng and Alice Y. Hom, eds., *Q & A: Queer in Asian America* (Philadelphia: Temple University Press, 1998); Chris Friday, *Organizing Asian American Labor: The Pacific Coast Canned-Salmon Industry, 1870–1942* (Philadelphia: Temple University Press, 1994); Russell Leong, ed., *Asian American Sexualities: Dimensions of the Gay and Lesbian Experience* (New York: Routledge, 1996); Jennifer Ting, "Bachelor Society: Deviant Heterosexuality and Asian American Historiography," in *Privileging Positions: The Sites of Asian American Studies,* edited by Gary Y. Okihiro, Marilyn Alquizola, Dorothy Fujita Rony, and K. Scott Wong (Pullman: Washington State University Press, 1995); and Jennifer Ting, "The Power of Sexuality," *Journal of Asian American Studies* 1, no. 1 (1998): 65–82.

56. Leong, "Home Bodies and the Body Politic," p. 11.

57. Kitty Tsui, "chinatown talking story," in *The Words of a Woman Who Breathes Fire* (Iowa City: Spinsters Ink, 1983).

CHAPTER 8: BECOMING MOM CHUNG

1. Chung, "Autobiography."

2. Jespersen argues that three events in 1931—the Japanese invasion of Manchuria, the publication of Pearl Buck's novel *The Good Earth,* and the widely reported conversion of China's President Chiang Kai-shek to Christianity—combined to elicit support for the plight of China. T. Christopher Jespersen, *American Images of China, 1931–1949* (Stanford, Calif.: Stanford University Press, 1996), p. xx.

3. Chung, "Autobiography."

4. Ibid.

5. Hilda Sidaras, "Woman Doctor Tells How She Chose 1,000 Service Men as Her 'Sons'," *Miami Daily News,* 1 April 1946, 7-A.

6. U.S. Navy, "Mom Chung Here for Air Show," press release, Chung Collection, box 6, folder 1.

7. Chung, "Autobiography"; and "Kiwi," *American Magazine,* November 1941.

8. Chung, "Autobiography."

9. Ibid.

10. Although Chung lived apart from her most of her siblings, she felt partially responsible for their education and welfare. After her siblings married, they most likely increased their financial and emotional separation from Chung as they focused their energies on their own families. Most of her siblings stayed in Southern California, but two of her sisters, Flo and V., moved to San Francisco.

11. Chung, "Autobiography."

12. Joseph J. Corn, *The Winged Gospel: America's Romance with Aviation, 1900–1950* (New York: Oxford University Press, 1983).

13. Amelia Earhart became a public figure after flying across the Atlantic in 1928 as part of a three-person crew. As the only woman on board and the first to cross the Atlantic, she achieved instant fame. However, she felt unworthy of the publicity until she repeated Lindbergh's feat as a solo pilot in 1932. Susan Ware, *Still Missing: Amelia Earhart and the Search for Modern Feminism* (New York: W. W. Norton, 1993).

14. Ibid., p. 36.

15. Cheung obtained the license in 1931. Yung, *Unbound Feet: A Social History of Chinese Women in San Francisco* (Berkeley and London: University of California Press, 1995), p. 162.

16. *San Francisco: The Bay and Its Cities* (New York: Hastings House, 1940), p. 500.

17. Mel Scott, *The San Francisco Bay Area: A Metropolis in Perspective* (Berkeley and London: University of California Press, 1959), pp. 218–21.

18. Susan Ware estimates that 500,000 out of 125 million Americans were flying in the early 1930s, a low number reflecting the prohibitive costs as well as the fears associated with flight. See Ware, *Still Missing,* p. 68.

19. Ware estimates that "no more than five hundred women held pilots' licenses in the early 1930s compared with fifteen thousand men." Ibid., p. 80.

20. For a discussion of the body image of female pilots, see ibid.

21. Chan Dwight, #361, to Margaret Chung, 1 February 1945, Chung Collection, box 5, folder 3.

22. John F. McGinty, #149 to Chung, 2 November 1944, Chung Collection, box 4, folder 9.

23. "'Mom, She's a Great Guy' to Her 465 Flying 'Sons': Dr. Margaret Chung, Chinese American, Keeps Close Watch over Brood: Each Wear Buddha," Chung Scrapbook, Chung Collection, box 10.

24. Helen Rich, "1000 Hero 'Sons' in Service Honor San Francisco 'Mom,'" Chung Scrapbook, Margaret Chung Collection, box 10, folder 7.

25. Chung, "Biography of Sons," Chung Collection, box 1, folder 2.

26. Chung, "Autobiography."

27. Paul Starr, *The Social Transformation of American Medicine: The Rise of a Sovereign Profession and the Making of a Vast Industry* (New York: Basic Books, 1982), p. 270.

28. Ibid., p. 271.

29. Yung, *Unbound Feet,* p. 183.

30. Chung, "Autobiography."

31. Ibid. The brackets indicate that Chung wrote the material by hand, but that it was not contained in the typed version.

32. Yong Chen, *Chinese San Francisco, 1850–1943: A Trans-Pacific Community* (Stanford, Calif.: Stanford University Press, 2000); Him Mark Lai, "The Kuomintang in Chinese American Communities before World War II," in *Entry Denied: Exclusion and the Chinese Community in America, 1882–1943,* edited by Sucheng Chan (Philadelphia: Temple University Press, 1991), pp. 170–212; L. Eve Armentrout Ma, "Chinatown Organizations and the Anti-Chinese Movement, 1882–1914," in *Entry Denied,* pp. 147–69; Victor G. Nee and Brett de Bary Nee, *Longtime Californ': A Documentary Study of an American Chinatown* (Palo Alto, Calif.: Stanford University Press, 1972); Shih-Shan Henry Tsai, *The Chinese Experience in America* (Bloomington: Indiana University Press, 1986); K. Scott Wong and Sucheng Chan, eds., *Claiming America: Constructing Chinese American Identities during the Exclusion Era* (Philadelphia: Temple University Press, 1998); K. Scott Wong, "War Comes to Chinatown: Social Transformation and the Chinese of California," in *The Way We Really Were: The Golden State in the Second Great War,* edited by Roger W. Lotchin (Urbana: University of Illinois Press, 2000), pp. 164–86; Renqiu Yu, *To Save China, To Save Ourselves: The Chinese Hand Laundry Alliance of New York* (Philadelphia: Temple University Press, 1992).

33. Gloria Heyung Chun, *Of Orphans and Warriors: Inventing Chinese American Culture and Identity* (New Brunswick, N.J.: Rutgers University Press, 2000), p. 27.

34. Andrew Lee to Chen Chung Loh, 4 May 1933, Chung Collection, box 2, folder 2.

35. "Noted Chinese Woman Doctor Offers Her Aid," *San Francisco Chronicle,* 17 August 1937.

36. Him Mark Lai, "Sprouting Wings on the Dragon," *East/West News,* 19 May 1988.

37. Yung, *Unbound Feet,* pp. 161–62.

38. Ibid., pp. 99–100 and 223–77; and Yung, "The Social Awakening of Chinese American Women as Reported in *Chung Sai Yat Po,* 1900–1911," in *Unequal Sisters: A Multicultural Reader in U.S. Women's History,* edited by Ellen Carol DuBois and Vicki L. Ruiz (New York: Routledge, 1990), pp. 195–207.

39. Yung, *Unbound Feet,* p. 231–32. The Women's Patriotic Club and the New Life Association attracted middle-class immigrant women. Working-class immigrant women joined the Women's War Zone Refugee Relief Committee and the Women's Council. The Patriotic Club and Women's Council were more critical of Chiang Kai-shek and the KMT. For American-born women, the young joined the Chinese YWCA, the business and professional women in their thirties participated in the Square and Circle Club. The Fidelis Coteri attracted "well-to-do matrons in their fifties." All seven women's organizations operated under the guidance of the male-dominated Chinese War Relief Association (CWRA).

40. Ibid., p. 233.

41. Ibid., p. 238.

42. Pearl Kwok, interview with author, 16 February 1996, Los Angeles.

43. I thank David Henkins for this insight. Linda Gordon makes a similar argument, asserting that the "whiteness" of the adopted child helps "whiten" the adopted parents. Linda Gordon, *The Great Arizona Orphan Abduction* (Cambridge, Mass.: Harvard University Press, 1999).

44. Henry Beckett, "'Mom' to 493 U.S. Fliers: Margaret Chung's 'Family' Spread Out," *New York Post*, 25 February 1942, Chung Scrapbook, Chung Collection.

45. Lowe, "Dr. Chung, the Doctor," box 128, PLP. I thank Jennifer Gee for bringing this source to my attention.

46. Ibid.

47. Rhea Talley, "One Beautifies Millions, One Mothers Thousands," *Louisville Courier-Journal*, n.d., Chung Scrapbook, Chung Collection.

48. Gertrude Atherton, *My San Francisco: A Wayward Biography* (Indianapolis: Bobbs-Merrill, 1946), p. 272.

49. Betty Hynes, "Distinguished Chinese Doctor Visits the Capital: Dr. Chung Here from the Coast for Brief Stay," 3 October 1942, Chung Scrapbook, Chung Collection.

50. Bob Poon, "Poo-Poo," *Chinese Digest,* 19 June 1936, p. 7.

51. Yung, *Unbound Feet,* p. 240.

52. For information about the Rice Bowls, see Yung, *Unbound Feet,* pp. 239–40. Lim P. Lee, a longtime Chinatown community member, recalls that Chung co-initiated the Rice Bowl Festival with Paul Smith, Night Chief of Police Captain Bennett, and Albert K. and W. Jack Chow. Lim P. Lee, "The Rice Bowl Parties 1938–40," *Asian Week,* 17 March 1989, p. 7.

53. Gladys Ng Gin, "Cocktail Waitress, 'That's What Happens When You're Illiterate,'" in *Unbound Voices: A Documentary History of Chinese Women in San Francisco,* by Judy Yung (Berkeley and London: University of California Press, 1999), p. 325.

54. Chung, "Autobiography." Chung's involvement in recruiting pilots for what would become known as the Flying Tigers is as yet unconfirmed by other sources. She explained that her activities were so secret that even the "Central Aircraft Company, which was the agency for sending the men out . . . [did not know] I was sending in recruits." Even General Claire Chennault, the head of the Flying Tigers and one of Chung's sons, did not know of her role. In fact, Flying Tiger Dick Rossi, another son, denies her involvement in his recruitment. Despite the lack of supporting evidence, the details that she recounts suggest the possibility of truth.

55. Ibid.

CHAPTER 9: A MODEL FAMILY AT WAR

1. Approximately 1 million African Americans, 350,000 Mexican Americans, 30,000 Japanese Americans, 20,000 Native Americans, and 12,000 Chinese Americans served in the military during World War II. See Allan Bérubé,

Coming Out under Fire: The History of Gay Men and Women in World War Two (New York: The Free Press, 1990); D'Ann Campbell, *Women at War with America: Private Lives in a Patriotic Era* (Cambridge, Mass.: Harvard University Press, 1984).

2. Karen Anderson, *Wartime Women: Sex Roles, Family Relations, and the Status of Women during World War II* (Westport, Conn.: Greenwood Press, 1981); William H. Chafe, *The American Woman: Her Changing Social, Economic, and Political Roles, 1920–1970* (New York: Oxford University Press, 1972), and *The Paradox of Change: American Women in the Twentieth Century* (New York: Oxford University Press, 1991); Susan M. Hartmann, *The Home Front and Beyond: American Women in the 1940s* (Boston: Twayne Publishers, 1982); Maureen Honey, *Creating Rosie the Riveter: Class, Gender, and Propaganda during World War II* (Amherst: University of Massachusetts Press, 1984); Leila J. Rupp, *Mobilizing Women for War: German and American Propaganda, 1939–1945* (Princeton, N.J.: Princeton University Press, 1978).

3. Perry R. Duis, "No Time for Privacy: World War II and Chicago's Families," in *The War in American Culture: Society and Consciousness during World War II,* edited by Lewis A. Erenberg and Susan E. Hirsch (Chicago: University of Chicago Press, 1996): pp. 17–45; Robert B. Westbrook, "'I Want a Girl, Just like the Girl that Married Harry James': American Women and the Problem of Political Obligation in World War II," *American Quarterly* 42, no. 4 (December 1990): 587–614; and Robert B. Westbrook, "Fighting for the American Family: Private Interests and Political Obligation in World War II," in *The Power of Culture: Critical Essays in American History,* edited by Richard Wightman Fox and T.J. Jackson Lears (Chicago: University of Chicago Press, 1993): 195–221.

4. Roger W. Lotchin, *Fortress California 1910–1961: From Warfare to Welfare* (New York: Oxford University Press, 1992).

5. Robert Mayer, *San Francisco: A Chronological and Documentary History, 1542–1970* (Dobbs Ferry, N.Y.: Oceana Publications, 1974), p. 44.

6. Marilynn S. Johnson, *The Second Gold Rush: Oakland and the East Bay in World War II* (Berkeley and London: University of California Press, 1993), p. 8; Arthur Verge, "Daily Life in Wartime California," in *The Way We Really Were: The Golden State in the Second Great War,* edited by Roger W. Lotchin (Urbana: University of Illinois Press, 2000), p. 20.

7. Sigrid Arne, "'Mom' Chung: A One-Woman Flyers' Recruiting Force," *Boston Daily Globe,* 3 February 1942.

8. Julia Cooley Altrocchi, *The Spectacular San Franciscans* (New York: E.P. Dutton and Co., 1949), p. 359.

9. Ted Friend and Dorothy Friend, "This Is the Life: Dr. Chung Cooks in Large Quantities," Chung Scrapbook, Chung Collection.

10. "Tex" to Chung, 28 August 1944, Chung Collection, box 4, folder 6.

11. Rascal to Chung, 13 August 1944, Chung Collection, box 4, folder 6.

12. Russ Bath to Chung, 14 December 1944, Chung Collection, box 4, folder 10.

13. Harry Carr, "The Lancer," *Los Angeles Times,* 23 July 1934.

14. Friend and Friend, "This Is the Life."

15. John Kuo Wei Tchen, *New York before Chinatown: Orientalism and the Shaping of American Culture, 1776–1882* (Baltimore: John Hopkins University Press, 1999).

16. Samuel Gompers and Herman Gutstadt, "Meat versus Rice: American Manhood against Asiatic Coolieism—Which Shall Survive?" originally published by the American Federation of Labor and printed as Senate Document 137 (1902), reprinted by Asiatic Exclusion League (San Francisco: 1908).

17. F.F. Gill to Chung, 19 February 1943, Chung Collection, box 3, folder 7. Big Game is an annual football competition between cross-bay rivals Stanford and Berkeley. Gill, an all-American football player, attended Berkeley.

18. Peggy Pascoe, *Relations of Rescue: The Search for Female Moral Authority in the American West, 1874–1939* (New York: Oxford University Press, 1990), p. 108.

19. Harry Byrone, "Press Release," 8 July 1944, Chung Collection, box 6, folder 4.

20. R.E. Randall to Chung, 4 February 1945, Chung Collection, box 5, folder 3.

21. Captain E.A. Byron to Chung, 19 November 1943, Chung Collection, box 3, folder 14.

22. E. Valencia to Chung, 10 June 1944, Chung Collection, box 4, folder 5.

23. Elmer Awl and B.F. Johnson to Chung, n.d., Chung Collection, box 3, folder 3.

24. Chuck to Chung, 4 October 1944, Chung Collection, box 4, folder 8.

25. Bill Baldwin to Chung, 23 October 1944, Chung Collection, box 4, folder 8.

26. Vincent Turner, interview with author, Los Angeles, 26 June 2001.

27. Again, my thanks to David Henkins for this interpretation.

28. Sigrid Arne, "'Mom' Chung: A One-Woman Flyers' Recruiting Force," *Boston Daily Globe,* 3 February 1942.

29. Ibid.

30. Chuck to Chung, 18 August 1944, Chung Collection, box 2, folder 4.

31. Ritchie Siau to Chung, 1 December 1944, Chung Collection, box 4, folder 9.

32. John W. Dower, *War without Mercy: Race and Power in the Pacific War* (New York: Pantheon Books, 1986).

33. Barry Urdang to Chung, 5 May 1943, Chung Collection, box 4, folder 1.

34. George Stimmel Jr. to Chung, 9 November 1944, Chung Collection, box 4, folder 9.

35. #523 to Chung, 22 November 1942, Chung Collection, box 3, folder 5.

36. #575 to Chung, 24 January [year n.d.], Chung Collection, box 3, folder 6.

37. In a speech celebrating the accomplishments of the Fighting Two, Chung credited the squadron with "506 Jap planes destroyed and 50,000 tons of enemy shipping sunk." Margaret Chung, "Speech," 31 October 1944, printed in *The Odyssey of Fighting Two,* by Thomas L. Morrissey (1945), p. 203.

38. Harry Byrne, "Press Release," 8 July [year n.d.], Chung Collection, box 6, folder 4.

39. Lin Yutang, "Chinese Nationalism and Anti-Nipponism," *New York Times Magazine,* reprinted in *Chinese Digest,* December 1937, p. 7.

40. William Hoy, "The Passing of Chinatown: Fact or Fancy," *Chinese Digest,* 31 January 1936, p. 11.

41. Ibid.

42. Yung, *Unbound Feet,* p. 235.

43. Ibid.

44. Bill and Marian Got, interview with author, 5 April 1997, San Jose, California. More research needs to be conducted to understand the full dynamics of Japanese American and Chinese American relations during the 1930s and 1940s. No doubt a range of opinions existed within the Chinese American community regarding internment.

45. *Time,* 22 December 1941, p. 33, quoted in Ronald Takaki, *Strangers from a Different Shore: A History of Asian Americans* (Boston: Little, Brown, 1989), p. 370.

46. Clifford Yip, interview with author, 17 November 1995, Mountain View, California.

47. Campbell, *Women at War with America,* p. 7. One popular opinion study, conducted two months after the bombing of Pearl Harbor, revealed that fewer women (36 percent) than men (57 percent) supported war against Japan.

48. Campbell, *Women at War with America,* p. 5.

49. Duis, "No Time for Privacy," pp. 17–45.

50. Bastard 642 to Chung, 20 November 1944, Chung Collection, box 4, folder 9.

51. Pat Robert A. May Williaman to Chung, 23 January 1945, Chung Collection, box 5, folder 2.

52. Craig G. Clark, telephone interview with author, 5 April 2002; and Guy Clark, telephone interview with author, 9 April 2002.

53. U.S. Navy, "Mom Chung Here for Air Show," press release, Chung Collection, box 6, folder 1.

54. Amy Bentley, *Eating for Victory: Food Rationing and the Politics of Domesticity* (Urbana: University of Illinois Press, 1998), pp. 31, 60.

55. Bentley, *Eating for Victory,* p. 48.

56. Clayton R. Koppes, "Hollywood and the Politics of Representation: Women, Workers, and African Americans in World War II Movies," in *The Home-Front War: World War II and American Society,* edited by Kenneth Paul O'Brien and Lynn Hudson Parsons (Westport, Conn.: Greenwood Press, 1995), pp. 29–30.

57. Evelyn Nakano Glenn, *Issei, Nisei, War Bride: Three Generations of Japanese American Women in Domestic Service* (Philadelphia: Temple University Press, 1986).

58. Floyd Bennett Aviation Post 333, American Legion, "Newsletter," Chung Collection, box 6, folder 1.

59. In several key respects, Chung's role as a wartime hostess replicated that of diplomatic wives. Cynthia Enloe notes that these well-educated and

politically skilled women focused their energies on complementing their husbands' duties by serving as hostesses, by fostering a "congenial environment," by "creating an atmosphere where men from different states can get to know one another 'man to man'." Among diplomatic wives, a commonly understood hierarchy or chain of command existed with the wife of the highest ranking diplomat. As Enloe explains, "The conduct of diplomacy relied on an embassy's senior women being able to mobilize the skills and labor of more junior women." Like these women, Chung upheld the belief that female contributions should focus on the traditional tasks of physically and emotionally nurturing men. She was different from these women in that she was not a wife, she had a career, and she was racially different from her diplomat and military sons. As a woman doctor of Chinese ancestry who chose not to marry, she was an unlikely candidate to serve as the head mother to the central constituents of the American state. Cynthia Enloe, *Bananas, Beaches and Bases: Making Feminist Sense of International Politics,* rev. ed. (Berkeley and London: University of California Press, 2000), pp. 97, 110.

60. La Verne Bradley, "San Francisco: Gibraltar of the West Coast," *National Geographic Magazine* 83, no. 3 (March 1943): 296–98. By the time of her death, Chung estimated the worth of her collection to be over $1 million.

61. Helen Rich, "Greatest Mother's Day Tribute: 1000 Hero 'Sons' in Service Honor San Francisco 'Mom,'" 14 May [year n.d.], Chung Scrapbook, Chung Collection.

62. Eleanor Grant Rigby, Oral History, Interviewed by Etta Belle Kitchen, 19 July 1970, Palo Alto, California, transcript published in *The Waves in World War II,* vol. 2 (Annapolis, Md.: U.S. Naval Institute, 1979), pp. 58–59.

63. Benedict Anderson, *Imagined Communities: Reflections on the Origin and Spread of Nationalism,* rev. ed. (London: Verso, 1991).

CHAPTER 10: CREATING WAVES

1. Cynthia Enloe, *Maneuvers: The Internal Politics of Militarizing Women's Lives* (Berkeley and London: University of California Press, 2000); Linda K. Kerber, *No Constitutional Right to Be Ladies* (New York: Hill and Wang, 1998).

2. Leisa D. Meyer, *Creating GI Jane: Sexuality and Power in the Women's Arm Corps during World War II* (New York: Columbia University Press, 1996), p. 14.

3. Joy Bright Hancock, *Lady in the Navy: A Personal Reminiscence* (Annapolis, Md.: Naval Institute Press, 1972), p. 48.

4. While the one thousand pilots in the Women Air Service Pilots (WASPs) participated as civilians, other women became official members of the military.

5. Meyer, *Creating GI Jane,* pp. 11–32.

6. Ibid., pp. 33–50.

7. Ibid., pp. 23–31.

8. Chung, "Autobiography."

9. Ibid.

10. Ibid.

11. Passages in the remainder of the paragraph are quoted from Mel Maas to Chung, 16 April 1942, Chung Collection, box 6, folder 5.

12. Albert B. Chandler to Chung, 18 March 1942, Chung Collection, box 3, folder 2.

13. Chung, "Autobiography."

14. Ibid.

15. "Diary," vol. 28, 22 June 1942, and vol. 29, 12 April 1943, Melvin Joseph Maas Papers, 1912–1968, Minnesota Historical Society, Manuscript Division, St. Paul, P1530, box 11.

16. Hancock, *Lady in the Navy*, p. 49. The Bureau of Navigation became the Bureau of Naval Personnel, the department that eventually sponsored the legislation. Also see Susan H. Godson, *Serving Proudly: A History of Women in the U.S. Navy* (Annapolis, Md.: U.S. Naval Institute Press, 2001).

17. Hancock, *Lady in the Navy*, p. 51.

18. Ibid., pp. 54–55.

19. Chung, "Autobiography."

20. Ibid.

21. United States Senate, 1942, Committee on Naval Affairs, *Women's Auxiliary Naval Reserve: Hearings on S. 2527*, 77th Congress, 2nd session.

22. Ibid., p. 14.

23. Hancock, *Lady in the Navy*, p. 55.

24. Mel Maas to Chung, 18 March 1942, quoted in "Autobiography." The original bill did restrict the duration of women's service to "six months after the termination of war." Hancock, *Lady in the Navy*, p. 55.

25. Chung, "Autobiography."

26. Hancock, *Lady in the Navy*, p. 55.

27. "Memo," Bureau of Naval Personnel (RG 24), General Correspondence 1941–45, box 2329, folder 4, National Archives, College Park, Maryland.

28. Margaret Chung to Edith Stallings, 1 July 1943, Joy Bright Hancock Papers, box 4, folder 10, Hargrett Rare Book and Manuscript Library, University of Georgia, Athens.

29. Ibid.

30. Ibid.

31. Margaret Chung to Melvin Maas, 22 April 1942, quoted in "Autobiography."

32. Melvin Maas to Chung, n.d., quoted in "Autobiography."

33. L. E. Denfeld to Chung, 2 May 1942, Chung Collection, box 6, folder 5.

34. In addition to Mildred McAfee, other advisory council members included Virginia C. Gildersleeve (dean of Barnard College); Ada Comstock (president of Radcliffe College); Mrs. Thomas S. Cates (wife of the president of the University of Pennsylvania); Meta Glass (president of Sweet Briar College); Alice M. Baldwin (dean of Women's College, Duke University); Alice C. Lloyd (dean of women, University of Michigan); Mrs. Malbone Graham (professor, author, and lecturer of Santa Monica, California); "History," Bureau of Naval Personnel, Assistant Chief of Naval Personnel for Women, National Archives, College Park, Maryland, box 4, folder 29. Hereafter cited as ACNP.

35. Meyer, *Creating GI Jane*, p. 66.

36. Meyer, *Creating GI Jane*.

37. Raymond Willis to Randall Jacobs, 25 June 1942, Bureau of Naval Personnel, GC, box 2330, folder 6.

38. Randall Jacobs to Willis, 27 June 1942, Bureau of Naval Personnel, GC, box 2330, folder 6.

39. Tova Petersen Wiley, Oral History, Interviewed by Etta-Belle Kitchen, 28 September 1969, in *The Waves in World War II*, vol. 2 (Annapolis, Md.: U.S. Naval Institute Press, 1979).

40. L.E. Denfeld to Basilio J. Valdes, 5 November 1942, Bureau of Naval Personnel, General Correspondence 1941–45, box 2331A, folder 1.

41. T.F. Darden, "Memorandum for the Chief of Naval Personnel," 5 November 1943, box 4, folder 30, ACNP.

42. Tova Petersen Wiley, "Memorandum to Assistant Chief of Personnel," box 4, folder 30, ACNP.

43. As late as January 1945, the Office of Strategic Services cautioned against granting "American citizens of Chinese origin . . . full security privileges." Edwin M. Martin, "Memorandum to Dr. William L. Langer," 22 January 1945, United States Office of Strategic Services, RG 226, "Far East IV," box 4, folder 7, National Archives, College Park, Maryland.

44. K. Scott Wong, "War Comes to Chinatown: Social Transformation and the Chinese of California," in *The Way We Really Were: The Golden State in the Second Great War*, edited by Richard W. Lotchin (Urbana: University of Illinois Press, 2000), p. 175.

45. Yung, *Unbound Feet*, p.256.

46. Meyer, *Creating GI Jane*.

47. L.B. Nichols to Mr. Tolson, 9 October 1940, United States Department of Justice, Federal Bureau of Investigation, "Dr. Margaret Chung" file, no. 65–35400.

48. District Intelligence Officer, Twelfth Naval District to Director of Naval Intelligence, "Report on Margaret Chung," 1 March 1945, "Margaret Chung" file, Department of the Navy.

49. Edith Stallings to Captain Weld, 6 June 1945, Joy Bright Hancock Papers, Hargrett Rare Book and Manuscript Library, University of Georgia, Athens, box 4, folder 10.

50. The historical party affiliations of Asian Americans need further study. Ron Takaki mentions the formation of Japanese American Democratic Clubs in the San Francisco Bay Area during the 1930s; *Strangers from a Different Shore: A History of Asian Americans* (Boston: Little, Brown, 1989), p. 221. See also Jo Freeman, *A Room at a Time: How Women Entered Party Politics* (Lanham: Rowman & Littlefield, 2000).

51. Susan M. Hartmann, *The Home Front and Beyond: American Women in the 1940s* (Boston: Twayne Publishers, 1982), pp. 31–32. The Marine Corps Women's Reserve (MCWR) enlisted 23,000 and the Coast Guard's SPARs (*Semper paratus*—always ready) recruited 13,000. In addition, 74,000 served in the Army and Navy Nurse Corps, and a small number of female doctors received commissions into the medical corps.

52. Margaret Chung to Stallings, 1 July 1943.

CHAPTER 11: "I'LL WAIT ON YOU FOREVER"

1. Hilda Sidaras, "Woman Doctor Tells How She Chose 1,000 Service Men as Her 'Sons'," *Miami Daily News,* 1 April 1946.

2. Margaret Chung to Sophie Tucker, 29 March 1945, Sophie Tucker Scrapbooks Collection, no. 10,957, New York Public Library, Performing Arts Branch. Hereafter cited as Tucker Scrapbooks.

3. Tucker was a prodigious saver. Her scrapbooks even contain letters from fans requesting autographs.

4. Michael Freedland, *Sophie: The Sophie Tucker Story* (London: Woburn, 1978), p. 211.

5. June Sochen, "From Sophie Tucker to Barbra Streisand: Jewish Women Entertainers as Reformers," in *Talking Back: Images of Jewish Women in American Popular Culture,* edited by Joyce Antler (Hanover, N.H.: Brandeis University Press and University Press of New England, 1998), p. 69. Between 1880 and World War I, approximately 2 million Jews immigrated to the United States. Susan A. Glenn, *Daughters of the Shtetl: Life and Labor in the Immigrant Generation* (Ithaca, N.Y.: Cornell University Press, 1990), p. 2.

6. Michael Rogin, *Blackface, White Noise: Jewish Immigrants in the Hollywood Melting Pot* (Berkeley and London: University of California Press, 1996, p. 16.

7. Robert Fyne, *The Hollywood Propaganda of World War II* (Lanham, Md.: Scarecrow Press 1997); Lary May, "Making the American Consensus: The Narrative of Conversion and Subversion in World War II Films," in *The War in American Culture: Society and Consciousness during World War II,* edited by Lewis A. Erenberg and Susan E. Hirsch (Chicago: University of Chicago Press, 1996).

8. Thomas Doherty, *Projections of War: Hollywood, American Culture, and World War II* (New York: Columbia University Press, 1993), pp. 60 and 7.

9. Roy Hoopes, *When the Stars Went to War: Hollywood and World War II* (New York: Random House, 1994).

10. Ernest Giglio, *Here's Looking at You: Hollywood, Film, and Politics* (New York: Peter Lang, 2000).

11. Mariko Tse, "Made in America." Research Project for East West Players on Chinese in Southern California. Unpublished paper, June 1979, p. 12.

12. Bessie Jeong, Oral History," interviewed by Suellen Cheng and Munson Kwok. 17 December 1981 and 17 October 1982, in *Southern California Chinese American Oral History Project,* Department of Special Collections, University Research Library, University of California, Los Angeles.

13. In her study of female athletes, Susan K. Cahn argues that women who threaten the gender hierarchy by excelling in traditionally masculine activities are pressured to emphasize their femininity. Susan K. Cahn, *Coming on Strong: Gender and Sexuality in Twentieth-Century Women's Sport* (New York: Free Press, 1994).

14. Elaine Tyler May, *Homeward Bound: American Families in the Cold War Era* (New York: Basic Books, 1988), p. 42.

15. Ibid.

16. Thomas Cripps, *Hollywood's High Noon: Moviemaking and Society before Television* (Baltimore: John Hopkins University Press, 1997).

17. Elizabeth Peck Hutchins, interview with author, 11 October 1995, San Ramon, California.

18. "Noted Chinese Woman Doctor Seeks to Aid China," 1937, Chung Scrapbook, Chung Collection.

19. Chung described their daily interaction in a series of letters to Tucker. See Chung to Tucker, 4, 5 January 1944, Tucker Scrapbooks, no. 10,950.

20. "Clipping," *San Francisco Call-Bulletin,* 17 November 1943, Chung Scrapbook, Chung Collection.

21. Chung to Tucker, 5 January 1944, Tucker Scrapbooks, no. 10,950.

22. Norman Clerk, telephone interview with author, 14 August 2001, Mt. Shasta, California.

23. Barbara Bancroft, "Creating Homes for Real Living: Dr. Chung's Decorative Furnishings Express Her," newspaper article provided by Betsy Bingham Davis.

24. Chung to Tucker, notes dated 13, 14, 17, 19 January 1945, Tucker Scrapbooks, no. 10,955. These notes were most likely attached to a series of birthday presents.

25. Chung to Tucker, 25 December 1947, Tucker Scrapbooks, no. 10,980.

26. Chung to Tucker, dated "Your last evening here in S.F.," Tucker Scrapbooks, no. 10,950.

27. Allan Bérubé discovered that gay men in the military also used song lyrics, originally intended to express heterosexual love, to suggest same-sex desire. For example, one male recruit sang "I Love My Man" to indicate his sexual orientation. Allan Bérubé, *Coming Out under Fire: The History of Gay Men and Women in World War Two* (New York: The Free Press, 1990).

28. Chung to Tucker, 17 January 1945, Tucker Scrapbooks, no. 10,955.

29. [Chung] to Tucker, n.d., Tucker Scrapbooks, no. 10,950.

30. Martha Vicinus, "Distance and Desire: English Boarding School Friendships, 1870–1920," in *Hidden from History: Reclaiming the Gay and Lesbian Past,* edited by Martin Bauml Duberman, Martha Vicinus, and George Chauncey Jr. (New York: New American Library, 1989), pp. 212–29, quotation on p. 224.

31. Estelle B. Freedman, "'The Burning of Letters Continues:' Elusive Identities and the Historical Construction of Sexuality," *Journal of Women's History* 9, no. 4 (1998): 185.

32. The use of religious and maternal language to express romantic longing represents a different strategy from the concept of "private lesbianism" suggested by Elizabeth Lapovsky Kennedy. She has argued for the possibility of women who "considered themselves lesbians but were completely private . . . about their erotic love for women." In contrast, Chung may not have embraced a lesbian identity, even in private, but instead fashioned alternative means to express her romantic desire for women. See Elizabeth Lapovsky Kennedy, "'But we would never talk about it': The Structures of Lesbian Discretion in South Dakota, 1928–1933," in *Inventing Lesbian Cultures in America,* edited by Ellen Lewin (Boston: Beacon Press, 1996), p. 18.

33. I thank Pamela Paxton for pointing out the ethnic and religious implications of Ruth's decision to follow Naomi.

34. Karen Garling Sickel, interview with author, Palo Alto, California, 17 September 1996.

35. Sophie Tucker, *Some of These Days* (Garden City, N.Y.: Doubleday, Doran and Co., 1945), p. 58.

36. Ibid., p. 33.

37. Ibid., p. 61.

38. Ibid., p. 33.

39. Sochen, "From Sophie Tucker to Barbra Streisand," p. 72.

40. Rogin, *Blackface, White Noise,* pp. 109, 111.

41. Tucker, *Some of These Days,* p. 35.

42. Karen Brodkin, *How Jews Became White Folks and What That Says about Race in America* (New Brunswick, N.J.: Rutgers University Press, 1998); and Matthew Frye Jacobson, *Whiteness of a Different Color: European Immigrants and the Alchemy of Race* (Cambridge, Mass.: Harvard University Press, 1998).

43. Tucker, *Some of These Days,* p. 63.

44. Chung to Tucker, 10 April 1955, Tucker Scrapbook, no. 15,850.

45. Henry Yu, "Mixing Bodies and Cultures: The Meaning of America's Fascination with Sex between 'Orientals'" and 'Whites'," in *Sex, Love, Race: Crossing Boundaries in North American History,* edited by Martha Hodes (New York: New York University Press, 1999), p. 447.

46. Elizabeth Peck Hutchins, interview with author, 11 October 1995, San Ramon, California.

47. "Launching Program, S.S. Grinnell Victory," 1945, in Tucker Scrapbooks, no. 10,956.

48. Bill Hodges to Tucker, Tucker Scrapbooks, no. 10,956.

49. Bérubé, *Coming Out under Fire;* Neil Okrent, "Right Place Wong Time: Why Hollywood's First Asian Star, Anna May Wong, Died a Thousand Movie Deaths," *Los Angeles Magazine,* May 1990, pp. 84+. Anthony W. Lee argues that the ability to perform, which "involve[s] role-playing, passing, masquerade, fantasy, and pantomime," facilitates opportunities to experiment with gender, sexual, and racial identities. Anthony W. Lee, *Picturing Chinatown: Art and Orientalism in San Francisco* (Berkeley and London: University of California Press, 2001), p. 285.

50. Nan Alamilla Boyd, "Homos Invade S.F.! San Francisco's History as a Wide-Open Town," in *Creating a Place for Ourselves: Lesbian, Gay, and Bisexual Community Histories,* edited by Brett Beemyn (New York: Routledge, 1997), p. 75.

51. Bill Wildey, telephone interview with author, 9 November 1999.

52. Bérubé, *Coming Out under Fire,* p. 125.

53. Ibid., p. 114.

54. Lillian Faderman, *Odd Girls and Twilight Lovers: A History of Lesbian Life in Twentieth-Century America* (New York: Columbia University Press, 1991), p. 181. For histories of the San Francisco gay and lesbian communities, see Susan Stryker and Jim Van Buskirk, *Gay by the Bay: A History of Queer*

Culture in the San Francisco Bay Area (San Francisco: Chronicle Books, 1996), pp. 22–27; and Faderman, *Odd Girls,* pp. 107 and 175–87.

55. Elaine Tyler May, "Rosie the Riveter Gets Married," in *The War in American Culture: Society and Consciousness during World War II,* edited by Lewis A. Erenberg and Susan E. Hirsch (Chicago: University of Chicago Press, 1996), p. 138.

56. Ibid.

57. Bérubé, *Coming Out under Fire,* p. 70.

58. Tucker, *Some of These Days,* p. 253.

59. Eric Garber, "A Spectacle in Color: The Lesbian and Gay Subculture of Jazz Age Harlem," in *Hidden from History: Reclaiming the Gay and Lesbian Past,* edited by Martin Bauml Duberman, Martha Vicinus, and George Chauncey Jr. (New York: New American Library, 1989), p. 326.

60. Chung to Tucker, 24 December 1945, Tucker Scrapbooks, no. 10,966.

EPILOGUE: "THERE WILL NEVER BE ANOTHER MOM CHUNG"

1. Margaret Chung to Halsey, 14 August 1945, William Frederick Halsey Jr. Papers, General Correspondence, box 4, August 1945, Library of Congress, Manuscript Division.

2. "Officer Biography Sheet" and "Rear Admiral William Sterling Parsons, United States Navy," William Sterling Parsons Papers, Library of Congress, box 2; and Thomas Parrish, ed., "William Sterling Parsons," *The Simon and Schuster Encyclopedia of World War II* (New York Simon and Schuster, 1978), p. 481.

3. "Dr. Chung Decorated by Chinese," *San Francisco Chronicle,* 5 June 1945; "Symbol," *San Francisco Chronicle,* 6 June 1945; Daisy Chinn, "Women of Initiative," *San Francisco Chinatown on Parade* (San Francisco: Chinese Chamber of Commerce, 1961), p. 64. Chung seldom adopted children of Chinese ancestry. She worked with Chinatown residents for professional and political reasons. However, her uneasy position in the community discouraged her from extending social invitations to her house. In fact, Chinese American military officer Richard Young, who attended one of Chung's Sunday parties in the company of a white friend, an American Air Force officer, sensed that she felt uncomfortable with him and tried to ignore his presence. She made no special attempts to talk with him, spending most of her time with white guests, some of whom she was meeting for the first time. Although Chung felt awkward with Chinese Americans, she enjoyed developing relationships with elite figures from China. Richard Young, interview with author, 15 November 1995, Palo Alto, California.

4. Chung, "Autobiography."

5. Ibid., pp. 244–45.

6. Beginning in 1942, Chung advertised her medical office hours as 2 to 4 P.M. daily. *San Francisco Directory,* 1942.

7. *San Francisco Directory,* 1951 and 1931.

8. Angelo J. Rossi, "Memo to Chung," 1 March 1943, Chung Collection, box 2, folder 8.

9. Chung, "China's View of the Present," *Journal of the National Association of Deans of Women* 5, no. 3 (March 1942): 107.

10. Madame Chiang Kai-shek to Chung, 29 December 1950, 25 August 1951, 18 November 1951, and 15 January 1952, Chung Collection, box 2, folder 2. It is unclear whether Chung ever visited Taiwan.

11. Chiang to Chung, 18 November 1951.

12. Arleigh A. Burke to Chung, 27 August 1951, Chung Collection, box 5, folder 6.

13. Hilda Sidaras, "Woman Doctor Tells How She Chose 1,000 Service Men as Her 'Sons'," *Miami Daily News,* 1 April 1946.

14. Randy Carol Balano, letter to author, 12 March 2000; Patricia Ward Wallace, *Politics of Conscience: A Biography of Margaret Chase Smith* (Westport, Conn.: Praeger, 1995), p. 72; Janann Sherman, *No Place for a Woman: A Life of Senator Margaret Chase Smith* (New Brunswick, N.J.: Rutgers University Press, 2000), pp. 58–72.

15. "Around the Town at Night with Syd Goldie," Chung Scrapbook.

16. Robert O'Brien, "San Francisco," Chung Scrapbook.

17. Charles Lockwood, "Diary," 1954, Charles Andrews Lockwood Papers, box 2, Library of Congress, Manuscript Division. Lockwood served as the commander of the U.S. Pacific Fleet's submarine forces during World War II.

18. "Dr. Chung, War Flyers' 'Mom,' Dies," *San Francisco Chronicle,* 6 January 1959.

19. Michael Freedland, *Sophie: The Sophie Tucker Story* (London: Woburn Press, 1978), p. 211.

20. Sophie Tucker, "Trees for Israel: The Sophie Tucker Forest," Dorothy Siu Papers, private collection, Los Angeles.

21. Eleanor Page, "Colorful Lots Are 'Sons' of Dr. Margaret Chung: Former Chicagoan Is Proud of Every Last One," *Chicago Tribune,* n.d., and Judith Cass, "Recorded at Random," Chung Scrapbook. Chung previously owned a German shepherd named Lady.

22. "Kiwi," *American Magazine* (November 1941), p. 85.

23. Chung, "Handwritten Notes to Autobiography."

24. Margaret Chung to Nimitz, n.d., Chester W. Nimitz Papers, Series 2, "C" 1946–1950, Operational Archives, Naval Historical Center, Washington, D.C.

25. Chung Scrapbook. For an analysis of Stanwyck's portrayal as the white female object of desire in *The Bitter Tea of General Yen* (1933), see Gina Marchetti, *Romance and the "Yellow Peril": Race, Sex, and Discursive Strategies in Hollywood Fiction* (Berkeley and London: University of California Press, 1993).

26. T. Christopher Jespersen, *American Images of China, 1931–1949* (Palo Alto, Calif.: Stanford University Press, 1996).

27. Shirley Jennifer Lim makes a similar argument in "Girls Just Wanna Have Fun: The Politics of Asian American Women's Public Culture, 1930–1960," PhD diss., University of California, Los Angeles, 1998.

28. Like Ling, Chung was drawn to figures in the underworld. She not only had a penchant for "queer" speakeasies, Chung also became friends with actress

Virginia Hill, the girlfriend of Bugsy Siegel. In fact, one sensationalist biography of Siegel describes Chung as "a shadowy character who was just as intimate with . . . the kings of the underworld." Dean Jennings, *We Only Kill Each Other: The Life and Bad Times of Bugsy Siegel* (Englewood Cliffs, N.J.: Prentice-Hall, 1967).

29. *Real Heroes,* no. 9 (February/March 1943), pp. 9–14.

30. Bert Hansen, "Medical History for the Masses: How American Comic Books Celebrated Heroes of Medicine in the 1940s," *Bulletin of the History of Medicine* (spring 2004), pp. 148–91. My thanks to Bert Hansen for sharing his research with me prior to its publication.

31. *Real Heroes,* no. 1 (September 1941), p. 1.

32. Karen Janis Leong, "The China Mystique: Mayling Soong Chiang, Pearl S. Buck and Anna May Wong in the American Imagination," PhD diss., University of California, Berkeley, 1999.

33. Confidential Memo on Dr. Margaret Chung, 12 October 1953, "Dr. Margaret Chung File," United States Department of Justice, no. 65–35400.

34. Passport application, "Chung, Margaret Jessie," United States Department of State.

35. See Christina Klein, "Adoption and the Cold War Commitment to Asia," in *Cold War Constructions : The Political Culture of United States Imperialism, 1945–1966,* edited by Christian G. Appy (Amherst: University of Massachusetts Press, 2000), pp. 34–66.

36. Lockwood, "Diary," 26 September 1958.

37. Mrs. Nimitz, "Diary," 8 January 1959, Chester W. Nimitz Papers.

38. "Dr. Margaret Chung," *San Francisco News,* 9 January 1959, photograph and caption in the private collection of Rodney Low, San Francisco.

39. City and County of San Francisco, Department of Health, "Certificate of Death for Margaret J. Chung," no. 122. Harold I. Griffith, MD, signed the certificate on 7 January 1959.

40. Mrs. Nimitz, "Diary," 8 January 1959, Chester W. Nimitz Papers.

41. Lockwood, "Diary," 10 January 1959.

Bibliography

PRIMARY SOURCES

Manuscripts and Archival Collections

Addams, Jane, Memorial Collection. University of Illinois at Chicago, Department of Special Collections.

American Medical Women's Association. Medical College of Pennsylvania, Archives and Special Collections, Philadelphia.

American Red Cross. Record Group 200. National Archives, College Park, Maryland.

Chandler, Albert B., Collection. University of Kentucky, Lexington.

Chicago Medical Society, Chicago.

Chinese Historical Society. San Francisco Collection. Asian American Studies Collection, Ethnic Studies Library, University of California, Berkeley.

Chung, Margaret, Collection. Asian American Studies Collection, Ethnic Studies Library, University of California, Berkeley.

———, File. Santa Barbara Historical Society, Santa Barbara.

Culbertson, Margaret, Biographical File. Presbyterian Historical Society, Philadelphia.

Gidlow, Elsa, Papers. Gay and Lesbian Historical Society of Northern California, San Francisco.

Halsey, William Frederick Jr., Papers. Library of Congress, Manuscript Division.

Hancock, Joy Bright, Papers. Hargrett Rare Book and Manuscript Library, University of Georgia, Athens.

Hearst Collection. Newspaper Files. University of Southern California Library, Regional History Center, Department of Special Collections, Los Angeles.

Kankakee State Hospital Collection. Kankakee Historical Society, Kankakee, Illinois.

Leong, Charles, Collection. Asian American Studies Collection, Ethnic Studies Library, University of California, Berkeley.

Lockwood, Charles Andrews, Papers. Library of Congress, Manuscript Division.

Loo, Richard, Collection. "King of Chinatown" Film Script. American Heritage Center, University of Wyoming, Laramie.

Lowe, Pardee, Papers. Hoover Institution of War, Revolution and Peace, Stanford University, Stanford, California.

Maas, Melvin Joseph, Papers. Minnesota Historical Society, Manuscript Division, St. Paul.

Medical College of Pennsylvania Collection. The Medical College of Pennsylvania Archives, Philadelphia.

Ng Family Papers. Private Collection. Bakersfield, California.

Nimitz, Chester W., Papers. Operational Archives, U.S. Naval Historical Center, Washington, D.C.

Parsons, William Sterling, Operational Archives, U.S. Naval Historical Center, Washington, D.C.

———, Papers. Library of Congress.

Presbyterian Church, Commission on Ecumenical Mission and Relations. Secretaries' Files. Record Group 81. Presbyterian Historical Society, Philadelphia.

———, U.S.A. Board of Foreign Missions. Secretaries' Files, 1829–1895. Record Group 31. Presbyterian Historical Society, Philadelphia.

Roosevelt, Eleanor, Papers. Hyde Park, New York.

Roosevelt, Franklin Delano, Papers. Hyde Park, New York.

Siu, Dorothy, Papers. Private Collection. Los Angeles.

Tucker, Sophie, Collection. American Jewish Archives, Cincinnati.

———. Collection. Museum of the City of New York.

———. Scrapbooks. New York Public Library, Performing Arts Branch, New York.

Van Hoosen, Bertha. Biography File. Chicago Historical Society.

———, Collection. University of Illinois at Chicago, Department of Special Collections.

———, File. Medical College of Pennsylvania, Archives and Special Collections, Philadelphia.

———, Papers. Bentley Historical Library, University of Michigan, Ann Arbor.

Willis, Raymond, Collection. Indiana State Library, Indianapolis.

Interviews and Personal Communications

Berkeley Chinese Community Church Senior Center, Members. Conversation with author. 6 July 1999. Berkeley, California.

Bingham, Dick. Interview by author. 31 October 1996. San Francisco.

"Born in Los Angeles—Reared in Oriental Fashion." Oral History. In *Orientals and Their Cultural Adjustment: Interviews, Life Histories, and Social Adjustment Experiences of Chinese and Japanese of Varying Backgrounds and Length of Residence in the United States*. Nashville: Social Science Institute, Fisk University, 1946.

Bratton, Angelique. Interview by author. 25 February 1996. Los Angeles.

Cheng, Suellen, and Munson Kwok. Interviews by author. 6 February 1996. Los Angeles.

Chew, Loni. Interview by author. 2 August 1999. Alameda, California.

Chung, Bill. Interview by author. 27 January 1996. San Diego.

Chung, Lucile. Interview by author. 28 January 1996. Vista, California.

Chung, Roger. Interview by author. 29 November 1995. Concord, California.

Clark, Craig. Telephone Interview by author. 5 April 2002. Seaside California.

Clark, Guy. Telephone Interview by author. 9 April 2002. Seaside, California.

Clerk, Norman. Telephone Interview by author. 14 August 2001. Mt. Shasta, California.

Davis, Betsy Bingham. 24 September 1996. Telephone Interview by author. Portland, Oregon.

Eymann, Eleanor, and Kenneth Eymann. Telephone Interview by author. Santa Rosa, California.

Flowers, Bob. Telephone Interview by author. 24 September 2002. San Diego.

Gambarano, Elmo. Interview by author. 12 February 1996. Los Angeles.

Garling, John. Interview by author. 26 September 1996. Hillsborough, California.

Got, Bill, and Marian Got. Interviews by author. 5 April 1997. San Jose, California.

Greenwood, Roberta S. Letter to author. 28 October 1997.

Hall, James. "Summary of Interview." Conducted by Philip Choy and Him Mark Lai. 23 August 1970. Belmont, California.

Hutchins, Elizabeth Peck. Interview by author. 11 October 1995. San Ramon, California.

Jeong, Bessie. Oral History. Interviewed by Suellen Cheng and Munson Kwok. 17 December 1981 and 17 October 1982. In *Southern California Chinese American Oral History Project*. Department of Special Collections, University Research Library, University of California, Los Angeles.

Jung, Edmund. Interview with author. 21 July 1999. San Francisco.

Kwok, Pearl. Interview by author. 16 February 1996. Los Angeles.

Lee, Jane, and William Lee. Conversations with author. 13 April 1997. Oakland, California.

Lee, Leland. Interview by author. 17 February 1996. Pasadena, California.

Lee, Robert G. Conversation with author. Summer 1999. Palo Alto, California.

Leung, Vera. Interview by author. 31 November 1995. Palo Alto, California.

Lew, Lillie. Interview by author. 14 January 1996. Fresno, California.

Low, Rodney. Interviews by author. 31 November 1995, 20 December 1997, and 2 January 1998. San Francisco, California.

Mixer, Pat Chung, and Harry Mixer. Interviews by author. 28 January 1996. Vista, California.

Rigby, Eleanor Grant. Oral History. Interviewed by Etta Belle Kitchen. 19 July 1970. Palo Alto, California. In *The Waves in World War II*. Vol. 2. Annapolis, Md.: Naval Institute Press, 1979.

Rossi, Dick. Interview by author. 17 November 1996. Fallbrook, California.

Sewall, Dick, and Barbara Sewall. Interviews by author. 16 November 1996. Corona, California.

Sickel, Karen Garling. Interview by author. 17 September 1996. Palo Alto, California.

Siu, Dorothy. Oral History. Interviewed by Jean Wong. 12 January 1979 and 6 November 1980. In *Southern California Chinese American Oral History Project*. Department of Special Collections, University Research Library, University of California, Los Angeles.

Siu, Gilbert. Conversation with author. 24 June 2001. Los Angeles.

Siu, Gilbert, and Kay Siu. Interviews by author. 3 February 1996. Corona, California.

Smith, Gail Dormer. Interviews by author. 14 February 1996 and 21 February 1996. Santa Barbara.

Square and Circle Club, Members. Conversation with author. 17 July 1999. San Francisco.

Turner, Vincent. Interview by author. 26 June 2001. Los Angeles.

Wildey, Bill. Telephone Interview by author. 9 November 1999. Oklahoma City.

Wiley, Tova Petersen. Oral History. Interviewed by Etta-Belle Kitchen. 28 September 1969. In *The Waves in World War II*. Vol. 2. Annapolis, Md.: Naval Institute Press, 1979.

Wong, Betty. Interview by author. 21 July 1999. San Francisco.

Yep, Doris. Interview by author. 4 December 1995. Palo Alto, California.

Yip, Clifford. Interview by author. 17 November 1995. Mountain View, California.

Yip, Clifford, Dorothy Yip, and Ray Yip. Conversation with author. 23 July 1999. Mountain View, California.

Young, Richard. Interview by author. 15 November 1995. Palo Alto, California.

Government Documents

California Public Utilities Commission. Railroad Hospital Reports, 1917–1922. California State Archives.

California State Board of Medical Examiners. Department of Consumer Affairs. Deceased Physicians Files. California State Archives, Sacramento.

Chicago Municipal Court. Annual Reports, 1917–1920. Chicago Historical Society.

Cook County. *Charity Service Reports*, 1917–1919.

Illinois State. *Blue Book*, 1917–1918.

Illinois Board of Administration. Record Group 351. Illinois Office of the Secretary of State, Archives Division, Springfield.

Illinois Department of Mental Health. Employment Records. Illinois Office of the Secretary of State, Archives Division, Springfield.

Illinois Department of Public Welfare. Record Group 206. Minutes of Meetings. Illinois Office of the Secretary of State, Archives Division, Springfield.

Illinois Eastern Hospital for the Insane, Kankakee State Hospital, Kankakee Developmental Center. Record Group 258. Illinois Office of the Secretary of State, Archives Division, Springfield.

Illinois Institute for Juvenile Research. Record Group 266. Illinois Office of the Secretary of State, Archives Division, Springfield.

Illinois State Board of Health. Record Group 352. Illinois Office of the Secretary of State, Archives Division, Springfield.

Illinois State Civil Service Commission, Department of Personnel. Record Group 216. Illinois Office of the Secretary of State, Archives Division, Springfield.

Los Angeles County. Death Certificates.

———. Index to Register of Voters, Pasadena City, 1920, 1922.

San Francisco, City and County of. Department of Health. "Certificate of Death for Margaret J. Chung," no. 122.

San Francisco, Port of. Office of Collector of Customs. "Chinese Merchants Santa Barbara." 22 August 1894. Santa Barbara Historical Society.

Ventura County. Superintendent of Schools Office. Promotion Record. 1898–1902.

United States Bureau of the Census. Washington, D.C. Various years.

United States Department of Justice. Federal Bureau of Investigation. "Dr. Margaret Chung File," no. 65-35400.

United States Department of State. Division of Far Eastern Affairs. Record Group 59. National Archives, College Park, Maryland.

———. Passport Records for Margaret Jessie Chung.

United States Navy. Bureau of Aeronautics. General Correspondence, 1943–1945. Record Group 72. National Archives, College Park, Maryland.

———. Bureau of Medicine and Surgery. Record Group 52. National Archives, College Park, Maryland.

———. Bureau of Naval Personnel. General Correspondence 1941–45. Record Group 24. National Archives, College Park, Maryland.

———. Bureau of Naval Personnel. Assistant Chief of Naval Personnel for Women. National Archives, College Park, Maryland.

———. Naval Criminal Investigative Service. Margaret Chung Files.

———. Office of Naval Intelligence. Administrative Correspondence, 1942–1946. Record Group 38. National Archives, College Park, Maryland.

———. Twelfth Naval District. General Correspondence, 1945. Record Group 181. National Archives, Pacific Sierra Region, San Bruno, California.

United States Office of Strategic Services. Record Group 226. National Archives, College Park, Maryland.

United States Senate. Committee on Naval Affairs. *Women's Auxiliary Naval Reserve: Hearings on S. 2527.* 77th Congress, 2nd session (1942).

Other Published Primary Sources

Adler, Herman M. *Cook County and the Mentally Handicapped: A Study of the Provisions for Dealing with Mental Problems in Cook County, Illinois.* New York: National Committee for Mental Hygiene, Inc., 1918.

———. "The Juvenile Psychopathic Institute and the Work of the Division of the Criminologist." *The Institution Quarterly* 9, no. 1 (31 March 1918): 6–10.

Altrocchi, Julia Cooley. *The Spectacular San Franciscans*. New York: E.P. Dutton and Co.,1949.

American Medical Directory. Chicago: American Medical Association, 1938.

Arne, Sigrid. "'Mom' Chung: A One-Woman Flyers' Recruiting Force." *Boston Daily Globe*, 3 February 1942.

Atherton, Gertrude. *My San Francisco: A Wayward Biography*. Indianapolis: Bobbs-Merrill, 1946.

Bainbridge, Lucy S. *Woman's Medical Work in Foreign Missions*. New York: Women's Board of Foreign Missions of the Presbyterian Church, 1886.

Beckett, Henry. "'Mom' to 493 U.S. Fliers: Margaret Chung's 'Family' Spread Out." *New York Post*, 25 February 1942.

Bowen, Louise de Koven. *Growing Up with a City*. New York: Macmillan, 1926.

Boyington, Gregory. *Baa Baa Black Sheep*. New York: Putnam, 1958.

Bradley, La Verne. "San Francisco: Gibraltar of the West Coast." *National Geographic Magazine* 83, no. 3 (March 1943): 296–98.

Brown, Charlotte Blake. "Obstetric Practice among the Chinese in San Francisco." *Pacific Medical and Surgical Journal* (July 1883): 15–21.

The California Legionnaire (San Francisco).

California Medicine (San Francisco).

Carr, Harry. "The Lancer." *Los Angeles Times*, 23 July 1934.

Chicago City Directory, 1917–1919.

Chicago Medical Directory, 1916–1919.

Chicago Medical Society. *Official Bulletin*, 1916–1919.

The Chinese Digest (San Francisco).

Chinn, Daisy. "Women of Initiative." *San Francisco Chinatown on Parade*. San Francisco: Chinese Chamber of Commerce, 1961.

Chung, Margaret. "China's View of the Present." *Journal of the National Association of Deans of Women* 5, no. 3 (March 1942): 106–8.

———. "Our Golden Girl." *Fabulous Las Vegas Magazine*, 17 October 1953.

Cook County Hospital. *Annual Reports*. Chicago, 1918.

The Daily Southern Californian (University of Southern California, Los Angeles), 1912–1915.

The Dawning. San Francisco: Chinese Hospital Medical Staff Archives, 1978.

Detwiler, Justice B., ed. *Who's Who in California: A Biographical Directory 1928–1929*. San Francisco: Who's Who Publishing Company, 1929.

Doyle, Helen MacKnight. *A Child Went Forth*. New York: Gotham House, 1934.

Eastman, Charles A. *From the Deep Woods to Civilization: Chapters in the Autobiography of an Indian*. Boston: Little, Brown, and Co., 1920.

Edwards, William A. "In the Days of Pon Sue." *Noticias* 13, no. 4 (Autumn, 1967).

Fluckey, Eugene B. *Thunder Below! The USS Barb Revolutionizes Submarine Warfare in World War II*. Urbana: University of Illinois, 1992.

Following the Dawn. San Francisco: Chinese Hospital Medical Staff Archives, 1979.

Gardner, Mabel E. "Bertha Van Hoosen, M.D.: First President of the American Medical Women's Association." *Journal of the American Medical Women's Association* 5, no. 10 (October 1950): 413–14.

Gidlow, Elsa. *Elsa: I Come with My Songs.* San Francisco: Booklegger Press, 1986.

Ginjee, T. J., and Howard H. Johnson. "San Francisco's First Chinese Hospital." *The Modern Hospital,* October 1925: 283–85.

Gompers, Samuel, and Herman Gutstadt. "Meat versus Rice: American Manhood against Asiatic Coolieism—Which Shall Survive?" Originally published by the American Federation of Labor and Printed as Senate Document 137 (1902). Reprint. San Francisco: Asiatic Exclusion League, 1908.

Grigg, Bessie. *Directory of Medical Women.* Cincinnati and Newpark, Ky.: Elizabeth Press, 1945, 1949, and 1952.

Hancock, Joy Bright. *Lady in the Navy: A Personal Reminiscence.* Annapolis, Md.: Naval Institute Press, 1972.

Henley, W. Ballentine, and Arthur E. Neelley, eds. *Cardinal and Gold: A Pictorial and Factual Record of the Highlights of Sixty Years of Progress on the Southern California Campus with Views and News of Some of the 70,000 Students Who Played Their Part in the Growth of a Great University, 1880–1940.* Los Angeles: General Alumni Association, University of Southern California, 1939.

History of Medicine and Surgery and Physicians and Surgeons of Chicago. Chicago: Biographical Publishing Corporation, 1922.

History of Santa Barbara and Ventura Counties, California. 1883. Reprint. Berkeley, Calif.: Howell-North Books, 1961.

"Hospital's History in Chinatown." *Asian Week,* 19 May 1989.

Houde, Mary Jean, and John Klasey. *Of the People: A Popular History of Kankakee County.* Chicago: General Printing Company, 1968.

"How to Tell Japs from the Chinese." *Life,* 19 December 1941, 14.

"How to Tell Your Friends from the Japs." *Time,* 22 December 1941, 33.

Hudgens, K. B. "Across the River: A Brief History of Kankakee Developmental Center." Unpublished paper, Kankakee (Illinois) Historical Society, 1976.

The Institution Quarterly (Springfield, Illinois), 1917–1920.

Jeter, Helen Rankin. *The Chicago Juvenile Court.* U.S. Department of Labor, Children's Bureau, Publication no. 104. Washington: Government Printing Office, 1922.

Kankakee (Illinois) City Directory.

"Kiwi." *American Magazine,* November 1941.

Kao, George. *San Francisco Chinatown in 1950.* Hong Kong: Chinese University Press, 1988.

Kostelanetz, Andre, with Gloria Hammond. *Echoes: Memoirs of Andre Kostelanetz.* New York: Harcourt Brace Jovanovich, 1981.

Lee, Lim P. "The Rice Bowl Parties 1938–40." *Asian Week,* 17 March 1989, p. 7.

Leung, Louise. "Chinatown Woman Noted for Surgery." *San Francisco News,* 7 November 1929.

Los Angeles City Directory, 1902–1922.

Los Angeles County Medical Association. *Bulletin,* 1918–1922, 1924, 1959.

Lui, Garding. *Inside Los Angeles Chinatown.* Los Angeles, 1948.

Medical California. San Francisco: California Medical Association, 1923.

Medical Care of Industrial Workers. New York: National Industrial Conference Board, Inc., 1926.

Mendian, Rose V. "Bertha Van Hoosen: A Surgical Daughter's Impressions." *Journal of American Medical Women's Association* (April 1965).

Morrissey, Thomas L. *The Odyssey of Fighting Two.* 1945.

The Occident, 1888, 1890.

Occidental Leaves. San Francisco, 1893.

O'Gara, Gerald J. "Interesting Westerners: The Ministering Angel of Chinatown." *Sunset,* December 1924, pp. 28–29.

Okrent, Neil. "Right Place, Wong Time: Why Hollywood's First Asian Star, Anna May Wong, Died a Thousand Movie Deaths." *Los Angeles Magazine,* May 1990, pp. 84+.

Pasadena City Directory, 1920–1926.

Phillips, Michael James. *History of Santa Barbara County, California: From Its Earliest Settlement to the Present Time.* Chicago: S. J. Clarke Publishing Co., 1927.

Puckett, Pearl P. "She's Mom to Two Thousand American Flyers." *Independent Woman,* January 1946.

Radke, Shirley. "We Must Be Active Americans." *Christian Science Monitor,* 3 October 1942.

Real Heroes. No. 1, September 1941. No. 9, February/March 1943.

San Francisco: The Bay and Its Cities. New York: Hastings House, 1940. Rev. ed., 1947.

The San Francisco Chronicle.

San Francisco City Directory, 1921–1959.

Santa Barbara City Directory, 1888, 1893, and 1897. Santa Barbara Historical Society.

The Santa Barbara News Press.

Satterlee, Helen. "The Story of a Persevering Chinese Girl Who Reached the Heights of Surgical Fame." *Los Angeles Times Sunday Magazine* (25 June 1939).

Scholten, Paul, and Collin P. Quock. "Chinese Hospital: The Legacy of the Tung Wah Dispensary." *San Francisco Medicine* (May 1990): 29–31.

Selby, C. D. *Studies of the Medical and Surgical Care of Industrial Workers.* Treasury Department, United States Public Health Service, Public Health Bulletin no. 99. Washington: Government Printing Office, 1919.

Sidaras, Hilda. "Woman Doctor Tells How She Chose 1,000 Service Men as Her 'Sons'." *Miami Daily News,* 1 April 1946.

The Society of Medical History of Chicago. *Bulletin,* 1924.

Southern California Practitioner, 1913–1920.

The Southern California Trojan (University of Southern California, Los Angeles), 1915–1916.

Storke, Yda Addis. *A Memorial and Biographical History of the Counties of Santa Barbara, San Luis Obispo and Ventura, California.* Chicago: Lewis Publishing Company, 1891.

A Struggle for Excellence: One Hundred Years of the Los Angeles County Medical Association, 1871–1971. Los Angeles County Medical Association, 1971.

Thompson, Mary Harris. "The Chicago Hospital for Women and Children." In *In Memoriam, Mary Harris Thompson,* edited by Maria S. Iberne. Chicago: Board of Managers, 1896.

Tsui, Kitty. "chinatown talking story." In *The Words of a Woman Who Breathes Fire.* Iowa City: Spinsters, Ink, 1983.

Tucker, Sophie. *Some of These Days.* Garden City, N.Y.: Doubleday, Doran and Co., 1945.

Tyroler, A. "The Santa Fe Hospital in Los Angeles Provides a Practical Cause for Thanksgiving." *The Santa Fe Magazine* 20, no. 12 (November 1926): 21–25.

University of Southern California. *Bulletin, College of Liberal Arts Year Book, 1906–1916.*

———. *El Rodeo, 1908–1917.*

USC Medicine 33, no. 2 (1985).

Van Hoosen, Bertha. *Petticoat Surgeon.* Chicago: Pellegrini & Cudahy, 1947.

———. "Travel Letters through the Orient: Personal Observations and Experiences of Dr. Bertha Van Hoosen." *Medical Women's Journal* 30, no. 3 (March 1923): 76–78.

Wicher, Edward Arthur. *The Presbyterian Church in California, 1849–1927.* New York: Crafton Press, 1927.

Woman's Foreign Missionary Society of the Presbyterian Church of the Pacific Coast, *Reports of the Occidental Board.* San Francisco, 1874–1920.

Woon, Basil. *San Francisco and the Golden Empire.* New York: Harrison Smith and Robert Haas, 1935.

Yetzler, Carl. "San Bernardino Proud to Be a Railroad City." *San Bernardino Sun-Telegram.* Clipping found in San Bernardino Public Library.

SECONDARY SOURCES

Abbott, Elizabeth Lee. "Dr. Hu King Eng, Pioneer." In *The Life, Influence and the Role of the Chinese in the United States, 1776–1960.* San Francisco: Chinese Historical Society of America, 1976.

Allen, Joseph R. "Dressing and Undressing the Chinese Woman Warrior." *Positions* 4, no. 2 (1996): 343–79.

Almaguer, Tomás. *Racial Fault Lines: The Historical Origins of White Supremacy in California.* Berkeley and London: University of California Press, 1994.

Alpern, Sara, Joyce Antler, Elisabeth Israels Perry, and Ingrid Winther Scobie, eds. *The Challenge of Feminist Biography: Writing the Lives of Modern American Women.* Urbana: University of Illinois Press, 1992.

Amerasia Journal: Dimensions of Desire 20, no. 1 (1994).

Anderson, Benedict. *Imagined Communities: Reflections on the Origin and Spread of Nationalism.* Rev. ed. London: Verso, 1991.

Anderson, Karen. *Wartime Women: Sex Roles, Family Relations, and the Status of Women during World War II*. Westport, Conn.: Greenwood Press, 1981.

Asian Women United of California, ed. *Making Waves: An Anthology of Writings by and about Asian American Women*. Boston: Beacon Press, 1989.

Baker, Paula. "The Domestication of Politics: Women and American Political Society, 1780–1920." In *Unequal Sisters: A Multicultural Reader in U.S. Women's History*. New York: Routledge, 1990.

Balakrishnan, Gopal, ed. *Mapping the Nation*. London: Verso, 1988.

Barrett, James R., and David Roediger. "Inbetween Peoples: Race, Nationality and the 'New Immigrant' Working Class." *Journal of American Ethnic History* 16, no. 3 (spring 1997): 3–44.

Bentley, Amy. *Eating for Victory: Food Rationing and the Politics of Domesticity*. Urbana: University of Illinois Press, 1998.

Bentz, Linda. "The Overseas Chinese of Ventura." Honors thesis. University of California, Los Angeles, 1994.

Bérubé, Allan. *Coming Out under Fire: The History of Gay Men and Women in World War Two*. New York: The Free Press, 1990.

Bodnar, John. *The Transplanted: A History of Immigrants in Urban America*. Bloomington: Indiana University Press, 1985.

Bonner, Thomas Neville. *Medicine in Chicago, 1850–1950: A Chapter in the Social and Scientific Development of a City*. 1957. Reprint. Urbana: University of Illinois Press, 1991.

———. *To the Ends of the Earth: Women's Search for Education in Medicine*. Cambridge, Mass.: Harvard University Press, 1992.

Bost, Martha Douglas. "History of Mary Thompson Hospital, 1865–1973." Unpublished paper, December 1973. Chicago Historical Society.

Boyd, Nan Alamilla. "Homos Invade S.F.! San Francisco's History as a Wide-Open Town." In *Creating a Place for Ourselves: Lesbian, Gay, and Bisexual Community Histories*, edited by Brett Beemyn. New York: Routledge, 1997.

———. "Sex Tourism and the Emergence of Lesbian Communities in San Francisco's Historic North Beach District: 1933–1960." Unpublished Paper. Berkshire Conference on the History of Women, Rochester, New York, June 1999.

Bradley, Glenn Danford. *The Story of the Santa Fe*. Boston: Gorham Press, 1920.

Brandes, Stuart D. *American Welfare Capitalism, 1880–1940*. Chicago: University of Chicago Press, 1970.

Brodkin, Karen. *How Jews Became White Folks and What That Says about Race in America*. New Brunswick, N.J.: Rutgers University Press, 1998.

Brown, Victoria Bissell. "The Fear of Feminization: Los Angeles High Schools in the Progressive Era." In *Gender and American Law: The Impact of the Law on the Lives of Women*, edited by Karen J. Maschke. New York: Garland Publishing, Inc. 1997.

———. "Golden Girls: Female Socialization in Los Angeles, 1880 to 1910." PhD diss., University of California, San Diego, 1985.

Bryant, Keith L. Jr. *History of the Atchison, Topeka and Santa Fe Railway*. New York: Macmillan, 1974.

Bullough, Vern L., and Bonnie Bullough. *Cross Dressing, Sex, and Gender.* Philadelphia: University of Pennsylvania Press, 1993.

Burton, Margaret E. *Women Workers of the Orient.* New York: The Woman's Press, 1919.

Butler, Judith. "Performative Acts and Gender Constitution: An Essay in Phenomenology and Feminist Theory." In *Performing Feminisms: Feminist Critical Theory and Theatre.* Baltimore: John Hopkins University Press, 1990.

Cahn, Susan K. *Coming on Strong: Gender and Sexuality in Twentieth-Century Women's Sport.* New York: Free Press, 1994.

Camarillo, Albert. *Chicanos in a Changing Society: From Mexican Pueblos to American Barrios in Santa Barbara and Southern California, 1848–1930.* Cambridge, Mass.: Harvard University Press, 1979.

Campbell, D'Ann. *Women at War with America: Private Lives in a Patriotic Era.* Cambridge, Mass.: Harvard University Press, 1984.

Chafe, William H. *The American Woman: Her Changing Social, Economic, and Political Roles, 1920–1970.* New York: Oxford University Press, 1972.

———. *The Paradox of Change: American Women in the Twentieth Century.* New York: Oxford University Press, 1991.

Chan, Sucheng. *Asian Americans: An Interpretive History.* Boston: Twayne Publishers, 1991.

———. "The Exclusion of Chinese Women, 1870–1943." In *Entry Denied: Exclusion and the Chinese Community in America, 1882–1943,* edited by Sucheng Chan. Philadelphia: Temple University Press, 1991.

———. *This Bitter-Sweet Soil: The Chinese in California Agriculture, 1860–1910.* Berkeley and London: University of California Press, 1986.

Chaudhuri, Nupur, and Margaret Strobel, ed. *Western Women and Imperialism: Complicity and Resistance.* Bloomington: Indiana University Press, 1992.

Chauncey, Jr., George. "From Sexual Inversion to Homosexuality: The Changing Medical Conceptualization of Female 'Deviance.'" In *Passion and Power: Sexuality in History.* Philadelphia: Temple University Press, 1989.

Chen, Yong. *Chinese San Francisco, 1850–1943: A Trans-Pacific Community.* Stanford, Calif.: Stanford University Press, 2000.

Cheng, Suellen, and Munson Kwok. "The Golden Years of Los Angeles Chinatown: The Beginning." In *Chinatown Los Angeles: The Golden Years, 1938–1988.* Los Angeles: Chinese Chamber of Commerce, 1988.

Cherny, Robert W., and William Issel. *San Francisco: Presidio, Port and Pacific Metropolis.* San Francisco: Boyd and Fraser Publishing Company, 1981.

Chin, Soo-Young. *Doing What Had to Be Done: The Life Narrative of Dora Yum Kim.* Philadelphia: Temple University Press, 1999.

Chinese Historical Society of Southern California. *Linking Our Lives: Chinese American Women of Los Angeles.* Los Angeles: Chinese Historical Society of Southern California, 1984.

Chinn, Thomas W. *Bridging the Pacific: San Francisco Chinatown and Its People.* San Francisco: Chinese Historical Society of America, 1989.

Choy, Catherine Ceniza. "The Usual Suspects: Medicine, Nursing, and American Colonialism in the Philippines." *Hitting Critical Mass: A Journal of Asian American Cultural Criticism* 5, no. 2 (fall 1998).

Chun, Gloria Heyung. "'Go West . . . to China': Chinese American Identity in the 1930s." In *Claiming America: Constructing Chinese American Identities during the Exclusion Era,* edited by K. Scott Wong and Sucheng Chan. Philadelphia: Temple University Press, 1998.

————. *Of Orphans and Warriors: Inventing Chinese American Culture and Identity.* New Brunswick, N.J.: Rutgers University Press, 2000.

Cleland, Robert Glass. *The History of Occidental College, 1887–1937.* Los Angeles, 1937.

Corn, Joseph J. *The Winged Gospel: America's Romance with Aviation, 1900–1950.* New York: Oxford University Press, 1983.

Costin, Lela B. *Two Sisters for Social Justice: A Biography of Grace and Edith Abbott.* Urbana: University of Illinois Press, 1983.

Cott, Nancy F. "Across the Great Divide: Women in Politics before and after 1920." In *Women, Politics, and Change,* edited by Louise A. Tilly and Patricia Gurin. New York: Russell Sage Foundation, 1990.

————. *The Grounding of Modern Feminism.* New Haven, Conn.: Yale University Press, 1987.

————. "What's in a Name—The Limits of Social Feminism—or, Expanding the Vocabulary of Women's History." *Journal of American History* 76, no. 3 (December 1989): 809–29.

Cripps, Thomas. *Hollywood's High Noon: Moviemaking and Society before Television.* Baltimore: John Hopkins University Press, 1997.

Dasgupta, Shamita Das, ed. *A Patchwork Shawl: Chronicles of South Asian Women in America.* New Brunswick, N.J. : Rutgers University Press, 1998.

Davis, Madeline, and Elizabeth Lapovsky Kennedy. "Oral History and the Study of Sexuality in the Lesbian Community: Buffalo, New York, 1940–1960." In *Hidden from History: Reclaiming the Gay and Lesbian Past,* edited by Martin Bauml Duberman, Martha Vicinus, and George Chauncey Jr. New York: New American Library, 1989.

Davis, Mike. *City of Quartz.* New York: Vintage Books, 1990.

D'Emilio, John. *Sexual Politics, Sexual Communities: The Making of a Homosexual Minority in the United States, 1940–1970.* Chicago: University of Chicago Press, 1983.

D'Emilio, John, and Estelle B. Freedman. *Intimate Matters: A History of Sexuality in America.* New York: Harper and Row, 1988.

Doherty, Thomas. *Projections of War: Hollywood, American Culture, and World War II.* New York: Columbia University Press, 1993.

Dower, John W. *War without Mercy: Race and Power in the Pacific War.* New York: Pantheon Books, 1986.

Drachman, Virginia G. *Hospital with a Heart: Women Doctors and the Paradox of Separatism at the New England Hospital, 1862–1969.* Ithaca, N.Y.: Cornell University Press, 1984.

Duberman, Martin Bauml, Martha Vicinus, and George Chauncey Jr., eds. *Hidden from History: Reclaiming the Gay and Lesbian Past.* New York: New American Library, 1989.

Ducker, James H. *Men of the Steel Rails: Workers on the Atchison, Topeka and Santa Fe Railroad, 1869–1900.* Lincoln: University of Nebraska Press, 1983.

Duke, Donald, and Stan Kistler. *Santa Fe: Steel Rails through California.* San Marino, Calif.: A Golden West Book, 1963.

Duggan, Lisa. "The Trials of Alice Mitchell: Sensationalism, Sexology, and the Lesbian Subject in Turn-of-the-Century America." *Signs* 18, no. 4 (summer 1993): 791–814.

Duis, Perry R. "No Time for Privacy: World War II and Chicago's Families." In *The War in American Culture: Society and Consciousness during World War II,* edited by Lewis A. Erenberg and Susan E. Hirsch. Chicago: University of Chicago Press, 1996.

Eng, David L., and Alice Y. Hom, eds. *Q&A: Queer in Asian America.* Philadelphia: Temple University Press, 1998.

Enloe, Cynthia. *Bananas, Beaches and Bases: Making Feminist Sense of International Politics.* Rev. ed. Berkeley and London: University of California Press, 2000.

———. *Maneuvers: The Internal Politics of Militarizing Women's Lives.* Berkeley and London: University of California Press, 2000.

Espiritu, Yen Le. *Asian American Women and Men: Labor, Laws, and Love.* Thousand Oaks: Sage, 1997.

Etter-Lewis, Gwendolyn, and Michéle Foster, ed. *Unrelated Kin: Race and Gender in Women's Personal Narratives.* New York: Routledge, 1996.

Faderman, Lillian. *Odd Girls and Twilight Lovers: A History of Lesbian Life in Twentieth-Century America.* New York: Columbia University Press, 1991.

Fan, Tin-Chiu. "Chinese Residents in Chicago." PhD diss., University of Chicago, 1926.

Flemming, Leslie A. *Women's Work for Women: Missionaries and Social Change in Asia.* Boulder: Westview Press, 1989.

Fogelson, Robert M. *The Fragmented Metropolis: Los Angeles, 1850–1930.* Cambridge, Mass.: Harvard University Press, 1967.

Fong, Colleen, and Judy Yung. "In Search of the Right Spouse: Interracial Marriage among Chinese and Japanese Americans." *Amerasia Journal* 21, no. 3 (1995): 77–98.

Fong, Timothy P. *The Contemporary Asian American Experience: Beyond the Model Minority.* Upper Saddle River, N.J.: Prentice-Hall, 1998.

Freedland, Michael. *Sophie: The Sophie Tucker Story.* London: Woburn, 1978.

Freedman, Estelle B. "'The Burning of Letters Continues': Elusive Identities and the Historical Construction of Sexuality." *Journal of Women's History* 9, no. 4 (1998): 181–200.

———. *Maternal Justice: Miriam Van Waters and the Female Reform Tradition.* Chicago: University of Chicago Press, 1996.

————. "Separatism Revisited: Women's Institutions, Social Reform, and the Career of Miriam Van Waters." In *U.S. History as Women's History: New Feminist Essays*. Chapel Hill: University of North Carolina Press, 1995.

Freeman, Jo. *A Room at a Time: How Women Entered Party Politics*. Lanham, Md.: Rowman & Littlefield, 2000.

Friday, Chris. *Organizing Asian American Labor: The Pacific Coast Canned-Salmon Industry, 1870–1942*. Philadelphia: Temple University Press, 1994.

Fyne, Robert. *The Hollywood Propaganda of World War II*. Lanham, Md.: Scarecrow Press, 1997.

Garber, Eric. "A Spectacle in Color: The Lesbian and Gay Subculture of Jazz Age Harlem." In *Hidden from History: Reclaiming the Gay and Lesbian Past*, edited by Martin Bauml Duberman, Martha Vicinus, and George Chauncey Jr. New York: New American Library, 1989.

Garber, Marjorie. *Vested Interests: Cross-Dressing and Cultural Anxiety*. New York: Routledge, 1992.

Getis, Victoria. *The Juvenile Court and the Progressives*. Urbana: University of Illinois Press, 2000.

Giglio, Ernest. *Here's Looking at You: Hollywood, Film, and Politics*. New York: Peter Lang, 2000.

Gin, Gladys Ng. "Cocktail Waitress, 'That's What Happens When You're Illiterate.'" In *Unbound Voices: A Documentary History of Chinese Women in San Francisco*, edited by Judy Yung. Berkeley and London: University of California Press, 1999.

Ginzberg, Lori D. *Women and the Work of Benevolence: Morality, Politics, and Class in the Nineteenth-Century United States*. New Haven, Conn.: Yale University Press, 1990.

Glenn, Evelyn Nakano. *Issei, Nisei, War Bride: Three Generations of Japanese American Women in Domestic Service*. Philadelphia: Temple University Press, 1986.

Glenn, Susan A. *Daughters of the Shtetl: Life and Labor in the Immigrant Generation*. Ithaca, N.Y.: Cornell University Press, 1990.

Godfrey, Brian J. *Neighborhoods in Transition: The Making of San Francisco's Ethnic and Nonconformist Communities*. Berkeley and London: University of California Press, 1988.

Godson, Susan H. *Serving Proudly: A History of Women in the U.S. Navy*. Annapolis, Md.: Naval Institute Press, 2001.

Goossen, Rachel Waltner. *Women against the Good War*. Chapel Hill: University of Carolina Press, 1997.

Gordon, Linda. *The Great Arizona Orphan Abduction*. Cambridge, Mass.: Harvard University Press, 1999.

Gordon, Lynn D. *Gender and Higher Education in the Progressive Era*. New Haven, Conn.: Yale University Press, 1990.

Gray, Barbara Bronson. *120 Years of Medicine: Los Angeles County, 1871–1991*. Houston: Pioneer Publications, Inc.

Greenwood, Roberta S. "Chinatown in Ventura." *Gum Saan Journal* 7, no. 1 (June 1984): 1–11.

———. *Cultural Resources Impact Mitigation Program Los Angeles Metro Rail Red Line Segment 1.* Los Angeles: Los Angeles County Metropolitan Transportation Authority, 1993.

———. "The Overseas Chinese at Home: Life in a Nineteenth-Century Chinatown in California." *Archaeology* 31, no. 4 (September/October 1978): 42–49.

———. "Recovering Old Chinatowns." *Gum Saan Journal* 18, no. 2 (December 1995): 41–43.

Greenwood, Roberta S., and James J. Schmidt. "Data Recovery at the Soo Hoo Property, Ventura." Report. Pacific Palisades, Calif.: Greenwood and Associates, December 1993.

Halberstam, Judith. *Female Masculinity.* Durham, N.C.: Duke University Press, 1998.

Hamamoto, Darrell Y. *Monitored Peril: Asian Americans and the Politics of TV Representation.* Minneapolis: University of Minnesota Press, 1994.

Hansen, Bert. "American Physicians' 'Discovery' of Homosexuals, 1880–1900: A New Diagnosis in a Changing Society." In *Framing Disease: Studies in Cultural History,* edited by Charles E. Rosenberg and Janet Golden. New Brunswick, N.J.: Rutgers University Press, 1992.

———. "Medical History for the Masses: How American Comic Books Celebrated Heroes of Medicine in the 1940s." *Bulletin of the History of Medicine* (spring 2004): 148–91.

Harris, Carl V., Jarrell C. Jackman, and Catherine Rudolph, eds. *Santa Barbara Presidio Area 1840 to the Present.* Santa Barbara, Calif.: Presidio Research Center, 1993.

Hartmann, Susan M. *The Home Front and Beyond: American Women in the 1940s.* Boston: Twayne Publishers, 1982.

———. "Women's Organizations during World War II: The Interaction of Class, Race, and Feminism." In *Woman's Being, Woman's Place: Female Identity and Vocation in American History.* Boston: G.K. Hall & Co., 1979.

Hazlett, T. Lyle, and William W. Hummel. *Industrial Medicine in Western Pennsylvania, 1850–1950.* Pittsburgh: University of Pittsburgh Press, 1957.

Hellrigel, Maryann. "A Social History of Presidio Area Occupants 1900 to the Present." In *Santa Barbara Presidio Area 1840 to the Present,* edited by Carl V. Harris, Jarrell C. Jackman, and Catherine Rudolph. Santa Barbara, Calif.: Presidio Research Center, 1993.

Hendricks, Rickey. "Feminism and Maternalism in Early Hospitals for Children: San Francisco and Denver, 1875–1915." *Journal of the West* (July 1993): 61–69.

Hill, Patricia R. *The World Their Household: The American Woman's Foreign Mission Movement and Cultural Transformation, 1870–1920.* Ann Arbor: University of Michigan Press, 1985.

Hine, Darlene Clark. *HineSight: Black Women and the Re-construction of American History.* Brooklyn, N.Y.: Carlson Publishing, 1994.

Hirata, Lucie Cheng. "Free, Indentured, Enslaved: Chinese Prostitutes in Nineteenth-Century America." *Signs* (autumn 1979): 3–29.

Hofstadter, Richard. *Age of Reform.* New York: Knopf, 1955.

Hollinger, David A. *Science, Jews, and Secular Culture: Studies in Mid-Twentieth-Century American Intellectual History.* Princeton, N.J.: Princeton University Press, 1996.

Honey, Maureen. *Creating Rosie the Riveter: Class, Gender, and Propaganda during World War II.* Amherst: University of Massachusetts Press, 1984.

Hoopes, Roy. *When the Stars Went to War: Hollywood and World War II.* New York: Random House, 1994.

Hsu, Madeline Y. *Dreaming of Gold, Dreaming of Home: Transnationalism and Migration between the United States and South China, 1882–1943.* Stanford, Calif.: Stanford University Press, 2000.

Hunter, Jane. *The Gospel of Gentility: American Women Missionaries in Turn-of-the-Century China.* New Haven, Conn.: Yale University Press, 1984.

Iles, Teresa, ed. *All Sides of the Subject: Women and Biography.* New York: Teachers College Press, 1992.

Jacobson, Matthew Frye. *Whiteness of a Different Color: European Immigrants and the Alchemy of Race.* Cambridge, Mass.: Harvard University Press, 1998.

Jaffary, Stuart K. *The Mentally Ill and Public Provision for Their Care in Illinois.* Chicago: University of Chicago press, 1942.

Jayawardena, Kumari. *The White Woman's Other Burden: Western Women and South Asia during British Colonial Rule.* New York: Routledge 1995.

Jennings, Dean. *We Only Kill Each Other: The Life and Bad Times of Bugsy Siegel.* Englewood Cliffs, N.J.: Prentice-Hall, 1968.

Jennings, Margaret. "The Chinese in Ventura County." *Ventura County Historical Society Quarterly* 29, no. 3 (spring 1984): 3–31.

Jespersen, T. Christopher. *American Images of China, 1931–1949.* Palo Alto, Calif.: Stanford University Press, 1996.

Johnson, Marilynn S. *The Second Gold Rush: Oakland and the East Bay in World War II.* Berkeley and London: University of California Press, 1993.

Kao, George. "Tung Wah Hospital." In *Cathay by the Bay: San Francisco Chinatown in 1950.* Hong Kong: Chinese University Press, 1988.

Kennedy, Elizabeth Lapovsky. "'But we would never talk about it': The Structures of Lesbian Discretion in South Dakota, 1928–1933." In *Inventing Lesbian Cultures in America,* edited by Ellen Lewin. Boston: Beacon Press, 1996.

Kerber, Linda K. *No Constitutional Right to Be Ladies.* New York: Hill and Wang, 1998.

———. *Women of the Republic: Intellect, and Ideology in Revolutionary America.* Chapel Hill: University of North Carolina Press, 1980.

Kimm, Gregory. "This Remarkable Couple: The Story of Ng Hon Gim and Chin Mooie." Unpublished paper, 1995.

Klein, Christina. "Adoption and the Cold War Commitment to Asia." In *Cold War Constructions: The Political Culture of United States Imperialism, 1945–1966,* edited by Christian G. Appy. Amherst: University of Massachusetts Press, 2000.

Koppes, Clayton R. "Hollywood and the Politics of Representation: Women, Workers, and African Americans in World War II Movies." In *The Home-Front War: World War II and American Society,* edited by Kenneth Paul O'Brien and Lynn Hudson Parsons. Westport, Conn.: Greenwood Press, 1995.

Koven, Seth, and Sonya Michel. *Mothers of a New World: Maternalist Politics and the Origins of Welfare States.* New York: Routledge, 1993.

———. "Womanly Duties: Maternalist Politics and the Origins of the Welfare States in France, Germany, Great Britain, and the United States, 1880–1920." *American Historical Review* 95 (1990): 1076–1108.

Lai, Him Mark. "The Kuomintang in Chinese American Communities before World War II." In *Entry Denied: Exclusion and the Chinese Community in America, 1882–1943,* edited by Sucheng Chan. Philadelphia: Temple University Press, 1991.

———. "Sprouting Wings on the Dragon." *East/West News,* 19 May 1988.

Leavitt, Judith Walzer. "Birthing and Anesthesia: The Debate over Twilight Sleep." In *Mothers and Motherhood: Readings in American History,* edited by Rima D. Apple and Janet Golden. Columbus: Ohio State University Press, 1997.

Lee, Anthony W. *Picturing Chinatown: Art and Orientalism in San Francisco.* Berkeley and London: University of California Press, 2001.

Lee, Mary Paik. *Quiet Odyssey: A Pioneer Korean Woman in America,* edited by Sucheng Chan. Seattle: University of Washington Press, 1990.

Lee, Robert G. *Orientals: Asian Americans in Popular Culture.* Philadelphia: Temple University Press, 1999.

Leonard, Karen Isaksen. *Making Ethnic Choices: California's Punjabi Mexican Americans.* Philadelphia: Temple University Press, 1992.

Leong, Karen Janis. "The China Mystique: Mayling Soong Chiang, Pearl S. Buck and Anna May Wong in the American Imagination." PhD diss., University of California, Berkeley, 1999.

Leong, Russell. ed. *Asian American Sexualities: Dimensions of the Gay and Lesbian Experience.* New York: Routledge, 1996.

Lepore, Jill. "Historians Who Love Too Much: Reflections on Microhistory and Biography." *Journal of American History* 88, no. 1 (June 2001): 129–44.

Light, Ivan. "From Vice District to Tourist Attraction: The Moral Career of American Chinatowns, 1880–1940." *Pacific Historical Review* 43, no. 3 (1974): 367–94.

Lim, Shirley Jennifer. "Girls Just Wanna Have Fun: The Politics of Asian American Women's Public Culture, 1930–1960." PhD diss., University of California, Los Angeles, 1998.

Limerick, Patricia Nelson. *The Legacy of Conquest: The Unbroken Past of the American West.* New York: W. W. Norton, 1988.

Ling, Huping. *Surviving on the Gold Mountain: A History of Chinese American Women and Their Lives.* Albany: State University of New York Press, 1998.

Liu, Haiming. "The Resilience of Ethnic Culture: Chinese Herbalists in the American Medical Profession." *Journal of Asian American Studies* 1, no. 2 (1988): 173–91.

Lodwick, Kathleen L. *Educating the Women of Hainan: The Career of Margaret Moninger in China, 1915–1942*. Lexington: University Press of Kentucky, 1995.

Lotchin, Roger W. *Fortress California 1910–1961: From Warfare to Welfare*. New York: Oxford University Press, 1992.

Lou, Raymond. "The Chinese American Community of Los Angeles, 1870–1900: A Case of Resistance, Organization, and Participation." PhD diss., University of California, Irvine, 1982.

Luchetti, Cathy. *Medicine Women: The Story of Early-American Women Doctors*. New York: Crown Publishers, Inc., 1998.

Lui, Mary Ting Yi. "'The Real Yellow Peril': Mapping Racial and Gender Boundaries in New York City's Chinatown, 1870–1910." *Hitting Critical Mass: A Journal of Asian American Cultural Criticism* 5, no. 1 (spring 1998).

Lunbeck, Elizabeth. *The Psychiatric Persuasion: Knowledge, Gender, and Power in Modern America*. Princeton, N.J.: Princeton University Press, 1994.

Ma, L. Eve Armentrout. "Chinatown Organizations and the Anti-Chinese Movement, 1882–1914." In *Entry Denied: Exclusion and the Chinese Community in America, 1882–1943*. Philadelphia: Temple University Press, 1991.

Marchetti, Gina. *Romance and the "Yellow Peril": Race, Sex, and Discursive Strategies in Hollywood Fiction*. Berkeley and London: University of California Press, 1993.

Margadant, Jo Burr, ed. *The New Biography: Performing Femininity in Nineteenth-Century France*. Berkeley and London: University of California Press, 2000.

Marshall, James. *Santa Fe: The Railroad That Built an Empire*. New York: Random House, 1945.

Martin, Helen Eastman. *The History of the Los Angeles County Hospital (1878–1968) and the Los Angeles County-University of Southern California medical Center (1968–1978)*. Los Angeles: University of Southern California Press, 1979.

Mason, William. "The Chinese in Los Angeles." *Chinese Historical Society of America Bulletin* 4, no. 3 (March 1969).

May, Elaine Tyler. *Homeward Bound: American Families in the Cold War Era*. New York: Basic Books, 1988.

———. "Rosie the Riveter Gets Married." In *The War in American Culture: Society and Consciousness during World War II*, edited by Lewis A. Erenberg and Susan E. Hirsch. Chicago: University of Chicago Press, 1996.

May, Lary. "Making the American Consensus: The Narrative of Conversion and Subversion in World War II Films." In *The War in American Culture: Society and Consciousness during World War II*, edited by Lewis A. Erenberg and Susan E. Hirsch. Chicago: University of Chicago Press, 1996.

Mayer, Robert. *San Francisco: A Chronological and Documentary History, 1542–1970*. Dobbs Ferry, N.Y.: Oceana Publications, 1974.

McAfee, Ward. *California's Railroad Era, 1850–1911*. San Marino, Calif.: Golden West Books, 1973.

Mehr, Linda Harris. "The Way We Thought We Were: Images in World War II Films." In *The Way We Really Were: The Golden State in the Second Great War*, edited by Roger W. Lotchin. Urbana: University of Illinois Press, 2000.

Meites, Hyman L., ed. *History of the Jews of Chicago*. Chicago: Chicago Jewish Historical Society and Wellington Publishing, Inc., 1990. Facsimile of the original 1924 edition.

Mennel, Robert M. *Thorns and Thistles: Juvenile Delinquents in the United States, 1825–1940*. Hanover, N.H.: University Press of New England, 1973.

Meyer, Leisa D. *Creating GI Jane: Sexuality and Power in the Women's Arm Corps during World War II*. New York: Columbia University Press, 1996.

Meyerowitz, Joanne J. *Women Adrift: Independent Wage Earners in Chicago, 1880–1930*. Chicago: University of Chicago Press, 1988.

Milkman, Ruth. "Women's Work and the Economic Crisis: Some Lessons from the Great Depression." In *A Heritage of Her Own: Toward a New Social History of American Women*. New York: Simon and Schuster, 1979.

Morantz-Sanchez, Regina Markell. *Sympathy and Science: Women Physicians in American Medicine*. New York: Oxford University Press, 1985.

More, Ellen S. *Restoring the Balance: Women Physicians and the Profession of Medicine, 1850–1995*. Cambridge, Mass.: Harvard University Press, 1999.

Moy, Susan Lee. "The Chinese in Chicago: The First One Hundred Years, 1870–1970." Master's thesis, University of Wisconsin, Madison, 1978.

Muench, Christopher. "Chinese Medicine in America: A Study in Adaptation." *Caduceus* 4 (1988): 5–35.

Mumford, Kevin J. *Interzones: Black/White Sex Districts in Chicago and New York in the Early Twentieth Century*. New York: Columbia University Press, 1997.

Myrick, David F. *San Francisco's Telegraph Hill*. Berkeley, Calif.: Howell-North Books, 1972.

Nee, Victor G., and Brett de Bary Nee. *Longtime Californ': A Documentary Study of an American Chinatown*. Stanford, Calif.: Stanford University Press, 1972.

Nelson, Howard J. *The Los Angeles Metropolis*. Dubuque, Ia.: Kendall/Hunt Publishing Company, 1983.

Newton, Esther. "The Mythic Mannish Lesbian: Radclyffe Hall and the New Woman." In *Hidden from History: Reclaiming the Gay and Lesbian Past*, edited by Martin Bauml Duberman, Martha Vicinus, and George Chauncey Jr. New York: New American Library, 1989.

Ng, Vivien. "Looking for Lesbians in Chinese History." In *The New Lesbian Studies: Into the Twenty-First Century*, edited by Bonnie Zimmerman and Toni A.H. McNaron. New York: The Feminist Press, 1996.

Ngai, Mae N. "The Architecture of Race in American Immigration Law: A Reexamination of the Immigration Act of 1924." *Journal of American History* 86 (June 1999): 67–92.

Norton, Mary Beth. *Liberty's Daughters: The Revolutionary Experience of American Women, 1750–1800*. Boston: Little, Brown, 1980.

Okhiro, Gary Y. *Margins and Mainstreams: Asians in American History and Culture*. Seattle: University of Washington Press, 1994.

Parrish, Thomas, ed. *The Simon and Schuster Encyclopedia of World War II.* New York: Simon and Schuster, 1978.

Pascoe, Peggy. "Gender Systems in Conflict: The Marriages of Mission-Educated Chinese American Women, 1874–1939." In *Unequal Sisters: A Multicultural Reader in U.S. Women's History,* edited by Ellen Carol DuBois and Vicki L. Ruiz. New York: Routledge, 1990.

———. *Relations of Rescue: The Search for Female Moral Authority in the American West, 1874–1939.* New York: Oxford University Press, 1990.

Paxman, Marlys Elaine. "The Development of Medical Education at the University of Southern California." Master's thesis, University of Southern California, January 1966.

Peiss, Kathy. *Cheap Amusements: Working Women and Leisure in Turn-of-the-Century New York.* Philadelphia: Temple University Press, 1986.

Piedmonte, Richard. "The Chinese Presidio Community." In *Santa Barbara Presidio Area 1840 to the Present.* Santa Barbara, Calif.: Presidio Research Center, 1993.

Platt, Anthony M. *The Child Savers: The Invention of Delinquency.* 1969. Rev. ed. Chicago: University of Chicago Press, 1977.

Quan, Ella Yee. "Santa Barbara Chinatown: The Early Years." *Gum Saan Journal* 5, no. 2 (November 1982): 1–5.

Reagan, Leslie J. *When Abortion Was a Crime: Women, Medicine, and Law in the United States, 1867–1973.* Berkeley and London: University of California Press, 1997.

Renov, Michael. *Hollywood's Wartime Woman: Representation and Ideology.* Ann Arbor: UMI Research Press, 1988.

Robert, Dana L. *American Women in Mission: A Social History of Their Thought and Practice.* Macon, Ga.: Mercer University Press, 1996.

Rodgers, Daniel T. "The Promise of American History: Progress and Prospects." *Reviews in American History,* 10, no. 4 (December 1982): 113–32.

Roediger, David R. *The Wages of Whiteness: Race and the Making of the American Working Class.* New York: Verso Press, 1991.

Rogin, Michael. *Blackface, White Noise: Jewish Immigrants in the Hollywood Melting Pot.* Berkeley and London: University of California Press, 1996.

Rosenberg, Charles E. *The Care of Strangers: The Rise of America's Hospital System.* New York: Basic Books, Inc., 1987.

Rothman, David J. *Conscience and Convenience: The Asylum and Its Alternatives in Progressive America.* Boston: Little, Brown and Company, 1980.

Rothstein, William G. *American Medical Schools and the Practice of Medicine: A History.* New York: Oxford University Press, 1987.

Rupp, Leila J. *A Desired Past: A Short History of Same-Sex Love in America.* Chicago: University of Chicago Press, 1999.

———. "'Imagine My Surprise': Women's Relationships in Mid-Twentieth Century America." In *Hidden from History: Reclaiming the Gay and Lesbian Past,* edited by Martin Bauml Duberman, Martha Vicinus, and George Chauncey Jr. New York: New American Library, 1989.

———. *Mobilizing Women for War: German and American Propaganda, 1939–1945.* Princeton, N.J.: Princeton University Press, 1978.

Rury, John Leslie. "Women, Cities and Schools: Education and the Development of an Urban Female Labor Force, 1890–1930." PhD diss., University
of Wisconsin, Madison, 1982.

Said, Edward. *Orientalism*. New York: Vintage Books, 1979.

Sánchez, George J. *Becoming Mexican American: Ethnicity, Culture and
Identity in Chicano Los Angeles, 1900–1945*. New York: Oxford University
Press, 1993.

San Francisco Lesbian and Gay History Project. "'She Even Chewed Tobacco':
A Pictorial Narrative of Passing Women in America." In *Hidden from
History: Reclaiming the Gay and Lesbian Past*, edited by Martin Bauml
Duberman, Martha Vicinus, and George Chauncey Jr. New York: New
American Library, 1989.

The Santa Fe Trail: A Chapter in the Opening of the West. New York: Random
House, 1946.

Scharff, Virginia. *Taking the Wheel: Women and the Coming of the Motor Age*.
New York: The Free Press, 1991.

Schwarz, Henry G. ed. *Chinese Medicine on the Golden Mountain: An Interpretive Guide*. Seattle, Wash.: Wing Luke Memorial Museum, 1984.

Scott, Joan W. "The Evidence of Experience." *Critical Inquiry* 17 (summer
1991): 773–97.

Scott, Mel. *The San Francisco Bay Area: A Metropolis in Perspective*. Berkeley
and London: University of California Press, 1959.

See, Lisa. *On Gold Mountain: The One-Hundred-Year Odyssey of My Chinese-
American Family*. New York: Vintage Books, 1995.

Selleck, Henry B., and Alfred H. Whittaker. *Occupational Health in America*.
Detroit: Wayne State University Press, 1962.

Servin, Manuel P., and Iris Higbie Wilson. *Southern California and Its
University: A History of USC, 1880–1964*. Los Angeles: Ward Ritchie Press,
1969.

Shah, Nayan. "Cleaning Motherhood: Hygiene and the Culture of Domesticity
in San Francisco's Chinatown, 1875–1900." In *Gender, Sexuality and
Colonial Modernities*, edited by Antoinette Burton. London: Routledge,
1999.

———. *Contagious Divides: Epidemics and Race in San Francisco's
Chinatown*. Berkeley and London: University of California Press, 2001.

———. "San Francisco's 'Chinatown': Race and the Cultural Politics of Public
Health, 1854–1952." PhD diss., University of Chicago, 1995.

Sherman, Janann. *No Place for a Woman: A Life of Senator Margaret Chase
Smith*. New Brunswick, N.J.: Rutgers University Press, 2000.

Singh, Maina Chawla. *Gender, Religion, and "Heathen Lands": American
Missionary Women in South Asia, 1860s-1940s*. New York: Garland
Publishing, 2000.

Sitton, Tom, and William Deverell, eds. *Metropolis in the Making: Los Angeles
in the 1920s*. Berkeley and London: University of California Press,
2001.

Siu, Paul C.P. *The Chinese Laundryman: A Study of Social Isolation*, edited by
John Kuo Wei Tchen. New York: New York University Press, 1987.

Sklar, Kathryn Kish. *Florence Kelley and the Nation's Work: The Rise of Women's Political Culture, 1830–1900.* New Haven, Conn.: Yale University Press, 1995.

Smith, Icy. *The Lonely Queue: The Forgotten History of the Courageous Chinese Americans in Los Angeles.* Gardena, Calif.: East West Discovery Press, 2000.

Smith-Rosenberg, Carroll. "Discourses of Sexuality and Subjectivity: The New Woman, 1870–1936." In *Hidden from History: Reclaiming the Gay and Lesbian Past,* edited by Martin Bauml Duberman, Martha Vicinus, and George Chauncey Jr. New York: New American Library, 1989.

———. *Disorderly Conduct: Visions of Gender in Victorian America.* New York: Oxford University Press, 1985.

Sochen, June. "From Sophie Tucker to Barbra Streisand: Jewish Women Entertainers as Reformers." In *Talking Back: Images of Jewish Women in American Popular Culture,* edited by Joyce Antler. Hanover, N.H.: Brandeis University Press and University Press of New England, 1998.

Spaulding, Edward Selden. *A Brief Story of Santa Barbara.* Santa Barbara: Pacific Coast Publishing, 1964.

Starr, Paul. *The Social Transformation of American Medicine: The Rise of a Sovereign Profession and the Making of a Vast Industry.* New York: Basic Books, 1982.

Stryker, Susan, and Jim Van Buskirk. *Gay by the Bay: A History of Queer Culture in the San Francisco Bay Area.* San Francisco: Chronicle Books, 1996.

Swanson, Mark T. "From Spanish Land Grants to World War II: An Overview of Historic Resources at the Naval Air Weapons Station, Point Mugu, California." Report prepared for Naval Air Weapons Station, Point Mugu. Tucson: Statistical Research, 1994.

Suski, P.M. *My Fifty Years in America.* English Summary. 1960. Reprint. Hollywood: Hawley Publications, 1990.

Takaki, Ronald. *Strangers from a Different Shore: A History of Asian Americans.* Boston: Little, Brown, 1989.

Tchen, John Kuo Wei. *New York before Chinatown: Orientalism and the Shaping of American Culture, 1776–1882.* Baltimore: John Hopkins University Press, 1999.

Ting, Jennifer. "Bachelor Society: Deviant Heterosexuality and Asian American Historiography." In *Privileging Positions: The Sites of Asian American Studies,* edited by Gary Y. Okihiro, Marilyn Alquizola, Dorothy Fujita Rony, and K. Scott Wong. Pullman: Washington State University Press, 1995.

———. "The Power of Sexuality." *Journal of Asian American Studies* 1, no. 1 (1998): 65–82.

Tom, Kim Fong. "The Participation of the Chinese in the Community Life of Los Angeles." Master's thesis, University of Southern California, 1944. Reprint. San Francisco: R and E Research Associates, 1974.

Tong, Benson. *Susan La Flesche Picotte, M.D.: Omaha Indian Leader and Reformer.* Norman: University of Oklahoma Press, 1999.

Trachtenberg, Alan. *The Incorporation of America: Culture and Society in the Gilded Age.* New York: Hill and Wang, 1982.

Trauner, Joan B. "The Chinese as Medical Scapegoats in San Francisco, 1870–1905." *California History* 57, no. 1 (spring 1978): 70–87.

Tsai, Shih-Shan Henry. *The Chinese Experience in America.* Bloomington: Indiana University Press, 1986.

Tse, Mariko. "Made in America." Research Project for East West Players on Chinese in Southern California. Unpublished paper, June 1979.

Verge, Arthur. "Daily Life in Wartime California." In *The Way We Really Were: The Golden State in the Second Great War,* edited by Roger W. Lotchin. Urbana: University of Illinois Press, 2000.

Vicinus, Martha. "Distance and Desire: English Boarding School Friendships, 1870–1920." In *Hidden from History: Reclaiming the Gay and Lesbian Past,* edited by Martin Bauml Duberman, Martha Vicinus, and George Chauncey Jr. New York: New American Library, 1989.

———, ed. *Lesbian Subjects: A Feminist Studies Reader.* Bloomington: Indiana University Press, 1996.

Vospan, Max, and Lloyd P. Gartner. *History of the Jews of Los Angeles.* Philadelphia: Jewish Publication Society of America, 1970.

Wagner-Martin, Linda. *Telling Women's Lives: The New Biography.* New Brunswick, N.J.: Rutgers University Press, 1994.

Wallace, Patricia Ward. *Politics of Conscience: A Biography of Margaret Chase Smith.* Westport, Conn.: Praeger, 1995.

Walsh, Mary Roth. *"Doctors Wanted: No Women Need Apply": Sexual Barriers in the Medical Profession, 1835–1975.* New Haven, Conn.: Yale University Press, 1977.

Ware, Susan. *Beyond Suffrage: Women in the New Deal.* Cambridge, Mass.: Harvard University Press, 1981.

———. *Still Missing: Amelia Earhart and the Search for Modern Feminism.* New York: W. W. Norton, 1993.

Warren, Viola Lockhart. "The Old College of Medicine." Reprinted from *Historical Society of Southern California Quarterly* (December 1959–March 1960).

Weinstein, James. *The Corporate Ideal in the Liberal State.* Boston: Beacon Press, 1968.

Westbrook, Robert B. "Fighting for the American Family: Private Interests and Political Obligation in World War II." In *The Power of Culture: Critical Essays in American History,* edited by Richard Wightman Fox and T. J. Jackson Lears. Chicago: University of Chicago Press, 1993.

———. "'I Want a Girl, Just like the Girl That Married Harry James': American Women and the Problem of Political Obligation in World War II." *American Quarterly* 42, no. 4 (December 1990): 587–614.

Wiebe, Robert. *The Search for Order, 1877–1920.* New York: Hill and Wang, 1967.

Williams, Pierce. *The Purchase of Medical Care through Fixed Periodic Payment.* New York: National Bureau of Economic Research, Inc., 1932.

Wlodarski, Robert J. "A Brief History of Chinatown in Ventura." In *The Changing Faces of Main Street,* by Roberta S. Greenwood. Report for Redevelopment Agency, City of San Buenaventura, 1976.

Wong, Charles Choy. "Los Angeles Chinatown: A Public and Home Territory."
    In *The Chinese American Experience: Papers from the Second National
    Conference on Chinese American Studies.* San Francisco: Chinese Historical
    Society of America and the Chinese Culture Foundation of San Francisco,
    1980.
Wong, K. Scott. "War Comes to Chinatown: Social Transformation and the
    Chinese of California." In *The Way We Really Were: The Golden State in the
    Second Great War,* edited by Roger W. Lotchin. Urbana: University of
    Illinois Press, 2000.
Wong, K. Scott, and Sucheng Chan, eds. *Claiming America: Constructing
    Chinese American Identities during the Exclusion Era.* Philadelphia: Temple
    University Press, 1998.
Wu, Judy Tzu-Chun. "Was Mom Chung a 'Sister Lesbian'? Asian American
    Gender Experimentation and Interracial Homoeroticism." *Journal of
    Women's History* 13, no. 1 (spring 2001): 58–82.
Yanagisako, Sylvia. "Transforming Orientalism: Gender, Nationality, and Class
    in Asian American Studies." In *Naturalizing Power: Essays in Feminist
    Cultural Analysis,* edited by Sylvia Yanagisako and Carol Delaney. New
    York: Routledge, 1995.
Ye, Weili. "Crossing the Cultures: The Experience of Chinese Students in the
    U.S.A., 1900–1925." PhD diss., Yale University, 1989.
Yee, George, and Elsie Yee. "The Chinese and the Los Angeles Produce
    Market." *Gum Saan Journal* 9, no. 2 (December 1986): 4–17.
Yoshihara, Mary. "Women's Asia: American Women and the Gendering of
    American Orientalism, 1870s–WWII." PhD diss., Brown University, 1997.
Yu, Henry. "Mixing Bodies and Cultures: The Meaning of America's
    Fascination with Sex between 'Orientals" and 'Whites'." In *Sex, Love, Race:
    Crossing Boundaries in North American History,* edited by Martha Hodes.
    New York: New York University Press, 1999.
———. *Thinking Orientals: Migration, Contact, and Exoticism in Modern
    America.* New York: Oxford University Press, 2001.
Yu, Renqiu. *To Save China, to Save Ourselves: The Chinese Hand Laundry
    Alliance of New York.* Philadelphia: Temple University Press, 1992.
Yung, Judy. "The Social Awakening of Chinese American Women as Reported
    in *Chung Sai Yat Po,* 1900–1911." In *Unequal Sisters: A Multicultural
    Reader in U.S. Women's History,* edited by Ellen Carol DuBois and Vicki
    L. Ruiz. New York: Routledge, 1990.
———. *Unbound Feet: A Social History of Chinese Women in San Francisco.*
    Berkeley and London: University of California Press, 1995.
———. *Unbound Voices: A Documentary History of Chinese Women in San
    Francisco.* Berkeley and London: University of California Press, 1999.
Zhao, Xiaojian. *Remaking Chinese America: Immigration, Family, and
    Community, 1940–1965.* New Brunswick, N.J.: Rutgers University Press,
    2002.

Index

abortion, 99, 229–30n67. *See also* birth control; childbirth
actors, Chinese American, 80–83, 85, 189–90; gender presentation of, 173–74; as patients, 78–79; sexuality of, 181–82, 246n49; as surrogate family members, 1, 121, 127, 172–73. *See also* Hollywood
Adler, Herman, 67, 69, 72, 219n54
adoption: of Ah Yane (later Chung, Minnie), 12–16, 34, 60, 66, 106, 122, 205n7, 224n39; and Chung's surrogate family, 1–2, 119–95 (*see also* Fair-Haired Bastards; Golden Dolphins; Kiwis); ceremony, 124–25; during cold war, 185–89, 192–93; fraternal nature of, 122–27, 143–44; origins of, 119–22; and political networking, 155–69; and sexuality, 170–71, 174–83; during Sino-Japanese War, 127–36, 189–90; whiteness through, 127–28, 130–31, 237n43; surgical daughters, 60, 61, 122–23; transnational forms of, 193; World War II propaganda value of, 136–54, 172–73, 190–92. *See also* family, surrogate; maternalism; motherhood; Oriental Mammy
African Americans: in Chicago, 59, 83; in Los Angeles, 33, 34, 211n37; medical education of, 42, 43, 57, 213n12, 214n19; in military, 157, 161, 165–66, 237n1;

in Pasadena, 77; political affiliations of, 168; in San Francisco, 225n2
African American women: in domestic service, 150–51; entertainers, 151, 179, 182; in the military, 157, 161, 165–66; physicians, 42, 213n12; representations of, 151 (*see also* blackface)
Ah Yane (mother). *See* Chung, Minnie
American Federation of Labor (AFL), 141
American Medical Association (AMA), 43, 91, 93–94, 214n17
American Medical Women's Association (AWMA), 60, 62, 70
American Red Cross, 173, 185–86
antimiscegenation. *See* interracial sexuality; marriage
Ashwell, L. W., 152
assimilation, 3, 45–46, 178–80, 194. *See also* cultural identity; whiteness
Atchison, Topeka and Santa Fe Railroad, 73–76. *See also* hospitals, Santa Fe
Atherton, Gertrude, 132
athletics, 41, 80, 120, 123, 127, 141
autobiography, 188–89, 198, 204n7
automobiles, 105–6, 123, 231nn9,12
aviation, 123–24, 129, 134–35, 235n18. *See also* Fair-Haired Bastards; Fighting Two; military; pilots
Awl, Elmer, 143

Bancroft, Steven G., 120, 125–27, 133
Baldwin, Bill, 143
Bankhead, Tallulah, 1, 181

Compositor:	International Typesetting and Composition
Text:	10/13 Sabon
Display:	Sabon
Printer and binder:	Sheridan Books, Inc.